SOMATOSTATIN
Basic and Clinical Status

SERONO SYMPOSIA, USA

Series Editor: James Posillico

A Continuation Order Plan is available for this series. A continuation order will bring delivery of each new volume immediately upon publication. Volumes are billed only upon actual shipment. For further information please contact the publisher.

SOMATOSTATIN
Basic and Clinical Status

Edited by
Seymour Reichlin

Tufts University
Boston, Massachusetts

SPRINGER SCIENCE+BUSINESS MEDIA, LLC

Library of Congress Cataloging in Publication Data

International Conference on Somatostatin (1986: Washington, D.C.)
  Somatostatin: basic and clinical status.

  "Proceedings of the International Conference on Somatostatin, held May 6–8, 1986 in Washington, D.C."—T.p. verso.
  "Serono Symposia, USA"—Cover.
  Includes bibliographies and indexes.
  1. Somatostatin—Congresses. I. Reichlin, Seymour, 1924–   . II. Serono Symposia, USA. III. Title.
[DNLM: 1. Somatostatin—congresses. WK 515 I587s 1986]
QP572.S59I58 1986   612′.015756   87-7923
ISBN 978-1-4684-5328-7   ISBN 978-1-4684-5326-3 (eBook)
DOI 10.1007/978-1-4684-5326-3

Proceedings of the International Conference on Somatostatin,
held May 6–8, 1986, in Washington, D.C.

The views expressed in this volume are the responsibility of the named authors. Great care has been taken to maintain the accuracy of the information contained in the volume. However, neither Plenum Press, Serono Symposia, USA, nor the editors can be held responsible for errors or any consequences arising from the use of information contained herein.

Some of the names of products referred to in this book may be registered trademarks or proprietary names, although specific references to this fact may not be made; however, the use of a name without designation is not to be construed as a representation by the publisher or editors that it is in the public domain. In addition, the mention of specific companies or of their products or proprietary names does not imply any endorsement or recommendation on the part of the publisher or editors.

© 1987 Springer Science+Business Media New York
Originally published by Plenum Press, New York in 1987
Softcover reprint of the hardcover 1st edition 1987

SCIENTIFIC COMMITTEE

Seymour Reichlin, M.D., Ph.D., Chairman
Tufts University
Boston, MA

John Gerich, M.D.
Mayo Clinic
Rochester, MN

Richard H. Goodman, M.D., Ph.D.
Tufts University
Boston, MA

Yogesh C. Patel, M.D., Ph.D.
McGill University
Montreal, Canada

Roger Unger, M.D.
University of Texas
Dallas, TX

Klaus-Henning Usadel, M.D.
University of Heidelberg
Mannheim, West Germany

Tadataka Yamada, M.D.
University of Michigan
Ann Arbor, MI

ORGANIZING SECRETARIES

Ching Lau, Ph.D.
James T. Posillico, Ph.D.
Serono Symposia, USA
Randolph, MA

PREFACE

The discovery of hypothalamic factors that inhibited growth hormone secretion and of pancreatic factors that inhibited insulin secretion were the first clues to the existence of somatostatin. During the course of efforts to isolate growth hormone releasing factor, Krulich, McCann and Dhariwal found that hypothalamic extracts contained a potent inhibitor of growth hormone secretion. They postulated that growth hormone secretion was under a dual control system, one inhibitory and the other excitatory (1). In studies being carried out at about the same time, Hellman and Lernmark found a factor in pancreatic extracts that inhibited insulin secretion (2). They postulated that islet cell function was regulated by local hormonal factors. With the isolation and chemical characterization of somatostatin by Brazeau and colleagues (3), and the availability of relatively large amounts of the synthetic peptide for research, it has been possible to demonstrate that both predictions were true. Subsequent work revealed that somatostatin, as initially isolated (somatostatin 14), was but one of several related peptides, part of a multigene family, with tissue specific processing. Many of the details of biosynthesis and genetic control have been worked out, and this molecule has served many workers as a model gut-brain peptide for detailed study. The peptides are widely distributed in tissues and exert an extraordinary range of effects on most glandular secretions, both internal and external. Further, they are present in the central nervous system where they exert a number of physiological effects, and are present in the gastrointestinal tract where they regulate a number of functions. The development of potent analogues, with desirable properties, has led to new advances in the pharmacotherapy of endocrine and gastrointestinal disease.

The extraordinary range of distribution and actions of the somatostatin family of peptides continues to stimulate intense scientific interest and endeavor. Ongoing research has been reviewed in a number of publications (4-9), and three international symposia have been held on this topic: the first in 1977 in Freiberg, Germany (10), the second in 1981 in Athens, Greece (11), and the third in 1984 in Montreal, Canada (12). This International Conference on Somatostatin, which took place in Washington, DC, May 6-8, 1986, brought into focus the current status of knowledge in major areas of somatostatin research. The topics covered included the biosynthesis and processing of the peptide, mechanisms of action, an assessment of the role of somatostatin in central nervous system function and disease, the role of somatostatin in regulation of gastrointestinal function, and a critical summary of the current therapeutic uses of somatostatin and its analogues for the treatment of gastrointestinal bleeding, acromegaly, diabetes, and functioning gastrointestinal tumors. In addition to presenting an up-to-the-minute understanding of the current advances in somatostatin research, this volume captures the sense of excitement felt by leading investigators in the field.

REFERENCES

1. Krulich L, Dhariwal APS, McCann SM. Stimulatory and inhibitory effects of purified hypothalamic extracts on growth hormone release from rat pituitary in vitro. Endocrinology 1968; 83:783-90.
2. Hellman B, Lernmark A. Inhibition of the in vitro secretion of insulin by an extract of pancreatic A-1 cells. Endocrinology 1969; 84:1484-7.
3. Brazeau P, Vale W, Burgus R, et al. Hypothalamic peptide that inhibits the secretion of immunoreactive pituitary growth hormone. Science 1973; 179:77-9.
4. Gerich JE. Somatostatin. In: Brownlee M, ed. Handbook of diabetes mellitus. New York: Garland Publishing, Inc., 1981; 1:297-354.
5. Arimura A, Fishback JB. Somatostatin: regulation of secretion. Neuroendocrinology 1981; 33:246-56.
6. Gottesman IS, Mandarino LJ, Gerich JE. Somatostatin. In: Cohen M, Foa P, eds. Special topics in endocrinology and metabolism. New York: Alan R. Liss, 1982:177-243.
7. Reichlin S. Somatostatin. In: Krieger DT, Brownstein MJ, Martin JB, eds. Brain peptides. New York: John Wiley, 1983:711-52.
8. Reichlin S. Somatostatin. New Engl J Med 1983; 309:1495-1501, 1556-63.
9. Patel Y, Srikant C. Somatostatin. Annu Rev Physiol 1986; 48:551-67.
10. Gerich JE, Raptis S, Rosenthal J, eds. Somatostatin symposium. Metabolism 1978; 28:1129-1469.
11. Raptis S, Rosenthal J, Gerich JE, eds. 2nd international symposium on somatostatin. Germany: Attempto Verlag Tubingen GmbH, 1984.
12. Patel JC, Tannenbaum GS, eds. Somatostatin. New York: Plenum Press, 1985.

CONTENTS

III. ROLE OF SOMATOSTATIN IN NERVOUS SYSTEM FUNCTION AND

CONTROVERSIES IN SOMATOSTATIN RESEARCH

IV. SOMATOSTATIN IN GASTROINTESTINAL FUNCTION

V. CLINICAL APPLICATIONS

I. BIOSYNTHESIS AND PROCESSING

REGULATION AND DIVERSITY OF PEPTIDE HORMONE GENE EXPRESSION

Joel F. Habener

Laboratory of Molecular Endocrinology, Massachusetts
General Hospital and Howard Hughes Medical Institute
Harvard Medical School, Boston, Massachusetts 02114

During the past several years several fundamental advances have been made in our understanding of the cellular factors involved in the control of gene expression (1-4). Much of this new information has come from studies of the regulation of expression of genes encoding the polypeptide hormones. Our current conceptual views of the cellular regulation of gene expression indicate that extracellular signals consisting of small molecules such as amino acid transmitters, steroids, and thyroid hormones, or proteins such as peptide hormones, interact with the cell by high-affinity binding to receptor molecules located either in the plasma membrane (peptide hormone receptors) or in the cytoplasm (steroid or T-3 receptors) (5-7).

CELLULAR SIGNALLING IN THE REGULATION OF GENE EXPRESSION

The initial ligand-receptor interaction begins a cascade of events that leads to the transduction of information encoded in specific regulatory molecules to the nucleus where these molecules interact with the genome resulting in the expression of specific target genes (Fig. 1) (8). Based on our understanding of the steps that take place in the expression of the genetic information encoding polypeptide hormones it is likely that, in any given circumstance, the regulatory signals exert their actions on any one or more of the multiple steps of protein synthesis. These steps involve (i) the transcription of the genetic information from DNA into RNA in the form of RNA precursors (pre-mRNAs), (ii) the post-transcriptional processing of the pre-mRNAs to the mature protein-encoding mRNA, (iii) the transport of the mRNAs from the nucleus to the cytoplasm and (iv) subsequent translation of the mRNAs into peptide hormone precursors, preprohormones or prehormones, which are processed to the prohormone or hormone during the intracellular transport, segregation, and packaging of the hormones into secretory granules.

Another important process on which effector molecules act is that of secretion of hormone via fusion of granules to the plasma membrane and consequent exocytosis. Although it is generally believed that effectors are most often directly coupled via the signal-transduction pathways to the various steps in gene expression, it is also possible that circumstances exist where the process of secretion begins the signal-transduction cascade (9). That is, the depletion of intracellular stores

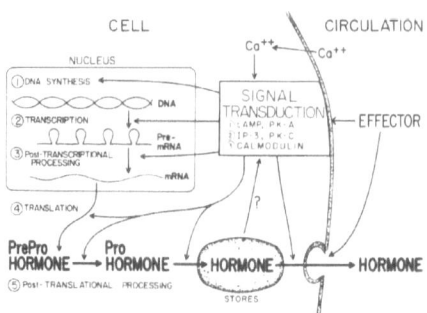

Fig. 1. Levels in gene expression at which potential regulation may take place in response to effector-mediated activation of specific signal-transduction pathways. Effectors may consist of peptide ligands, metabolites, catecholamines, etc., that interact with receptors on the plasma membrane. Arbitrarily, three signal transduction pathways are indicated: (i) cyclic AMP-dependent activation of protein kinase A, (ii) phospholipid synthesis and activation of protein kinase C, and (iii) Calmodulin-dependent processes. Fluxes of calcium, and hydrogen ions, are also important in signal transduction.

of hormone signals increased gene expression at levels of transcription, translation and/or posttranslational processing.

Information regarding the workings of the signal-transduction pathways has increased remarkably during the past decade. Although this process remains a black box, the box is getting smaller. At least three transduction pathways have been rather extensively elucidated: (1) cyclic AMP-dependent pathways involving the activation of the A group of protein kinases (8), (2) the protein kinase C-dependent pathway which involves the formation and processing of phospholipids (10), and (3) calmodulin-dependent pathways (11) (Fig. 1). In addition to these three signaling pathways others such as insulin-dependent pathways, exist but are less well understood.

For simplicity of discussion it is useful to describe the regulation of gene expression from two aspects: (i) identification and elucidation of the levels in gene expression in which biologic diversification takes place, and (ii) identification of the genetic and cellular factors that are necessary for the regulated expression of specific genes in specific cells. This latter aspect incorporates factors responsible for cell-specific gene expression, a situation that dictates the remarkable specificity of expression of certain genes only in certain cells, as well as the factors that participate in the metabolic regulation of genes, that is, the factors that turn up or down the expression of a gene in conditions in which the gene can be expressed in a specific cell phenotype.

GENERATION OF BIOLOGIC DIVERSIFICATION

Several different levels in gene expression provide the opportunity for the generation of biologic diversification (Fig. 2). As a first approximation one can consider the diversity of genes encoded in an animal genome. Genetic information encoded in molecules (RNAs, proteins) with

4

biologic utility tend to be multiplied within the genome over the course
of evolutionary time. For example, sequences encoding peptide hormones
which serve as informational molecules, in the sense of ligands that
interact with specific receptors resulting in the activation of a signal-
transduction pathway and subsequent gene expression in this target cell,
are often represented in multiple copies in the genome. This multiplicity
of gene copies constitutes what is known as supra-gene families encoding
structurally-related proteins. An example of such a multigenic family is
the glucagon gene family which includes not only glucagon but the structurally-related peptides, vasoactive intestinal peptide, gastric inhibitory peptide, secretin, growth hormone releasing hormone, the glucagon-
like peptides (encoded in the same transcriptional unit in which glucagon
is encoded), and many other glucagon-related genes yet to be discovered
(12). Other examples are the growth hormone gene family consisting of
growth hormone, prolactin, lactogen, and the newly-discovered placental
proliferins; the insulin-related sequences of insulin-like growth factors
and relaxin; and the family of beta subunits for the glycoprotein hormones
(13).

A second level of gene expression at which biologic diversification
takes place is that of the utilization of alternative splicing of RNA
precursors. It came as a surprise about a decade ago when it was discovered that genes encoding proteins are often interrupted by intervening
DNA (introns). Soon it became clear that the entire sequence of exons and
introns is transcribed into a single large RNA precursor which then
undergoes processing by splicing-out of introns and the knitting together
of the exons. At least two mechanisms are utilized to generate biologic
diversity at the level of RNA splicing; (i) alternative splice-sites and
(ii) exon-switching. Utilization of alternative splice-sites resulting in

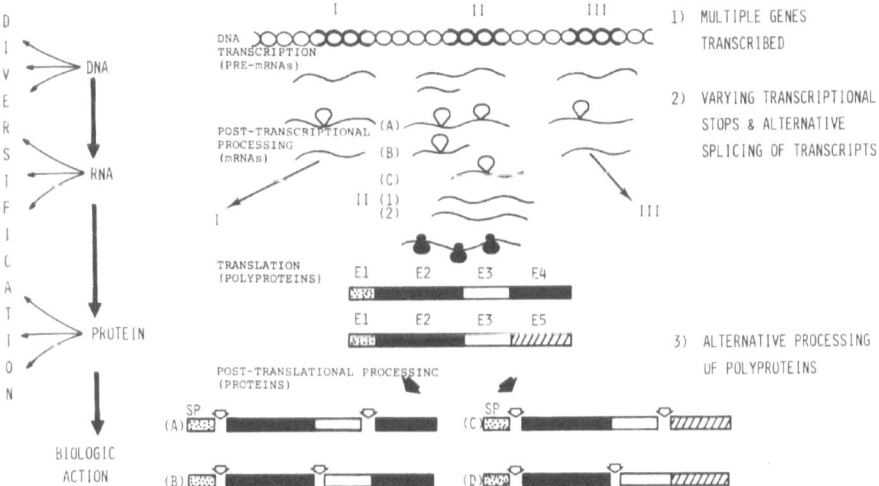

Fig. 2. Generation of biologic diversification at various
levels of gene expression. Flow of genetic information is from
DNA to RNA to protein. The existence of multiple genes (gene
duplication), alternative splicing of RNA precursors and alternative posttranslational processing of prohormones (polyproteins) may contribute to diversification and amplification of
the genetic repertoire of informational molecules in the form of
bioactive peptides.

the incorporation of segments of introns or exons in exons or introns, respectively. Recently, an alternative-splicing mechanism has been demonstrated to result in the utilization of a second reading-frame in the protein-coding sequence of the polynucleotide sequence. In the splicing of the primary transcript encoding the precursor gastrin-releasing peptide, at least two alternative splice-sites result in the reproduction of two mRNAs which utilize two entirely different reading frames within the carboxy-terminus of the precursor (14). Although the significance of this alternative utilization of reading-frames is presently unknown it points to the possibility that utilization of two, or even three, reading frames could provide entirely different genetic information from the identical DNA sequence. A second variation of this splicing of transcripts involves the substitution of exons. Thus a multi-exonic gene can be knit together in a chimeric fashion such that two messenger RNAs share several common exons and yet contain one or more different exons that may encode different functional domains. Examples of such alternate-exon-splicing are seen in the expression of the calcitonin (15), substance P/K (16), and bradykinin (17) genes. In the example of calcitonin, the messenger RNA encodes the sequence for the calcitrophic hormone calcitonin, whereas the identical precursor contains an exon encoding a calcitonin-related peptide gene in place of the calcitonin (15). This peptide appears to be a potent neuropeptide expressed in the central nervous system, where it is involved in olfaction and gustatory sensation and is also expressed in blood vessels where it serves as a potent vasodilator.

The third level of biologic diversification results from alternative processing of polyproteins. Without exception, all of the peptide hormones are encoded in large precursors which often contain within their protein-coding sequences the sequences of other potentially bioactive peptides (18). Alternative posttranslational processing is a highly-utilized level of genetic diversification. It is important to note that the final biologic action of programmed gene expression requires the precise proteolytic processing of the prohormone and modification of the peptide to provide the final bioactive product. Specific, unaltered amino-terminal and carboxy-terminal ends of peptides are almost always required for their expression of biologic actions on their specific receptors, and precursor-extensions at either ends of peptide most often lead to inactivation of the specific biologic activity. Therefore, alternative processing of a polyprotein or prohormone may take place in several patterns, leading to the liberation of specific bioactive peptides in one cell and another spectrum of bioactive peptides in yet another cell. Examples of such alternative posttranslational processing are seen in the polyprotein pro-opiomelanocortin which encodes, alternatively, the peptides ACTH and endorphins, or MSH and other cleaved peptides (19). Another example is the proglucagon, the precursor to glucagon, which contains in its coding sequences two additional peptides that are structurally related to glucagon (12). In the pancreas, the major peptide released is glucagon, whereas the glucagon-like peptides remain as biologically-inactive incompletely processed fragments of the precursor. In the intestine glucagon remains as part of a bio-inactive precursor, called enteroglucagon or glicentin, and the glucagon-like peptides are liberated from the precursor under conditions in which they presumably have important biologic actions (20).

Nature often uses combinatorial processes to generate biologic diversification. An example of such a combinatorial process is the genetic rearrangement of a relatively few genomic segments encoding the immunoglobulins resulting in the generation of an enormously diverse repertoire of immunoglobulin molecules (21). Likewise, one can envision that the combinations of diversification at the level of gene multiplication, alternative RNA splicing and alternative posttranslational process-

6

ing of protein precursors could, in varying combinations, lead to a wide
diversity of bioactive peptides.

DIVERSIFICATION OF THE EXPRESSION OF THE SOMATOSTATIN GENE

Biologic diversification in the expression of the somatostatin gene
appears to occur predominantly at the level of alternative posttranslational processing. With the exception of the piscine species (anglerfish,
catfish) (22,23) which have two or more somatostatin-encoding genes,
current evidence indicates that the rat (24,25) and human (26), and
perhaps other mammalian genomes, contain a single unique gene for somatostatin. The determinations of the complete nucleotide sequences of the
rat (24,25) and human (26) somatostatin genes indicate that they are
relatively simple genes consisting of two exons and a single intron. The
single intron interrupts the coding sequence of preprosomatostatin within
the middle of the amino-terminal peptide extension upstream from the
carboxy-terminal sequence which encodes the somatostatins 14 and 28 (Fig.
3). To date there is no experimental evidence to indicate alternative
splicing of the RNA precursor encoding preprosomatostatin. However, there
is striking conservation of the amino terminal sequence of the precursor
among fish, rat and human. The fish and mammalian prosomatostatin share
approximately 60 percent of their amino acid sequences in common (27), and
the rat sequence differs from the human prosomatostatin sequence in only
two amino acid substitutions within the amino-terminal extension sequence
(28). This high degree of conservation throughout eons of evolutionary
time strongly suggests the existence of a biologic function for the amino-
terminal extension of prosomatostatin, although no such biologic activity
has yet been identified.

ALTERNATIVE POSTTRANSLATIONAL PROCESSING OF PROSOMATOSTATIN

As a consequence of the decoding of the cDNA and genomic sequences
encoding the preprosomatostatins, it became evident that the two forms of
somatostatin that had been identified in intestinal and neural tissues,
namely, somatostatin-14 and somatostatin-28, an amino terminal extended
form of somatostatin-14, arise by alternative posttranslational processing
of the common prosomatostatin that is expressed in the different cell
types (29) (Fig. 4). In the pancreatic islets the predominant form of
somatostatin is liberated as the somatostatin-14, whereas in the intestine
the somatostatin-28 predominates. In the nervous system combinations of
somatostatin-14 and somatostatin-28 are liberated in specific regions of
the hypothalamus and extrahypothalamic brain. There is some evidence that
separate and distinct receptors exist for somatostatin-14 and somato-
statin-28.

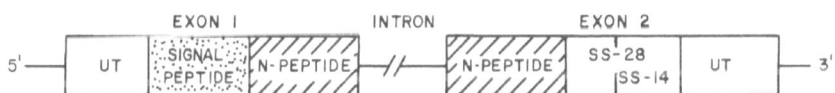

Fig. 3. Diagram of the somatostatin gene. The rat (24,25) and
human (26) genes share the identical topography and are 70-80%
similar in their nucleotide sequences. UT = untranslated tracts
of the mRNA; SS-14 and SS-28 indicate sequences of the somatostatin peptides of 14 and 28 amino acids, respectively.

7

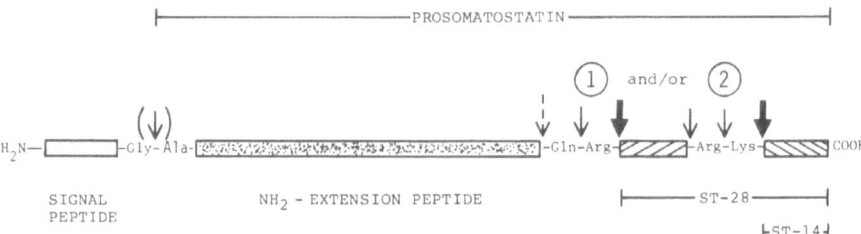

Fig. 4. Diagram of the structure of rat preprosomatostatin. The structures of the rat, human and fish preprohormones are similar. The N-terminal signal sequence required for entrance of the nascent polypeptide into the cisterna of the rough endoplasmic reticulum during amino acid polymerization, is cleaved at a Gly-Ala bond. The somatostatin peptides, somato-statin-28 (ST-28) and somatostatin-14 (ST-14) reside at the carboxyl end of the prohormone and are liberated from the prohormone by cleavages at the basic residues, Arginine and Arginine-Lysine. The prosomatostatin undergoes alternative processing at either (1) the Gln-Arg or the Arg-Lys sequence depending upon the specific cellular phenotype in which the somatostatin gene is expressed.

REGULATION OF PEPTIDE HORMONE GENE TRANSCRIPTION

As indicated earlier, the expression of specific genes could, in theory, be regulated at any one or more of several levels (Fig.1). Clearly, posttranscriptional RNA processing and posttranslational protein-processing are regulated with regard to the alternative patterns of processing that are observed in phenotypically different cells. This situation implies that there exist specific gene products involved in these regulatory processes. The major focus, however, in recent years has been on the molecular processes involved in the regulation of gene tran-scription (30). The factors that mediate gene transcription appear conceptually to fall into at least two classes: (i) Factors that lend inducibility or permissivity for the expression of a specific gene in a specific cell type, and (ii) the factors which serve as the metabolic inducers of gene transcription. Analyses of gene structure and function reveal that most genes encoding biologically important proteins are flanked by regulatory sequences that receive extra-genic signals trans-mitted by transacting factors that, in turn, transduce information through cis-acting mechanisms resulting in the activation of gene transcription (Fig. 5). For the most part, these signal-responsive regions of the gene reside in the 5' flanking sequences of genes but can also reside within introns or the coding or exons or even the 3' flanking region. These sequences are known as "regulatory response elements." The cis-acting regulatory response elements are termed "tissue-specific enhancers" when they serve permissive functions in allowing the expression of specific genes and "silencers" or repressors when they inhibit inducibility of expression of genes (31) (Fig. 6). Other regulatory-response elements serve as target sequences for the metabolic regulators such as thyroid hormones, or corticosteroids and require the presence and activation of tissue-specific enhancers (alternatively the absence of tissue-specific silencers) in order to function in response to metabolic signaling.

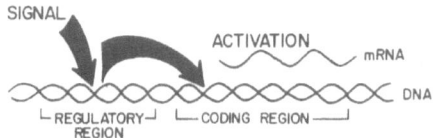

Fig. 5. Simplistic diagram depicting the concept of the activation of gene transcription. "Signals" consisting of transacting molecular complexes (proteins) impinge on "regulatory" regions of the gene, usually but not always, located in the 5' flanking region of the gene and send energy in cis to initiate the transcriptional processes for the synthesis of RNA from the template-coding region of the gene.

In many respects, the identification of regulatory-response elements flanking expressed genes fulfills a prediction and supports the hypothesis put forward by Davidson, Cohn and Britten over 20 years ago (32,33). These investigators discovered that mammalian genomes contain in addition to unique, single-copy DNA sequences, families of repetitive sequences that are reiterated throughout the genome. They proposed that in a qualitative sense, the genome contained genes encoding "constitutive" proteins consisting of structural proteins, enzymes, etc., that constitute the cellular architecture and serve metabolic functions of the cells, and in addition contained repetitive sequences which encode factors (RNAs, proteins) whose sole functions are to regulate other genes and serve as "integrating" sequences.

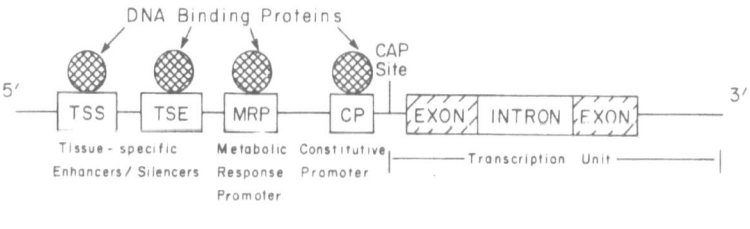

Fig. 6. Conceptual framework for the interactive process involved in gene regulation. To activate transcription of a transcription unit from the CAP site the specific interactions of a series of DNA binding proteins must occur with defined regulatory elements of the gene. For purposes of simplification the regulatory regions of the gene have been designated as constituative promoter (CP), metabolic response promoters (MRP) and tissue-specific enhancers (TSE), activators of gene transcription and tissue-specific silencers (TSS), repressors of gene transcription. Unique combinations of the presence or absence of specific DNA-binding proteins that interact with these DNA elements may confer the information requested for expression or non-expression of specific genes. The base-sequences shown at the bottom of the figure are conjectural inasmuch as some evidence indicates that sequences with those motifs may confer these categories of regulation to gene expression.

9

Indeed, the sequences of many of the regulatory-response elements are now known and consist of short (10 to 20 base pairs) sequences that exist in structurally homologous sets (34,35). They often have dyad symmetry, appear in sets of two or more, are independent of orientation, (3-5' or 5-3') and appear to have rather loose positional constraints inasmuch as that they may reside within several kilobases of the DNA surrounding the structural gene which they regulate. Current information indicates that these regulatory response elements serve as targets of interaction with regulatory proteins which are transacting DNA-binding proteins. One may conjecture that the genes encoding these transacting regulatory proteins may exist in families that are structurally related one to the other.

REGULATORY-RESPONSE ELEMENTS IN THE SOMATOSTATIN GENE

The somatostatin gene contains just such regulatory response elements (see chapters by Goodman and Dixon in this volume). Expression of the somatostatin gene is readily induced by factors that activate adenylate cyclase resulting in the formation of cyclic AMP. Mutational deletion analyses of the 5' sequences flanking the somatostatin gene reveal the presence of a cyclic AMP-response element which has the consensus motif of TGAGCTCAAGXXX. The sequence, or similar sequences, are found in many other genes that are responsive to cyclic AMP such as vasoactive intestinal peptide, glycoprotein hormone alpha subunit, prolactin, tyrosine hydroxylase, and phosphoenol pyruvate carboxy kinase. In addition to the presence of cyclic AMP-dependent metabolic-response elements there is also evidence that combinations of both tissue-specific enhancers and tissue-specific silencers reside in the further 5' flanking regions of the somatostatin gene.

SUMMARY

Based on these considerations of our current understanding of the molecular workings of the expression of genes, much excitement has been generated over the prospect of the eventual identification, isolation and structural characterization not only of the regulatory-response elements of the genes but of the regulatory genes themselves. It again appears that in her wonder nature has exploited the utilization of combinatorial functions to produce a complex set of regulatory processes from a relatively simple number of elements. One can imagine that the relatively small number of specific transacting regulatory factors (DNA binding proteins) could account for the specific regulation of a vastly large number of genes. The presence or absence of combinations of a few dozen positive and negative regulatory proteins interacting with the genes could conceivably account for the tissue-specific expression of the approximately 10^5-10^6 genes estimated to constitute the total informational repertoire of the mammalian genome.

ACKNOWLEDGMENTS

I thank Janice Canniff for typing the manuscript and Dr. Seymour Reichlin for the organization of this highly-informative symposium on the biology of the somatostatins.

REFERENCES

1. Brown DD. Gene expression in eukaryotes. Science 1981; 211:667-74.
2. Darnell JE. Variety in the level of gene control in eukaryotic

cells. Nature 1982; 297:365-71.

3. Alberts B, Bray D, Lewis J, Raff M, Roberts K, Watson JD. Molecular biology of the cell. New York: Garland, 1983.

4. Habener JF. Genetic control of hormone formation. In: Wilson J, Foster D, eds. Williams textbook of endocrinology. 7th ed. Saunders, 1985:9-32.

5. Baxter JD, Ivarie RD. Regulation of gene expression by glucocorticoid hormones: studies of receptors and responses in cultured cells. Recept Horm Action 1978; 2:251-84.

6. O'Malley B. Steroid hormone action in eukaryotic cells. J Clin Invest 1984; 74:307-12.

7. Hakanson R, Thorell J, eds. Biogenetics of neuro-hormonal peptides. Orlando, FL: Academic Press, 1985.

8. Cohen P. The role of protein phosphorylation in neural and hormonal control of cellular activity. Nature 1982; 296:613-20.

9. Rubin RP. The role of calcium in the release of neurotransmitter substances and hormones. Pharmacol Rev 1970; 22:389-428.

10. Berridge MJ, Irvine RF. Insositol triphosphate, a novel second messenger in cellular signal transduction. Nature 1984; 312:315-21.

11. Cheung WY. Calmodulin plays a pivotal role in cellular regulation. Science 1980; 207:19-27.

12. Heinrich G, Gros P, Habener JF. Glucagon gene sequence: four of six exons encode separate functional domains of rat pre-proglucagon. J Biol Chem 1984; 259:14082-7.

13. Dayhoff MO. In: Atlas of protein sequence and structure. Washington, DC: Nat Biomed Res Found, 1978; 5(suppl 3).

14. Spindel ER, Zilberberg MD, Habener JF, Chin WW. Two prohormones for gastrin-releasing peptides are encoded by two mRNAs differing by 19 nucleotides. Proc Natl Acad Sci USA 1986; 83:19-23.

15. Rosenfeld MG, Mermod JJ, Amara SG, et al. Production of a novel neuropeptide encoded by the calcitonin gene via tissue-specific RNA processing. Nature 1983; 304:129-36.

16. Nawa H, Kotani H, Nakanishi S. Tissue-specific generation of two preprotachykinin mRNAs from one gene by alternative RNA splicing. Nature 1984; 312:20-7.

17. Kitamura N, Takagaki Y, Furuto S, Tanaka T, Nawa H, Nakanishi S. A single gene for bovine high molecular weight and low molecular weight kininogens. Nature 1983; 305:545-9.

18. Habener JF, Lund PK, Jacobs W, Dee PC, Goodman RH. Polypeptide precursors of regulatory peptides. In: Rich DH, Gross E, eds. Peptides: synthesis, structure, function. Rockford, IL: Pierce Chem; 1981:457-69.

19. Chang ACY, Cochet M, Cohen SN. Structural organization of human genomic DNA encoding the pro-opiomelanocortin peptide. Proc Natl Acad Sci USA 1980; 77:4890-4.

20. Mojsov S, Heinrich G, Wilson IB, Ravazolla M, Orci L, Habener JF. Divestification of preproglucagon gene expression in pancreas and intestine occurs at the level of post-translational processing. J Biol Chem 1986 (in press).

21. Marx JL. Antibodies: getting their genes together. Science 1981; 217:1015-7.

22. Hobart P, Crawford R, Shen L, Pictet R, Rutter WJ. Cloning and sequence analyses of cDNAs encoding two distinct somatostatin precursors in the endocrine pancreas of anglerfish. Nature 1980; 288:137-41.

23. Magazin M, Minth CD, Funckes CL, Deschenes R, Tavianini MA, Dixon JE. Sequence of a cDNA encoding pancreatic presomatostatin-22. Proc Natl Acad Sci USA 1982; 79:5152-6.

24. Tavianini MA, Hayes TE, Magazin MD, Minth CD, Dixon JE. Isolation, characterization and DNA sequence of the rat somatostatin gene. J Biol Chem 1984; 259:11798-803.

25. Montminy MR, Goodman RH, Horovitch SJ, Habener JF. Primary structure of the gene encoding rat preprosomatostatin. Proc Natl Acad Sci USA 1984; 81:3337-40.

26. Shen L-P, Rutter WL. Sequence of the human somatostatin I gene. Science 1984; 224:168-71.

27. Shen L-P, Pictet RL, Rutter WL. Human somatostatin I: sequence of the cDNA. Proc Natl Acad Sci USA 1982; 79:4575-9.

28. Goodman RH, Aron DC, Roos BA. Rat pre-prosomatostatin. J Biol Chem 1983; 258:5570-3.

29. Reichlin S. Somatostatin. N Engl J Med 1983; 309:1495-1501.

30. Habener JF. Regulation of polypeptide-hormone biosynthesis at the level of the genome. Am J Physiol 1985; 249:C191-9.

31. Velcich A, Ziff E. Repression of activators. Nature 1984; 312:594-5.

32. Britten RJ, Davidson EH. Gene regulation for higher cells: a theory. Science 1969; 165:349-57.

33. Davidson EH, Britten RJ. Regulation of gene expression: possible role of repetitive sequences. Science 1979; 204:1052-9.

34. Reudelhuber T. Upstream and downstream control of eukaryotic genes. Nature 1984; 312:700-1.

35. Walker MD, Edlund T, Boulet AM, Rutter WJ. Cell-specific expression controlled by the 5'-flanking region of insulin and chymotrypsin genes. Nature 1983; 306:557-61.

2

STRUCTURE AND REGULATION OF THE RAT SOMATOSTATIN GENE

Jack E. Dixon, Timothy E. Hayes, Marie Tavianini,
Bernard A. Roos,* and Ourania Andrisani

Department of Biochemistry, Purdue University
West Lafayette, IN 47907

*Mineral Metabolism Laboratory, American Lake Veterans
Administration Medical Center, Tacoma, WA 98493

STRUCTURE AND ARCHITECTURE OF THE SOMATOSTATIN GENE

The function and structure of the polypeptide hormone somatostatin have been studied for a number of years in several species [see reviews] (1,2). The 14-residue form of somatostatin has been shown to be identical amongst all organisms examined. In addition, several other members of the somatostatin family have been identified, including a 28-residue somatostatin from the anglerfish (3) and a 22-residue somatostatin from the catfish (4,5). cDNAs have been isolated and sequenced which encode each of these peptides (3,6-12) and recently the gene encoding somatostatin-14 has been isolated from a human gene library by Shen and Rutter (13) and from a rat gene library both by Montminy et al. (14) and our laboratory (15). We have sequenced and analyzed the rat somatostatin gene in detail. The sequence of the gene is shown in Figure 1, and a schematic representation of the important structural features described below are outlined in Figure 2.

The transcriptional unit of the somatostatin gene includes exons of 238 and 367 base pairs (bp) separated by one intron of 621 bp. The intron is located between the codons for Gln (-57) and Glu (-56) of prosomatostatin. Analysis of the nucleotide sequence 5' to the start of transcription reveals a number of sequences which may be involved in the expression of somatostatin. A variant of the "TATA" box, TTTAAA, lies 26 bp upstream from the start of transcription, and a sequence homologous to the "CAAT" box (GGCTAAT) is 92 bp upstream from the transcription start. A long alternating purine-pyrimidine stretch, $(CT)_{25}$ which is similar to Z-DNA-forming sequences in other genes, lies 628 bp 5' to the transcription start and is flanked by small repeats. Hybridization analysis shows that this region is highly repeated in the genome and that homologous sequences are located approximately 2 kilobase pairs downstream from the poly(A) addition site. Southern hybridization of the lambda clone with probes derived from brain or liver poly(A+) RNA demonstrates that another transcribed sequence lies about 7 kilobase pairs downstream from the poly(A) addition site of the rat somatostatin gene. Southern blotting analysis of rat DNA suggests that a single gene is present which codes for the prohormone which is ultimately processed into somatostatin-14.

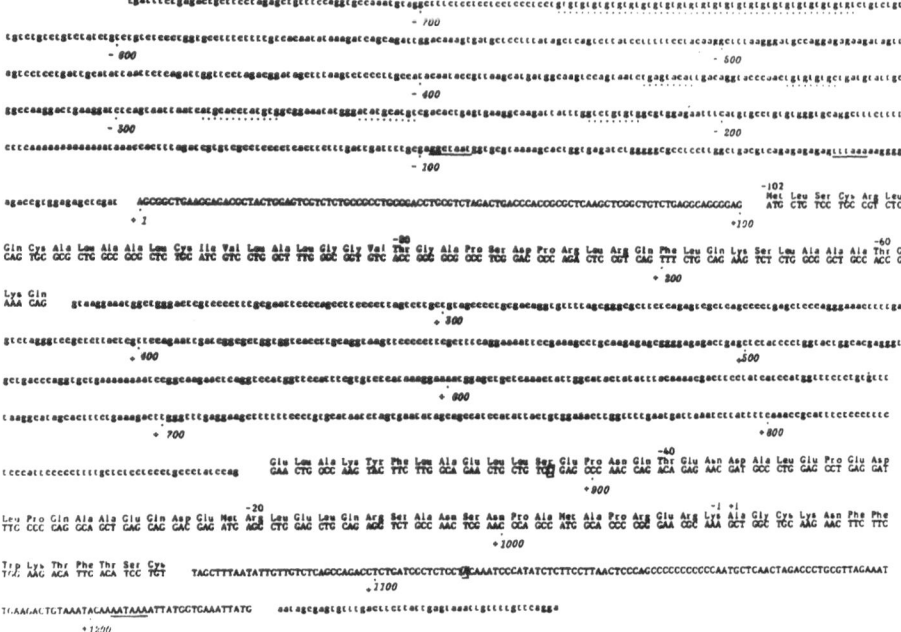

Fig. 1. DNA sequence of the rat somatostatin gene. Nucleotides found in mature messenger RNA are capitalized; nucleotides in flanking and intervening sequences are lower case. Nucleotides are numbered in *italics* with the start of transcription designated as +1. Amino acids are numbered with the first amino acid of somatostatin-p14 designated as +1. The TATA and CAAT boxes and the poly(A) addition site are underlined by solid lines. Alternating purine-pyrimidine sequences (potential Z DNA sequences) are underlined by dotted lines. Two changes in sequence from somatostatin cDNA are boxed.

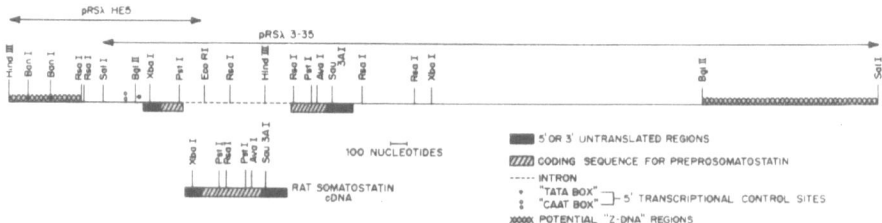

Fig. 2. Schematic comparison and structural features. Selected restriction sites are indicated on the composite map to facilitate alignment of the cDNA and gene. The extent of the two clones are indicated above the map. Location of introns, exons, and pertinent structural features are as shown.

The human gene also consists of two exons separated by an intron of 877 bp. The lambda phage harboring the human gene also contains repeated sequences but their nature and locations have not been determined, with the exception of an interrupted stretch of the repeated dinucleotide TG in the intron. The exon-intron junction is exactly in the same part in the rat and human genes. A comparison of the human and rat gene can be of some use in determining how the two genes have drifted evolutionarily and, by contrast, how well they have maintained important sequences. Implicit in the interpretation of such a comparison is the assumption that elements of organization and sequence or structure which are of importance at some level of function will be conserved across species lines. A diagrammatic comparison of the rat and human sequences is shown in Figure 3. The boxes represent identity of more than 75%, not counting small insertions added for optimization of alignment; gaps in the horizontal lines indicate breaks in nonhomologous regions for optimization of alignment. One of the most striking features of the comparison is that almost all of the sequences present in the mRNA are conserved. The two transcription initiation sites are 5 bp apart and are separated by nonhomologous sequences but except for a 9 bp stretch of nonhomology beginning 15 bp into the rat mRNA, the 5' untranslated regions are highly homologous. The translated sequences are 90% identical, as might be expected from the close relatedness of the two peptides. On the other hand, the introns show considerably less homology than the other transcribed sequences, indicating that a lack of drift between two regions is not necessarily an artifact of the relatedness of the two species. The lengths of the introns differ significantly (621 bp in the rat and 877 bp in the human gene) and alignment of homologous sequences in them requires the introduction of significant gaps. Twelve of 16 sequences between the blocks of homology in the intron require gaps of more than 5 bp to align the homologous sequences on either side. The largest such gap is 122 bp long and is near the middle of the intron. The blocks of homology comprise 46% of the intron, indicating the extent of drift in a presumably nonfunctional sequence. There are very short blocks of homology on the intron sides of the splice junctions (the intron begins with 7 identical bp at the 5' end and ends with a stretch of 12 out of 13 bp identical at the 3' end), indicating that only short sequences are needed to indicate the proper splice sites. The 3' untranslated sequences are less similar than those at the 5' end of the mRNA. There is a stretch of 7 identical bp past the codon for the C-terminal cysteine, but the two blocks of homology in the next 87 bp contain only 33 bp or about 38% of this segment. The final block of homology is much more similar. The 3' 56 bp are 93% identical and the 3' 36 bp are entirely identical, which is a surprising finding for a sequence in which the only recognized functional element is the 6 bp long AATAAA poly(A)-addition consensus signal. The conservation of such a long sequence hints at additional elements needed for a functional poly-(A)-addition signal.

In the process of studying the architecture of the rat somatostatin gene, Hayes and Dixon (16) have mapped and sequenced several repeated sequences which flank the gene and they also used several techniques to study DNA conformations within the gene. The work of Hayes and Dixon (16) has compared the sequence of the rat gene to the published sequence of the human gene, again with an eye toward potential variations in DNA conformation along the gene as well as how these variations might function in the regulation of gene expression. These investigators made the following observations in regards to DNA conformations in the rat gene: (a) the rat somatostatin gene is flanked both 5' and 3' by repeated elements with the sequence $(TG)_n$ and that these elements form Z-DNA in supercoiled plasmids; (b) the sequences adjoining the $(TG)_n$ elements interact with them at the B-DNA/Z-DNA junctions and influence Z-DNA formation there; (c) there is a 32 bp APP sequence in the human gene, which is in an analogous position to

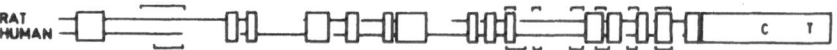

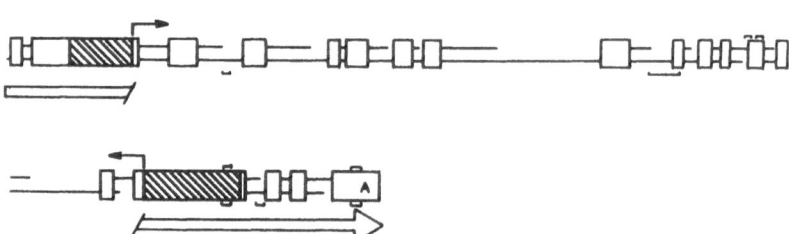

Fig. 3. Nucleotide sequence homology between the rat and human
somatostatin genes. Boxes indicate sequences which are at least
75% identical. Horizonal lines indicate nonhomologous sequences;
breaks in the horizontal lines indicate gaps introduced to op-
timize alignment of homologous sequences. The hatched boxes
represent translated sequences. The thick arrow marks sequences
which are present in the mature mRNA; the thin arrows mark the
boundaries of the introns. Brackets above or below the sequences
indicate the location and length of APP sequences. The locations
of the "CAAT" box, "TATA" box and AATAAA polyadenylation signal
are marked by the letters C, T and A, respectively.

the $(TG)_{25}$ tract upstream from the rat gene but whose sequence is not
homologous to it; and (d) in the region 5' to the transcribed sequences,
both the rat and human somatostatin genes contain short APP sequences
which are conserved between the two species with regard to their positions
in relation to the transcription initiation sites but not with regard to
their sequences.

CELL SPECIFIC REGULATION OF THE SOMATOSTATIN GENE

The expression of some eukaryotic genes is remarkably specific. An
individual gene may be highly expressed in one cell and almost completely
off in another. In addition, cells have the ability to selectively
regulate the levels of specific protein products. The factors which
govern cell specific expression are now under active investigation.

Our goal with regard to the somatostatin gene is to understand the
elements (promoter sequences and protein factors) involved in the expression and regulation of this promoter. We initially wanted to define the
sequences of the somatostatin promoter involved in the transcription of
this gene in endocrine and neuronally derived cells. In addition, we
planned to explore the mechanism of cell specific expression. Are there
particular sequences within the promoter that render the promoter cell
specific? We have utilized a neuronally derived cell line, CA-77, which
expresses the endogenous somatostatin gene to study the expression of the
somatostatin promoter. The CA-77 cell line takes up exogenous DNA by the
$CaPO_4$ co-precipitation technique poorly. However, utilizing electroporation DNA can be introduced into the CA-77 cell line.

16

In all of the experiments described below we have made use of a plasmid containing a "reporter gene." The reporter gene can produce the enzyme chloramphenicol acetyl transferase (CAT) (18). This enzyme can acetylate chloramphenicol in the presence of acetyl CoA, and the products of the reaction can easily be separated from the starting material on thin layer chromatography. The plasmid pCAT B contains the structural CAT gene and appropriate RNA splice sites, however it is incapable of expressing the CAT enzyme unless an appropriate promoter is cloned in front of the structural gene (Fig. 4). When sequences which harbor promoter activity are cloned in front of the CAT gene, the strength of that promoter can be determined indirectly by measuring CAT activity (18).

We have constructed a library of deletions of the somatostatin 5' regulatory region proceeding 3' from the HindIII site located 750 bp upstream from the start of transcription (15). An outline of how the deletions were carried out are shown in Figure 5. The method of DNA construction used here insured that no new plasmid sequences were positioned next to the somatostatin promoter, thus "false" promoter sites containing the plasmid could not selectively affect the expression of specific deletion-mutants. Figure 6 shows the results of a typical experiment where plasmids containing the somatostatin promoter fragment cloned in front of CAT gene were introduced into several cell lines. The CA-77 cell line synthesizes somatostatin, and thus the endogenous structural gene for somatostatin is "on." When the various plasmids harboring the somatostatin promoter were introduced into CA-77 cells, it is clear that both the 750 bp and 250 bp promoter actively "fire" the structural CAT gene. In contrast, neither plasmid construction is expressed in HeLa cells or a kidney cell line BSC 40. To insure that the transfections had proceeded properly, a plasmid harboring the Rous sarcoma viral (RSV) promoter cloned in front of CAT (pRSV CAT) was introduced into both HeLa and BSC 40 cell lines. From the results shown in Figure 6 it is evident that the RSV promoter is active in these cells, whereas the somatostatin promoter is inefficient in CAT gene expression, suggesting that cell specific factors are necessary for the transcriptional activity of this promoter. Utilizing additional deletions it is possible to show that only 70 bp of the somatostatin promoter are necessary for efficient expression

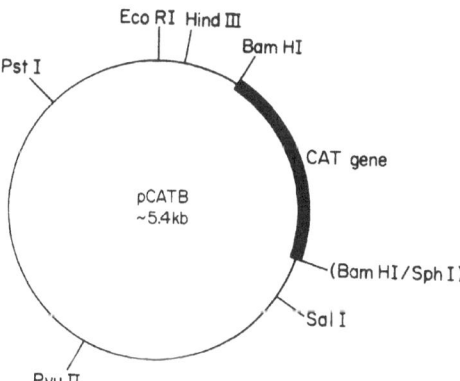

Fig. 4. The plasmid pCAT B. This plasmid is a derivative of pBR322 which contains the CAT structural gene and 3' polyadenylation and splice donor-acceptor sites from SV 40 T antigen.

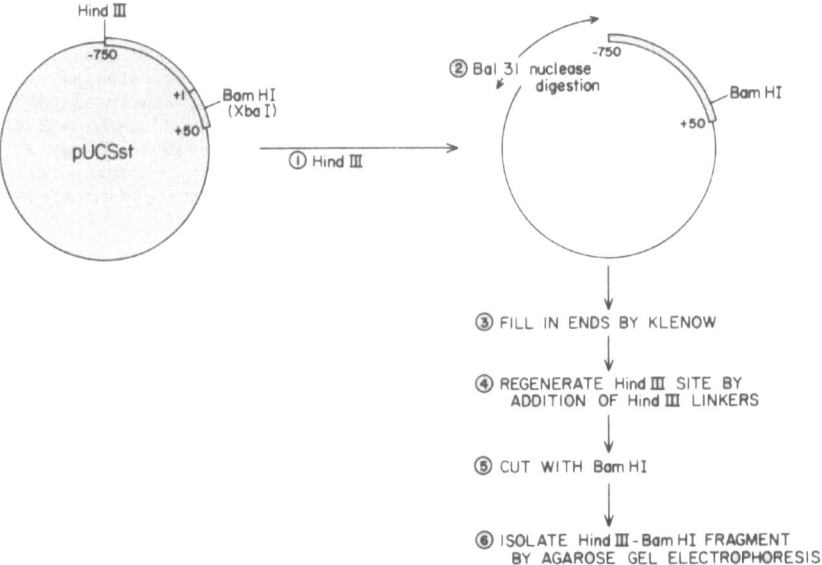

Fig. 5.   Construction of somatostatin promoter deletion mutants.
The plasmid pUC SST contains approximately 750 bp of the somatostatin promoter.   The plasmid was reacted with HindIII, followed
by Exo nuclease III digestion for various times.   HindIII
linkers were added and a HindIII-BamHI fragment removed and
cloned in front of the CAT structural gene.

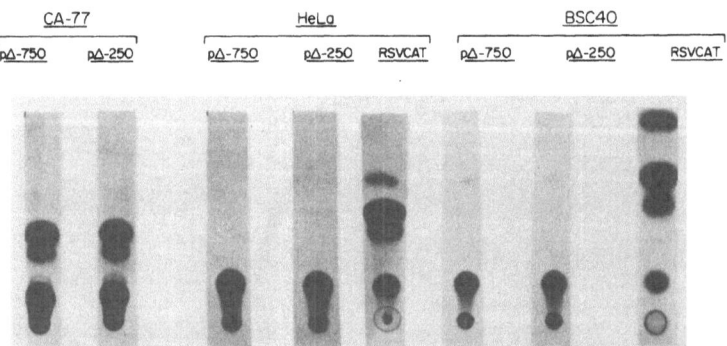

Fig. 6.   Cell specific expression of the rat somatostatin gene.
Three cell lines, CA-77, HeLa and BSC 40 were transfected with
the hybrid somatostatin-CAT plasmid containing either 750 or 250
bp of promoter DNA.   The three panels are autoradiograms of thin
layer chromatography.   The arrow denotes acetylated chloramphenicol resulting from the action of the acetyltransferase.   The
plasmid pRSV CAT was used as a control in all transfections
(only HeLa and BSC 40 results are shown).

in CA-77 cells. In contrast, transfection with plasmids containing only 43 bases of the somatostatin promoter are inactive. Thus the information necessary for cell specific expression of the rat somatostatin genes resides between nucleotides -70 and -43. It is also of interest that this region harbors sequences which modulate gene expression via cAMP regulation (see following manuscript, Goodman et al.).

REFERENCES

1. Reichlin S. Somatostatin. N Engl J Med 1983; 309:1495.
2. Vale W, Rivier C, Brown M. Regulatory peptides of the hypothalamus. Annu Rev Physiol 1977; 39:473.
3. Goodman RH, Jacobs JW, Chin WW, Lund PK, Dee PC, Habener JF. Somatostatin-28 encoded in a cloned cDNA obtained from a rat medullary thyroid carcinoma. Proc Natl Acad Sci USA 1980; 77:5869.
4. Oyama H, Bradshaw RA, Bates OJ, Permutt A. Amino acid sequence of catfish pancreatic somatostatin I. J Biol Chem 1980; 255:2251.
5. Andrews PC, Dixon JE. Isolation and structure of a peptide hormone predicted from an mRNA sequence: a second somatostatin from the catfish pancreas. J Biol Chem 1981; 256:8267.
6. Hobart P, Crawford R, Shen L-P, Pictet R, Rutter WJ. Cloning and sequence analysis of cDNAs encoding two distinct somatostatin precursors found in the endocrine pancreas of anglerfish. Nature (London) 1980; 288:137.
7. Taylor WL, Collier KJ, Deschenes RJ, Weith HL, Dixon JE. Sequence analysis of a cDNA coding for a pancreatic precursor to somatostatin. Proc Natl Acad Sci USA 1981; 78:6694.
8. Minth CD, Taylor WL, Magazin MA, Collier K, Weith HL, Dixon JE. The structure of cloned DNA complementary to catfish pancreatic somatostatin-14. J Biol Chem 1982; 257:10372.
9. Magazin M, Minth CD, Funckes CL, Deschenes R, Tavianini MA, Dixon JE. Sequence of a cDNA encoding pancreatic preprosomatostatin-22. Proc Natl Acad Sci USA 1982; 79:5152.
10. Goodman RH, Aron DC, Roos BA. Rat pre-prosomatostatin: structure and processing by microsomal membranes. J Biol Chem 1983; 258:5570.
11. Funckes CL, Minth CD, Deschenes R, Magazin M, Tavianini MA, Sheets M, Collier K, Weith HL, Aron DC, Roos BA, Dixon JE. Cloning and characterization of a mRNA-encoding rat preprosomatostatin. J Biol Chem 1983; 258:8781.
12. Shen L-P, Pictet RL, Rutter WJ. Human somatostatin I: sequence of the cDNA. Proc Natl Acad Sci USA 1982; 79:4575.
13. Shen L-P, Rutter WJ. Sequence of the human somatostatin I gene. Science 1984; 224:168.
14. Montminy R, Goodman RH, Horovitch SJ, Habener JF. Primary structure of a gene encoding rat pre-prosomatostatin. Proc Natl Acad Sci USA 1984; 81:3337.
15. Tavianini MA, Hayes TE, Magazin MD, Minth CD, Dixon JE. Isolation, characterization and DNA sequence of the rat somatostatin gene. J Biol Chem 1984; 259:11798.
16. Hayes T, Dixon JE. Z-DNA in the rat somatostatin gene. J Biol Chem 1985; 260:8145.
17. Birnbaum RS, Muszynski M, Roos BA. Tumor and plasma somatostatin-like immunoreactivity in transplantable rat medullary thyroid carcinoma. Cancer Res 1980; 40:4192.
18. Gorman CM, Moffat LF, Howard BH. Recombinant genomes which express chloramphenicol acetyltransferase in mammalian cells. Mol Cell Biol 1982; 2:1044.

3

REGULATION OF SOMATOSTATIN GENE EXPRESSION BY CYCLIC AMP

Richard H. Goodman, Gail Mandel, Kevin A. Sevarino, and
Marc R. Montminy*

Division of Molecular Medicine
Department of Medicine
Tufts-New England Medical Center, Boston, MA 02111
*Peptide Biology Laboratory, Salk Institute
La Jolla, CA 92037

The work of Sutherland, Rall, and colleagues in the 1950's firmly established the role of cyclic AMP as an important regulator of cellular processes. Cyclic AMP exerts profound effects on cytoskeletal assembly, intermediary metabolism, and cellular proliferation as well as on protein synthesis and secretion. More recently, cyclic AMP has been found to mediate the postsynaptic actions of some neurotransmitters. As a regulator of both protein synthesis and secretion, cyclic AMP could potentially play a central role in linking these two cellular processes. Such a linkage would assure that cells stimulated for secretion would also be stimulated for biosynthesis. Very little is known about how cyclic AMP regulates the biosynthesis of eukaryotic proteins.

This paper addresses the control of neuropeptide biosynthesis by cyclic AMP, an agent which stimulates secretion of many neuropeptides. We have focused on the peptide hormone somatostatin, whose biosynthesis and secretion has been extensively studied in several laboratories. We propose that the regulation of somatostatin biosynthesis by cyclic AMP is mediated through a specific genetic element located upstream from the somatostatin promoter. This element appears to be present in other neuropeptide genes that are regulated by cyclic AMP and consequently may be essential in a general way for stimulus-secretion-synthesis coupling in peptidergic neurons.

Many regulators of somatostatin secretion in neurons have been identified (for review see 1). Several somatostatin secretagogues, including some peptide hormones (vasoactive intestinal polypeptide, glucagon) and classical neurotransmitters (epinephrine), appear to act through a cyclic AMP-dependent pathway. Consequently, cyclic AMP-dependent mechanisms have been postulated to represent a common pathway for agents that influence somatostatin secretion.

In the following paper we have addressed two questions: Do agents that stimulate somatostatin secretion through cyclic AMP also regulate somatostatin biosynthesis and, if so, can specific elements within the somatostatin gene be identified that mediate the cyclic AMP-dependent regulation?

To determine whether cyclic AMP could mediate the coupling of somatostatin secretion to its biosynthesis, we initially asked whether somatostatin mRNA levels in primary cultures of diencephalic neurons were regulated by cyclic AMP. To perform these studies, we first prepared primary monolayer cultures of fetal (embryonic day 17) rat diencephalon. These cultures contain approximately 3% somatostatin-producing cells (2). Cells were maintained in culture for seven days and then were treated with 1 μM forskolin (a post-receptor activator of adenyl cyclase) or 30 mM KC1 for 1-4 hours. Somatostatin secretion was measured by radioimmunoassay, and somatostatin mRNA was extracted from the cells following the NP-40 method of Montminy, et al. (3).

RNA from the cultured cells was fractionated by electrophoresis on a denaturing agarose gel, transferred to nitrocellulose, and detected with an antisense somatostatin RNA hybridization probe. Preliminary studies had indicated that the level of sensitivity obtained using conventional nick-translated cDNA hybridization probes was not sufficient to allow us to detect somatostatin mRNA in the primary cultures. The antisense RNA probe was capable of detecting less than 1 pg of somatostatin mRNA. The construction of the antisense somatostatin RNA expression vector is depicted in Figure 1.

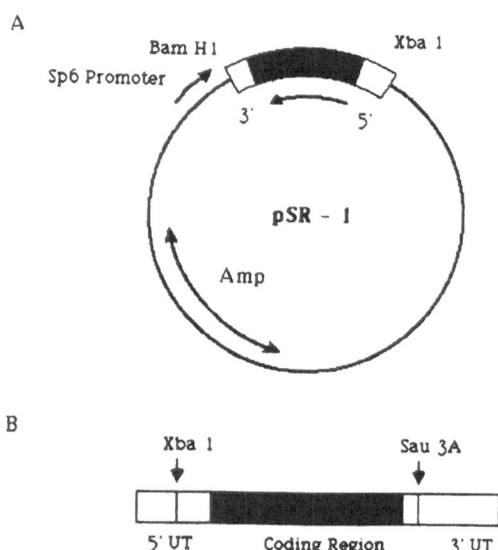

Fig. 1. (A) Structure of the somatostatin riboprobe vector, pSR-1. Bam H1 and Xba 1 indicate the sites of insertion of the somatostatin cDNA fragment into the pSP65 vector. The 5' to 3' orientation of the cDNA is shown with respect to the direction of transcription from the Sp6 promoter site. (B) Structure of the somatostatin cDNA. The Xba 1-Sau 3A fragment inserted into the pSP65 vector is delineated by arrows. 5'UT and 3'UT denote the 5' and 3' untranslated regions that flank the coding sequence.

Forskolin caused a two-fold increase in somatostatin secretion over a period of 4 hours, as shown in Figure 2. Somatostatin mRNA in the primary cultures increased approximately three- to four-fold over this period. Similar results were observed when the cells were treated with other agents that increase intracellular levels of cyclic AMP, such as cholera toxin or dibutyryl cyclic AMP. These results suggested that somatostatin mRNA accumulation might be coupled to secretion of the peptide. We considered two alternative hypotheses to explain these effects. The first, a cellular depletion model, proposed that somatostatin biosynthesis is regulated by intracellular levels of the neuropeptide. In this model, somatostatin secretion would be expected to stimulate mRNA accumulation by depleting intracellular stores. The second model proposed that cyclic AMP could independently stimulate somatostatin mRNA accumulation and peptide secretion. If the cellular depletion model was correct, we would expect that any somatostatin secretagogue would increase mRNA levels. We, therefore, measured somatostatin mRNA after treatment with 30 mM KCl, which stimulates somatostatin secretion but does not act through cyclic AMP (Fig. 2). KCl was as effective as forskolin in stimulating somatostatin secretion but had no effect on somatostatin mRNA levels. These results demonstrate that secretion of somatostatin can be uncoupled from mRNA accumulation, and that cyclic AMP probably stimulates somatostatin secretion and biosynthesis by independent pathways. To assure that KCl did not have a toxic effect on the diencephalic cells, we also measured somatostatin mRNA in cells treated with both forskolin and KCl. Somatostatin mRNA levels in these cells were no different from those in cells treated with forskolin alone, indicating that KCl does not have a toxic effect on mRNA accumulation.

As a first step toward characterizing the mechanism by which cyclic AMP regulates the biosynthesis of somatostatin, we introduced the cloned rat somatostatin gene into a foreign cell type, NIH 3T3 fibroblasts, which does not normally produce somatostatin. The expression vector for these studies, depicted in Figure 3, contains the somatostatin gene extending 750 base pairs upstream from the promoter to a site 3 kilobases downstream from the coding sequence. This construction is likely, therefore, to contain many of the sequences necessary for regulated expression of the somatostatin gene. Cells were transfected by the calcium phosphate tech-

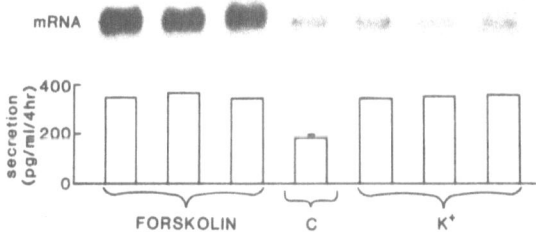

Fig 2. Stimulation of somatostatin mRNA accumulation and somatostatin secretion in primary cultures of diencephalic cells. The top of the figure shows an autoradiogram of a Northern blot containing cytoplasmic RNA from diencephalic cells hybridized with a ^{32}P-labeled somatostatin antisense RNA probe. The corresponding levels of somatostatin secretion from the individual cultures are shown at the bottom of the figure. Treatments with 1 μM forskolin, ethanol control, or 3 mM KCl are indicated.

nique (4) using the marker pSV2neo (5) which allows the selection of
stably transformed cells that have integrated the neomycin-resistant gene
into their genome. Stably transfected cells were grown in the presence of
400 μg/ml G418, a neomycin analog. The media from the antibiotic-selected
cell lines was assayed for immunoreactive somatostatin. Because the 3T3
fibroblasts secrete more than 95% of the peptides produced over 24 hours,
screening of the tissue culture media provided a very efficient method to
identify clones that expressed the foreign somatostatin gene. Stable
integration of the foreign gene into the genome of the 3T3 fibroblasts was
ultimately determined by Southern blotting analysis. This analysis
demonstrated that between 20 and 30 copies of the gene had integrated in a
head-to-tail fashion in the transfected cells.

To determine whether cyclic AMP could modulate expression of the
somatostatin gene in a heterologous cell type, we analyzed somatostatin
mRNA levels in three lines of transfected 3T3 cells. In each of the cell
lines, somatostatin mRNA levels increased after treatment with 1 μM
forskolin (Fig. 4). This increase in somatostatin mRNA occurred as early
as 1 hour after forskolin treatment, the earliest time tested. Levels of
immunoreactive somatostatin produced by the transfected cells were also
increased by forskolin. Somatostatin mRNA was not detectable in control
3T3 cells treated with forskolin. These studies indicate that the 4.2
kilobase somatostatin gene fragment in the expression vector D3pSal
contains all the sequences necessary for regulation by cyclic AMP.

NIH 3T3 cells, while good hosts for gene transfer experiments, are
not necessarily the best choice for studies of neuropeptide gene expression. Several neuroendocrine cell lines have been developed, for example,

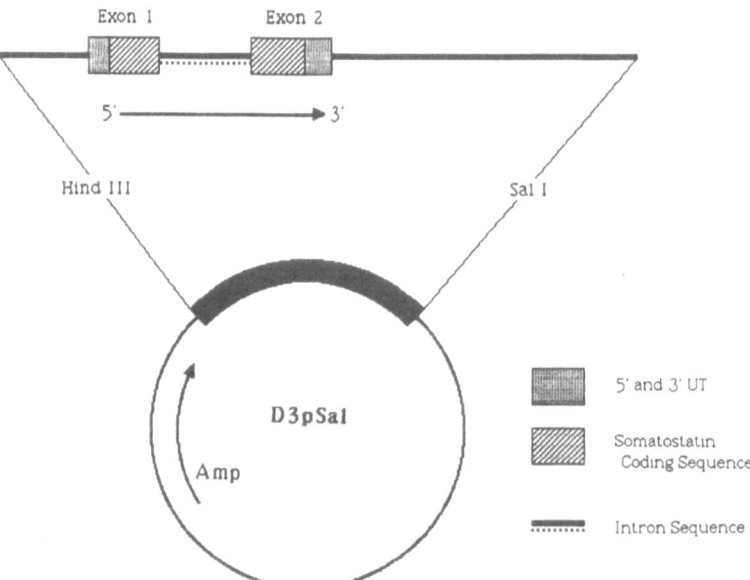

Fig. 3. Structure of the somatostatin gene expression vector
D3pSal. This plasmid contains the somatostatin gene extending
750 base pairs upstream from the promoter to a site 3 kilobases
downstream from the coding sequence. The two exons and single
intervening sequence are indicated.

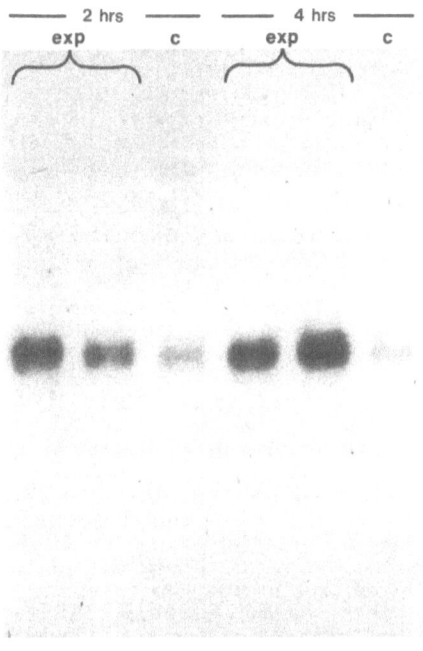

Fig. 4. Time course of forskolin-induced somatostatin mRNA accumulation in transfected 3T3 cells. This autoradiogram of a Northern blot depicts the amount of hybridizable somatostatin mRNA in either control (C) or 10^{-6} M forskolin (exp)-treated cells. Individual culture dishes containing 10^7 cells were harvested after 2 or 4 hours of treatment. This experiment was performed on a single transfected clone, D3pSal5. Other transfected 3T3 lines showed similar somatostatin mRNA induction in response to forskolin.

that probably contain many of the same membrane receptors and intracellular messenger systems normally involved in somatostatin regulation. Ideally, we would have performed our gene transfer experiments in a neuronal line that expresses the endogenous somatostatin gene. Unfortunately, neurons are particularly resistant to most gene transfer techniques. We, therefore, chose to use PC12 cells, derived from a rat pheochromocytoma (6) for further studies of somatostatin regulation.

The PC12 cell line provides a particularly good model for studies of cyclic AMP effects on neuropeptide gene transcription because cyclic AMP is known to regulate several genes normally expressed in PC12 cells. Additionally, mutant PC12 cell lines deficient in cyclic AMP-dependent protein kinases have been identified, allowing us to assess the role of these kinases in mediating the transcriptional effects of cyclic AMP on the somatostatin gene. PC12 cells also offer several technical advantages. They divide relatively rapidly in culture and can be selected with the neomycin analog G418. These cells can therefore be stably transfected by a variety of gene transfer techniques. After treatment with nerve growth factor, the cells develop a more differentiated phenotype, resembling mature sympathetic neurons. Cells can therefore be transfected with a foreign gene while in their undifferentiated, rapidly dividing state, then differentiated with nerve growth factor. PC12 cells do not normally produce somatostatin, eliminating problems of distinguishing between expression of the foreign and the endogenous gene.

Because PC12 cells are more difficult to transfect than 3T3 cells, we used electroporation to introduce the cloned rat somatostatin gene. This technique uses an electric current to produce small holes in the cell membrane and is more efficient than calcium phosphate precipitation for transfection of some cell lines (7). The somatostatin expression vector used in these studies extended from 250 base pairs upstream from the promoter to a site 4 kilobases downstream from the coding sequence. Cells were mixed with the cloned somatostatin gene and the selectable marker pSV2neo and were electroporated using a 3500 V, 0.9 MA shock. Antibiotic-resistant colonies were isolated after 2 to 3 weeks of selection, and somatostatin-expressing clones were detected by radioimmunoassay.

Somatostatin mRNA isolated from the transfected PC12 cells was identical in size to that found in normal somatostatin-producing cells (Fig. 5). For studies of gene regulation in foreign cells, it is also important to assure that the normal promoter signals are being used. We performed S1 nuclease mapping experiments to localize the transcriptional initiation site of the rat somatostatin gene in transfected PC12 cells. RNA from the medullary thyroid carcinoma cell line Ca-77 or one of the transfected PC12 cell lines was hybridized to a 5' end-labeled fragment of the cloned somatostatin gene, digested with S1 nuclease and analyzed on a denaturing polyacrylamide gel (Fig. 5). The size of the labeled DNA fragment protected by RNA from both cell lines was identical, indicating that the PC12 cells utilize the normal initiation signals in transcribing the foreign somatostatin gene.

Forskolin was used to examine the cyclic AMP-responsiveness of the foreign somatostatin gene expressed in PC12 cells. PC12 cells treated with 10 μM forskolin increased their level of somatostatin mRNA between 4 and 10-fold within 4 hours (Fig. 5). Wild-type PC12 cells treated with forskolin did not produce somatostatin. These findings confirmed our previous results using 3T3 fibroblasts but still did not identify the mechanism through which cyclic AMP stimulated somatostatin synthesis. Cyclic AMP could theoretically increase somatostatin mRNA levels through effects on transcriptional rate, mRNA precursor splicing, or mRNA stability.

To test the hypothesis that the regulation of somatostatin biosynthesis by cyclic AMP occurs at the transcriptional level and requires specific promoter sequences, we constructed a series of fusion genes containing portions of the somatostatin 5' flanking region linked to the bacterial marker enzyme chloramphenicol acetyltransferase (CAT) (Fig. 6). These fusion genes were introduced into PC12 cells by calcium phosphate precipitation and were tested in transient assays for their ability to respond to forskolin by increasing the level of CAT enzyme activity. CAT activity can be measured by determining the conversion of ^{14}C-chloramphenicol to mono- and diacetylated ^{14}C-chloramphenicol acetate, forms that can easily be separated by thin layer chromatography. Because CAT activity is not normally present in eukaryotic cells, all of the enzyme activity in the cell extracts is derived from the transfected fusion gene. An example of a CAT enzyme assay using a fusion gene that extended 750 bases in the 5' direction is shown in Figure 7. In this experiment, conversion of ^{14}C-chloramphenicol to ^{14}C-chloramphenicol acetate was increased 8-fold by

26

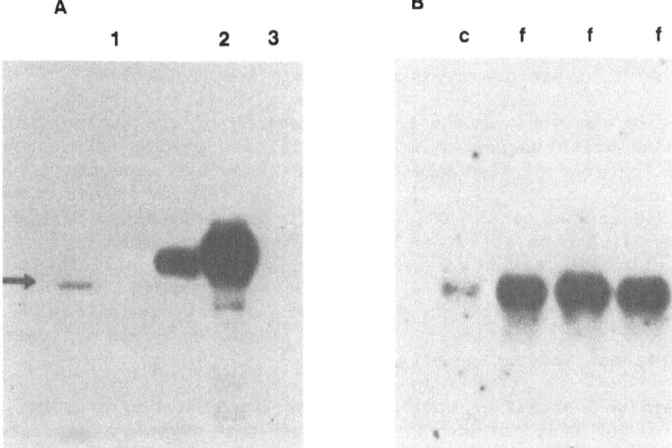

Fig. 5. (A) Localization of the transcriptional initiation site of the rat somatostatin gene in stably transfected PC12 cells and in Ca-77 rat medullary thyroid carcinoma cells. RNA from both cell lines was hybridized to a 5' end-labeled BssH2 fragment of the cloned somatostatin gene. The hybrid was digested with S1 nuclease and the products were analyzed on a denaturing 8% polyacrylamide gel. Lane 1 is an Hae 3-digested pBR322 size marker. Arrow indicates the position of a 123/124 bp doublet. Lanes 2 and 3 show the DNA fragments protected by mRNA from transfected PC12 and Ca-77 cells, respectively. (B) Effect of forskolin on somatostatin mRNA levels. Cytoplasmic RNA was prepared from stably transfected PC12 cells after treatment with either ethanol vehicle control (c) or 10 μM forskolin (f) for 4 hours. Three separate forskolin treatments are shown. One microgram of cytoplasmic RNA from each sample was electrophoresed, transferred to nitrocellulose, and hybridized to ^{32}P-labeled antisense somatostatin RNA.

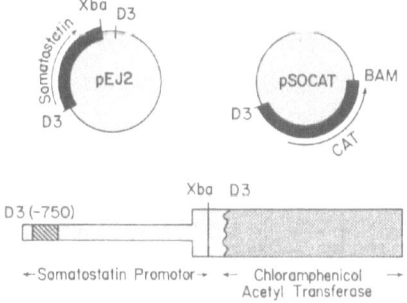

Fig. 6. Structure of the somatostatin-chloramphenicol acetyltransferase fusion gene. Hatched area within the somatostatin promoter represents region of Z-DNA.

forskolin. As a control for non-specific effects of forskolin, we also examined the activity of CAT genes under the control of a Rous sarcoma virus (RSV) or Simian virus 40 (SV40) promoters. CAT activity under the control of the viral promoters was not increased by forskolin.

By deleting portions of the promoter regions of the fusion genes, we could determine which sequences are essential for cyclic AMP-responsiveness. The structures of the deleted fusion genes are depicted in Figure 8. These genes contain 250, 71, or 48 bases of the somatostatin 5' flanking region linked to the CAT structural gene. Deletion of sequences upstream from -71 had no effect on cyclic AMP-responsiveness (Fig. 8). In contrast, cyclic AMP-responsiveness of a fusion gene containing only 48 bases of somatostatin 5' flanking sequences was markedly diminished. These results suggested that the 5' boundary of the somatostatin cyclic AMP-responsive element was located between 71 and 48 bases upstream from the transcriptional initiation site.

To determine whether a portion of the somatostatin promoter could confer cyclic AMP-responsiveness to a gene not normally regulated by cyclic AMP, we constructed the fusion gene depicted in Figure 9. In this construction, sequences between -60 and -29 of the somatostatin gene were ligated upstream from the SV40 promoter in the plasmid pA10-CAT2 (8). pA10-CAT2 contains the SV40 promoter without the enhancer sequences fused to the CAT structural gene. After treatment with forskolin, PC12 cells transfected with the somatostatin-SV40-CAT fusion gene increased their

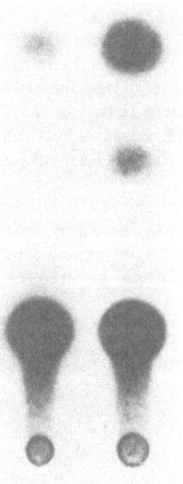

Fig. 7. CAT enzyme activity in PC12 cells transfected with the somatostatin-CAT fusion gene Δ (-750). Plates containing 10^6 cells were transfected with 40 μg of DNA and were treated for 48 hours with either ethanol vehicle (left) or 10 μM forskolin (right). Cell extracts were assayed for CAT activity by thin layer chromotography to separate acetylated forms (upper spots) from unreacted chloramphenicol.

28

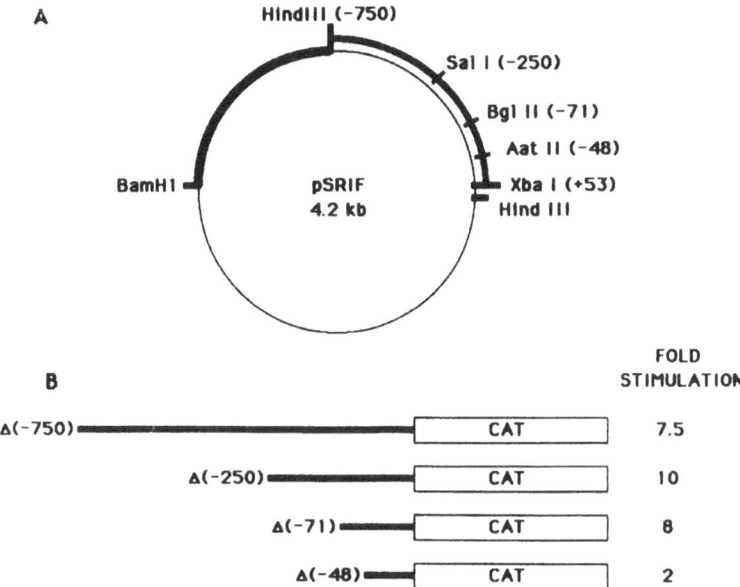

Fig. 8. Effect of forskolin on activity of somatostatin-CAT fusion genes. Fragments of the somatostatin 5' flanking region (A) were inserted upstream of the bacterial CAT gene. Four somatostatin-CAT constructions were prepared and analyzed for cAMP responsiveness after transfection into PC12 cells. (B) Fold-stimulation for each construction was calculated by dividing the percent conversion of (^{14}C)chloramphenicol to its acetylated forms in forskolin-treated samples by the percent conversion in control (ethanol-treated) samples.

level of CAT activity by 15-fold. Cells transfected with the parental vector pA10-CAT2 increased their level of CAT expression by only 1.5-fold after treatment with forskolin. When the somatostatin-SV40-CAT fusion gene was introduced into a mutant line of PC12 cells that lacks cyclic AMP-dependent protein kinase (Type 2) activity, CAT activity was not induced by forskolin. These results suggest that protein kinase (Type 2) activity is necessary for cyclic AMP's regulation of somatostatin gene expression.

Comparison of the cyclic AMP-responsive element within the somatostatin gene to sequences near the promoters of several other genes known to be regulated by cyclic AMP reveals a consensus sequence, 5'-TGACGTCA-3' (Table 1). Deletional analyses, similar to the studies we have described, have indicated that this consensus sequence may be involved in cyclic AMP-regulation of genes encoding vasoactive intestinal polypeptide (Tsukada, et al., submitted), proenkephalin (Comb, et al., in press), and phosphoenolpyruvate carboxykinase (9). Although the consensus sequence appears to be necessary, at least in some genes, for cyclic AMP-responsiveness, the sequence by itself is not sufficient for activity. Insertion of the consensus sequence alone into pA10-CAT2 does not confer cyclic AMP-responsiveness.

In summary, we have identified a region of the somatostatin gene that is required for regulation by cyclic AMP. This region is homologous to

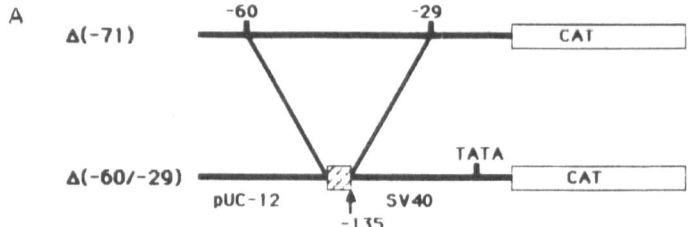

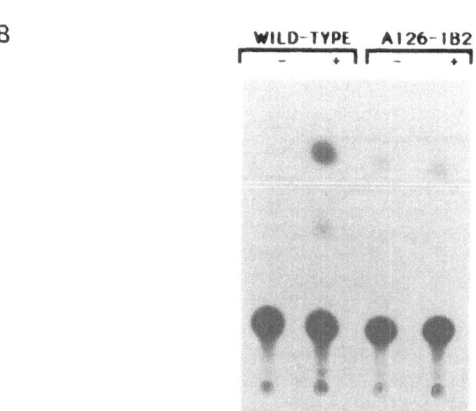

Fig. 9. Effects of forskolin on CAT activity of plasmid
Δ(-60/-29) in wild type and A126-1B2 cells. (A) A 30 bp
Nru 1-Dra 1 fragment from Δ(-71) was inserted into the Bg
12 site of pA10-CAT2, 135 bases upstream from the SV40
transcriptional initiation site. (B) Conversion of (^{14}C)-
chloramphenicol to acetylated forms in wild-type and A126-
1B2 cells after transfection with Δ(-60/-29). (+) indicates cells treated for 48 hours with 10 μM forskolin; (-)
indicates control cells treated with ethanol vehicle.

sequences in several other similarly regulated genes. Because cyclic AMP
can increase secretion of peptides from the regulated pathway of neuroendocrine cells, this cyclic AMP regulatory element may be important in
coordinating increases in secretion of specific peptides with increases in
peptide biosynthesis. It is likely that the cyclic AMP-regulatory element
identified in the promoter region of the somatostatin gene interacts with
DNA-binding proteins that are phosphorylated by cyclic AMP-dependent
protein kinase. The goal of future studies is to identify these DNA-
binding proteins, to determine how they are modified by cyclic AMP, and to
elucidate the mechanism by which they stimulate gene expression.

30

Table 1. Homology in 5'-flanking regions of genes containing
the somatostatin palindrome.

Gene	Sequence
Somatostatin*	TTGGCTGACGTCAGAGAGAGAG (−32)
PEPCK*	GCCCCTTACGTCAGAGGCGAGC (−74)
VIP*	TACTGTGACGTCTTTCAGAGCA (−60)
Parathyroid hormone	GGGAGTGACGTCATCT (−65)
Proenkephalin*	GGGCCTG CGTCAGC (−87)
α-Chorionic gonadotropin	AAAATTGACGTCATGG (−113)
C-fos*	CCCAGTGACGTAGGA (−57)
Cytomegalovirus enhancer	CCCATTGACGTCAATGGGAGTT (−124)
BLV LTR	GACAGAGACGTCAGCTGCCAGA (−144)
HTLV-II LTR	GGCCCTGACGTCCCTCCCCCCC (−162)
Intracisternal A particle	TCCCGTGACGTCATCTGGGG (−86)

Asterisks indicate genes that are known to be transcrip-
tionally regulated by cAMP. The position of the 3'-most
nucleotide is listed in parentheses at the end of each
sequence. PEPCK, phosphoenolpyruvate carboxykinase; BLV,
bovine leukemia virus; LTR, long terminal repeat; HTLV-II,
human T-cell leukemia virus type II.

ACKNOWLEDGMENTS

We thank A. B. Leiter, T. Tsukada, and J. S. Fink for helpful discussions and E. Goodman for editorial assistance. This work was supported by
NIH grants AM 31400 and P30 AM 39428.

REFERENCES

1. Reichlin S. Somatostatin. N Engl J Med 1983; 309:1495-501.
2. Delfs J, Robbins RJ, Connolly M, Dichter M, Reichlin S. Somatostatin
   production by rat cerebral neurons in dissociated cell culture.
   Nature 1980; 283:676-7.
3. Montminy MR, Low MJ, Tapia-Arancibia L, Reichlin S, Mandel G,
   Goodman RH. Cyclic AMP regulates somatostatin mRNA accumulation in
   primary diencephalic cultures and in transfected fibroblast cells. J
   Neurosci 1986; 6:1171-6.
4. Graham F, Van der Eb AJ. A new technique for the assay of human
   adenovirus 5 DNA. Virology 1973; 52:456-67.
5. Southern P, Berg P. Mammalian cell transformation with SV40 hybrid
   plasmid vectors. Mol Appl Genetics 1982; 1:327-33.
6. Tischler AS, Greene L. Nerve growth factor-induced process formation
   by cultured rat pheochromocytoma cells. Nature 1975; 258:341-2.

7. Potter H, Weir L, Leder P. Enhancer-dependent expression of human k immunoglobulin genes introduced into mouse pre-β lymphocytes by electroporation. Proc Natl Acad Sci USA 1984; 81:7161-5.
8. Laimins L, Gruss P, Pozzatti R, Khoury G. Characterization of the enhancer elements in the long terminal repeat of the Maloney murine sarcoma virus. J Virol 1984; 49:183-9.
9. Short JM, Wynshaw-Boris A, Short HP, Hanson RW. Characterization of the phosphenolpyruvate carboxykinase promoter regulatory region. J Biol Chem 1986; 261:9721-6.

4

PEPTIDES DERIVED FROM MAMMALIAN PROSOMATOSTATIN

Robert Benoit

The Montreal General Hospital Research Institute
Department of Medicine, McGill University
1650 Cedar Avenue, Montreal, Quebec H3G 1A4 Canada

Somatostatin is a tetradecapeptide known for its inhibitory action on the release of several hormones in addition to somatotropin (1,2). Results on the isolation and characterization of somatostatin-related peptides (3-9) as well as cloning and sequencing of the cDNA encoding the rat and human somatostatin precursors (10-12) are consistent: the bioactive core is contained in the cyclic ring present at the C-terminus of a unique preprohormone of 116 amino acids (Fig. 1).

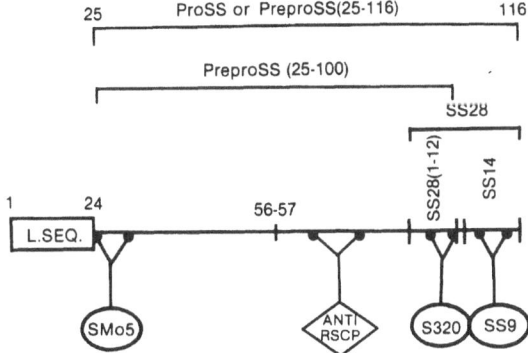

Fig. 1. Schematic diagram representing preprosomatostatin, a 116 amino acid polypeptide consisting of a leader sequence of 24 amino acids and of a prohormone of 92 amino acids (proSS). The whole prohormone corresponds to preproSS(25-116). Identified cleavage sites are at position 24-25, 56-57, 88-89 and at the basic pair ARG-LYS that separates SS28(1-12) and preproSS(25-100) from SS14. The recognition sites of the antibodies used in the present study as well as the rat somatostatin cryptic peptide (RSCP) sequence used by Goodman and co-workers are shown. Antiserum RB1563 used by Aron and co-workers (not shown) is similar to SMo5.

Information on the processing of preprosomatostatin leading to formation of the signal peptide and the prohormone was first provided by Goodman et al. who used microsomal enzymes to process the cell-free translation product of rat medullary thyroid carcinoma mRNA (11). Cleavage was shown to occur at position 24-25 of the precursor which corresponds to a GLY-ALA bond. The results of the characterization of rat preprosomatostatin(25-100) were in agreement with these findings (13): prosomatostatin is a 92 amino acid polypeptide (10-13) in which only two amino acid substitutions occurred between rodents and humans (Fig. 2). Since the whole prosomatostatin molecule itself is bioactive in vitro (14), what is the evidence for processing taking place before exocytosis? Are the peptides considered to be derived from prosomatostatin authentic post-translational products, products of catabolism or simply artifacts of extraction?

In this chapter we will summarize the data indicating that several peptides are derived from prosomatostatin and will put emphasis on those molecular forms that are derived from the NH_2-terminus of the prohormone.

SOMATOSTATIN-14 AND PEPTIDES CONTAINING SOMATOSTATIN-14 AT THEIR C-TERMINUS

Somatostatin-14

Since the original work on the identification of somatostatin-14 by Brazeau et al., the tetradecapeptide has consistently been the preponderant molecular form observed in most tissue extracts containing somato-

PROSOMATOSTATIN

H-Ala-Pro-Ser-Asp-Pro-Arg-Leu-Arg-Gln-Phe-Leu-Gln-Lys-Ser-Leu-

Ala-Ala-Ala-Thr-Gly-Lys-Gln-Glu-Leu-Ala-Lys-Tyr-Phe-Leu-Ala-Glu-

Leu-Leu-Ser-Glu-Pro-Asn-Gln-Thr-Glu-Asn-Asp-Ala-Leu-Glu-Pro-Glu-

Asp-Leu-Pro-Gln-Ala-Ala-Glu-Gln-Asp-Glu-Met-Arg-Leu-Glu-Leu-Gln-

Arg-Ser-Ala-Asn-Ser-Asn-Pro-Ala-Met-Ala-Pro-Arg-Glu-**Arg-Lys**-

Ala-Gly-Cys-Lys-Asn-Phe-Phe-Trp-Lys-Thr-Phe-Thr-Ser-Cys-OH

SS28

H-Ser-Ala-Asn-Ser-Asn-Pro-Ala-Met-Ala-Pro-Arg-Glu-Arg-Lys-

Ala-Gly-Cys-Lys-Asn-Phe-Phe-Trp-Lys-Thr-Phe-Thr-Ser-Cys-OH

SS14

H-Ala-Gly-Cys-Lys-Asn-Phe-Phe-Trp-Lys-Thr-Phe-Thr-Ser-Cys-OH

Fig. 2. Sequences of the three peptides derived from preprosomatostatin and containing the cyclic structure responsible for bioactivity: prosomatostatin, somatostatin-28 and the original tetradecapeptide somatostatin-14. The prosomatostatin structure shown here is that of rat prosomatostatin. In the human prohormone, ALA replaces THR at position 43 and SER replaces PRO at position 74.

statin-like immunoreactivity (1,15). No normal tissue has ever been shown to contain predominantly prosomatostatin. The only observation suggesting that somatostatin-14 may not be the ubiquitous molecular form described in biochemical studies is a surprising and yet unexplained finding: specific antibodies to somatostatin-14 cannot stain somatostatin cells in tissues such as the rat cerebral cortex. Yet if the fixed tissue is then acid extracted, it contains radioimmunoassayable somatostatin-14 measurable by specific RIA (Benoit, unpublished data).

The work of Patzelt et al. indicates that rat islet prosomatostatin is processed directly to somatostatin-14 by cleavage at a pair of basic amino acids (8). Moreover, an antibody population specific for the sequence ASN-PRO-ALA-MET-ALA-PRO-ARG-GLU-OH immediately preceding the ARG-LYS bond at position 101 and 102 of preprosomatostatin stains extensively somatostatin cells in brain and in pancreas (16,17). These observations indicate that somatostatin-14 is generated by cleavage of the classical basic pair that precedes it, as described previously for several peptide hormones and neuropeptides.

Somatostatin-28, Somatostatin-25 and
Somatostatin-20

Somatostatin-28 has been isolated and characterized in extracts of porcine gut and hypothalamus, in extracts of ovine and rat hypothalamus as well as in bovine retina (3-6,9,18,19). In all mammals studied so far, the same octacosapeptide structure is generated after cleavage of an Arg-Ser bond at position 88-89 of preprosomatostatin. Although not frequently reported, cleavage at a monobasic site has already been described for other precursors such as the one for arginine-vasopressin (20) in which an ARG-ALA bond is cleaved at position 108-109.

Somatostatin-28 is the preponderant molecular form derived from the precursor in the small intestine of the rat (21-24) and in the retina of certain species such as bovine and most probably guinea pig (18,25). It has been shown to be at least as potent as somatostatin-14 in most biological systems in which it was tested. In addition, an antibody population (S298) directed against the N-terminal portion of SS28 and which does not recognize N-terminally extended forms of SS28, detects immunoreactive material in somatostatin cell bodies and processes (16,26). Immunocytochemical and biochemical findings thus indicate that the Arg-Ser bond is cleaved during processing and that SS28 is an authentic endogenous molecule.

The early studies of Spiess et al. have raised some doubt on the existence of a precursor-product relationship between somatostatin-28 and somatostatin-14 in the hypothalamus (27). Subsequently Zingg and Patel observed that rat hypothalamic enzymes could process somatostatin-28 to somatostatin-14 (28). Pulse-chase studies performed with dispersed neonatal hypothalamic cells (29), with cerebral cortical cells from rat embryo (30) or with cultured pancreatic islets (15) have failed to demonstrate a precursor-product relationship. This was also the case in an in vivo study conducted by Van Itallie and Fernstrom in which ^{35}S-labelled cysteine was injected ICV into rats to study somatostatin biosynthesis (31). In rat cerebral cortex, however, Gluschankof and co-workers have recently identified a 90 kilodalton convertase which can process synthetic somatostatin-28 into somatostatin-28(1-12), somatostatin-14, free arginine and free lysine in vitro (32,33). These findings suggest that the convertase is also involved in the in vivo processing of the endogenous octacosapeptide. Results obtained after incorporation of tritiated phenylalanine in isolated rat dorsal root ganglia suggest that, in this tissue, somatostatin-28 is a precursor of somatostatin-14 (34).

We think that the precursor-product relationship as well as its importance may vary from one tissue to another or even at different stages of development. Isolation and characterization of the enzymes involved in the processing steps represent a stimulating new field in somatostatin research.

Somatostatin-25 and somatostatin-20 have been isolated from aged hypothalamic and intestinal tissue extracts (5,19). Their concentration is apparently lower than that of the octacosapeptide. We propose that these molecular forms be considered authentic natural products only if, using fresh tissue extracts, their presence is confirmed by isolation and characterization, by RIA determination, or by immunohistochemistry with specific antibodies.

Large Somatostatin-28 or 6K Somatostatin-28-like Peptide

Although unrecognized by many as a constituent of normal cerebral tissue, small amounts of a 6 kilodalton somatostatin-28-like peptide are present in rat brain extracts. This molecular form can be observed after gel permeation chromatography when using antibodies against somatostatin-28 (7) or when using centrally directed antibodies against somatostatin-14 (Fig. 1). In adult rat brain, it accounts for only 2.3% of total somatostatin-14-like immunoreactivity (Fig. 3) which is considerably less than the tetradecapeptide itself (77%), somatostatin-28 (14.3%) or even prosomatostatin (5.8%). Interestingly, relatively high levels of 6K SS28-like peptide have been observed in human fetal hypothalamic extracts of 14 weeks gestation (35). This molecular form decreases progressively during human fetal life and is no longer detectable at 22 weeks of gestation. Moreover, Low and co-workers have shown that processing of preprosomatostatin by transgenic mice carrying a metallothionein-somatostatin fusion gene leads predominantly to formation of a 6K SS14-like peptide in liver and kidney. Most of the somatostatin-14-like immunoreactivity in the plasma of these animals is a 6K peptide (36). This peptide has not been characterized nor do we possess information regarding its biological activity (if any). Since the whole prosomatostatin molecule has been shown to be bioactive in vitro (14), one would expect that the 6K SS28 is also bioactive. However, the absence of growth retardation observed by Low and co-workers in transfected mice with high circulating levels of this molecule suggests that it is not bioactive. It is conceivable that this 6K SS28 or 6K SS14-like peptide represents preprosomatostatin (57-116), a molecular form that would be generated after cleavage of a Leu-Leu bond (13).

SOMATOSTATIN-28(1-12) AND ITS N-TERMINALLY EXTENDED FORMS

Somatostatin-28(1-12) has been isolated and characterized (Fig. 4) in rat brain, rat pancreas and, more recently, in a human pancreatic somatostatinoma (26,37). It is present in somatostatin containing tissue in concentrations similar to those of the tetradecapeptide SS14. The dodecapeptide has no known biological function. It has been shown to be released from hypothalamic tissue both in vitro (38) and in vivo (39). Antibodies against somatostatin-28(1-12) are excellent probes for the study of the prosomatostatin system (17) and have often proven superior to antisomatostatin-14 sera for the visualization of nerve fibers and terminals (16,40,41).

The availability of an antibody population directed against the last 8 amino acids of somatostatin-28(1-12) has allowed us to (1) confirm the presence of high levels of the dodecapeptide in extracts of both the nervous and the digestive systems (42), and (2) characterize two peptides

36

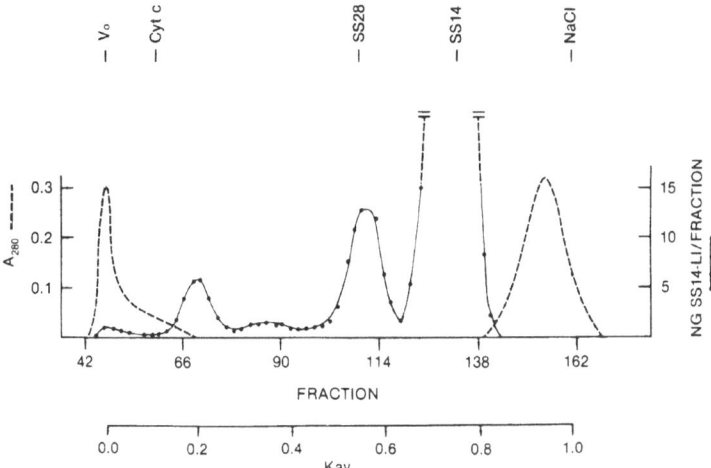

Fig. 3. Gel permeation chromatography (Sephadex G-75) of an acid extract of 3 rat brains (adults of ~300 g, both sexes, Sprague-Dawley, fed ad lib.). After rapid dissection, the brains were heated in 15 ml 2 M acetic acid containing 10 mg/L pepstatin, 10 mg/L PMSF and 30 mg/L bacitracin. Homogenization was done with a polytron followed by centrifugation at 50,000 x g for 30 min at 4°C. The pellet was homogenized with 10 ml of the extraction buffer and the homogenate centrifuged. The supernatants were combined and lyophilized. The dry material was dissolved in 12 ml 30% acetic acid, and spun at 50,000 x g for 30 min at 4°C. The supernatant was loaded onto a Sephadex column (113 x 4.8 cm) after adding 60 mg Pentex crystalline bovine serum albumin and 80 mg NaCl to it. For coating, 60 μl 0.5% albumin was added to each collecting tube. Somatostatin-14-like immunoreactivity was measured in every second fraction using SS9. Elution with 30% acetic acid, flow rate 30 ml/hr, fraction size 12 ml.

in brain extracts that contain somatostatin-28(1-12) at their C-terminus (13). The first of these peptides can be released in vitro from hypothalamic tissue along with somatostatin-28(1-12) and somatostatin-14 (43). It represents the whole prosomatostatin molecule without ARG-LYS-somatostatin-14 (Fig. 4), e.g., preprosomatostatin(25-100). The presence of this 76 amino acid peptide in several tissues implies that SS14 can be generated directly from prosomatostatin.

In addition to preprosomatostatin(25-100), we have partially characterized a 44 amino acid peptide from rat brain extracts (4.5K SS28(1-12)-like peptide). This peptide contains somatostatin-28(1-12) at its C-terminal end and is generated by cleavage of a Leu-Leu bond at position 56-57 of preprosomatostatin. Our initial studies on somatostatin-28(1-12)-like peptides showed that this molecular form accounted for up to 21% of the total SS28(1-12)-like immunoreactive material contained in certain brain extracts but was not secreted (7,43). It is now clear that when acid extraction is performed on frozen tissue using peptidase inhibitors (pepstatin 10 mg/L, PMSF 10 mg/L and bacitracin 30 mg/L), or if no defrosting precedes the extraction step, this molecular form is present in very low quantity in brain extracts (Fig. 5). Based on the very low amounts of 4.5K SS28(1-12)-like peptide present in fresh adult brain extracts (~8 ng per rat brain), it appears that any putative cleavage of the Leu-Leu bond in nervous tissue does not give rise to important molecular forms, at least as seen when using probes directed toward the C-terminus of the precursor.

IMMUNOREACTIVE MATERIAL DETECTED WITH AN ANTIBODY DIRECTED AGAINST THE CENTRAL REGION OF PROSOMATOSTATIN

Lechan et al. have generated an antibody against a synthetic fragment corresponding to preprosomatostatin 63-77, e.g., rat somatostatin cryptic peptide or RSCP which occupies the central region of the precursor (Fig. 1). This antibody stains somatostatin cells in brain as well as in pancreas (44,45). However, the brain levels of radioimmunoassayable RSCP are low when compared to those of somatostatin-14 (46). Chromatographic analysis of the RSCP-like immunoreactive material contained in a rat medullary thyroid carcinoma cell line indicates that it consists of pro-

SS28(1-12)

H-Ser-Ala-Asn-Ser-Asn-Pro-Ala-Met-Ala-Pro-Arg-Glu-OH

PREPRO SS (25-100)

25
H-Ala-Pro-Ser-Asp-Pro-Arg-Leu-Arg-Gln-Phe-Leu-Gln-Lys-Ser-Leu-

Ala-Ala-Ala-Thr-Gly-Lys-Gln-Glu-Leu-Ala-Lys-Tyr-Phe-Leu-Ala-Glu-

Leu-Leu-Ser-Glu-Pro-Asn-Gln-Thr-Glu-Asn-Asp-Ala-Leu-Glu-Pro-Glu-

Asp-Leu-Pro-Gln-Ala-Ala-Glu-Gln-Asp-Glu-Met-Arg-Leu-Glu-Leu-Gln-

Arg-Ser-Ala-Asn-Ser-Asn-Pro-Ala-Met-Ala-Pro-Arg-Glu-OH
100

PREPRO SS (25-56)

H-Ala-Pro-Ser-Asp-Pro-Arg-Leu-Arg-Gln-Phe-Leu-Gln-Lys-Ser-Leu-Ala

Ala-Ala-Ala-Gly-Lys-Gln-Glu-Leu-Ala-Lys-Tyr-Phe-Leu-Ala-Glu-Leu-OH
(Thr)

PREPRO SS (57-100)

H-Leu-Ser-Glu-Pro-Asn-Gln-Thr-Glu-Asn-Asp-Ala-Leu-Glu-Pro-Glu-

Asp-Leu-Pro-Gln-Ala-Ala-Glu-Gln-Asp-Glu-Met-Arg-Leu-Glu-Leu-Gln-

Arg-Ser-Ala-Asn-Ser-Asn-Pro-Ala-Met-Ala-Pro-Arg-Glu-OH

Fig. 4. Sequences of 4 prosomatostatin derived peptides characterized in tissue extracts. These peptides do not contain somatostatin. So far, no biological role has been ascribed to these molecules. SS28(1-12), preproSS(25-100) and preproSS(57-100) have been identified in rat tissue extracts (13,26). PreproSS(25-56) or "proSS 1-32" has been fully characterized in upper porcine gut (49). The 32 amino acid peptide of porcine origin contains an alanine at position 19 instead of the threonine that should theoretically be present in the murine 32 amino acid homologue. Only low amounts of preproSS(25-56) and preproSS(57-100) are present in brain.

somatostatin and an 8 kilodalton molecule (47). The 8 kilodalton RSCP-like peptide does not contain somatostatin-14 and its exact structure remains to be elucidated.

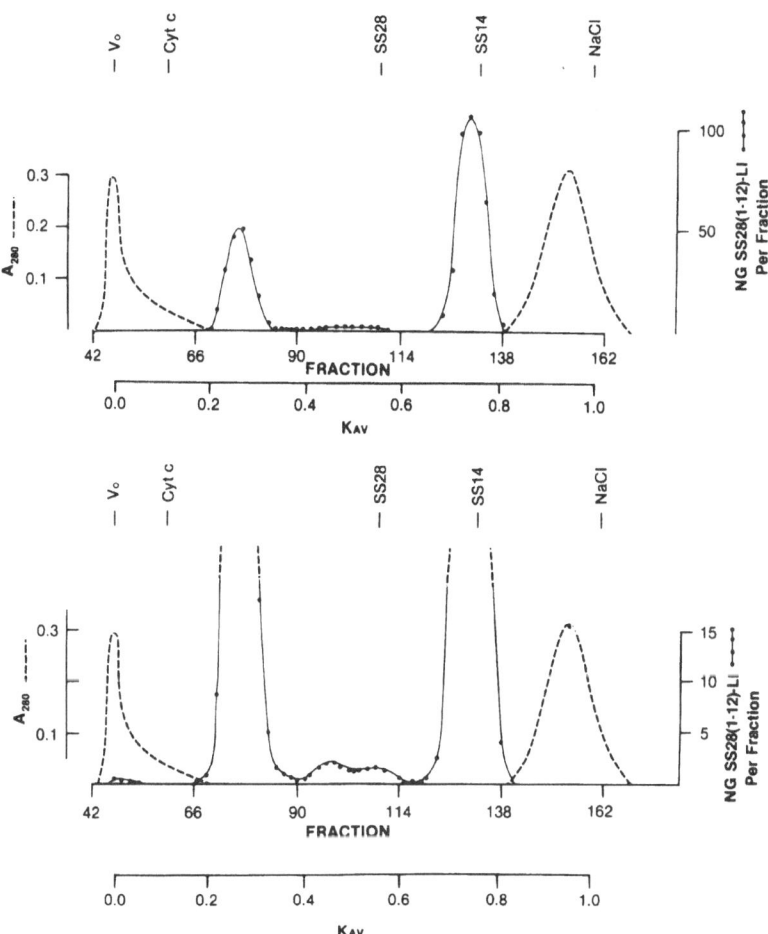

Fig. 5. Gel permeation chromatography (Sephadex G-75) of an acid extract of 3 rat brains as described in Fig. 3 with the same enzyme inhibitors. In the upper panel, somatostatin-28(1-12)-like immunoreactivity is measured using S320. Only two peaks of immunoreactivity are clearly present. In the lower panel, using a more sensitive scale, a third peak can be seen which has two components. The first component eluted from the column (fractions 90-103) is compatible with a peptide of ca 4.5 kilodaltons and totals 8 ng per adult rat brain. The second component corresponds to unidentified somatostatin-28(1-12)-like material.

PEPTIDES DERIVED FROM THE N-TERMINAL REGION OF PROSOMATOSTATIN

Studies Using Tumor Cells Originating from the
Neural Crest

Recently, Aron et al. have produced an antibody by immunizing with the first 13 amino acids present at the N-terminus of prosomatostatin (47). The radioimmunoassay developed with the N-terminally directed antibody has allowed these investigators to identify two peptides in acid extracts of a somatostatin secreting medullary thyroid carcinoma (CA77 rat MTC cell line). The most abundant of the two is a 4K prosomatostatin N-terminal peptide which is apparently not secreted by the CA77 cells (48). However, the other peptide is an 8 kilodalton molecule which can be released by calcium or glucagon. It is also RSCP immunoreactive and does not contain somatostatin-14. It is still unclear if the 8 kilodalton peptide corresponds to preprosomatostatin(25-100), to preprosomatostatin-(25-88) or to a closely related entity.

Studies Performed on Normal Rat Brain

We have developed a radioimmunoassay for the N-terminal region of prosomatostatin in which the first antibody has been raised against preprosomatostatin(25-33)-TYR conjugated to bovine serum albumin (SMo5, Fig. 1). Acid extracts of several tissues from the nervous and the digestive system contain apparently low levels of preprosomatostatin(25-33)-like immunoreactive material (preproSS(25-33)-LI). The hypothalamus contains the highest level of preproSS(25-33)-LI in the nervous system, i.e., 9.1 ± 1.4 mg per 100 mg wet wt (± SEM). The distribution in the extra-hypothalamic brain is rather uniform (Fig. 6).

Several extraction procedures can be used to analyze the molecular forms of preproSS(25-33)-LI material present in tissue extracts: (1) heating of tissue in 2 M acetic acid (90°C) during 15 min immediately after dissection, followed by homogenization (Polytron, 10 ml acetic acid per g tissue); (2) same procedure as in 1, except that the acetic acid contains pepstatin 20 mg/L, PMSF 20 mg/L and bacitracin 50 mg/L; (3) freezing of tissue in liquid nitrogen immediately after dissecting, lyophilization and storage at -20°C for less than two weeks, heating of tissue during 15 min in 2 M acetic acid containing the same enzyme inhibitors as in 2 and homogenization (Polytron); (4) freezing in liquid nitrogen immediately after dissection, lyophilization, storage at -20°C for less than two weeks, heating of tissue for 10 min in 0.05 M sodium phosphate pH 7.7 (10 ml per g wet tissue) and homogenization without peptidase inhibitor; (5) freezing in liquid nitrogen, storage at -20°C for 10 months, lyophilization of tissue, homogenization with a polytron in cold (0°C) 2 M acetic acid containing pepstatin 30 mg/L, PMSF 30 mg/L and bacitracin 250 mg/L. If any one of these five procedures is followed for brain extraction, gel chromatography of the extract will reveal three zones of preproSS(25-33)-LI material. The first peak which elutes from the column contains the largest amount of immunoreactive product and is clearly heterogeneous. The most important component of this peak elutes at a position compatible with a peptide of 6.2 kilodaltons (Fig. 7). When resolution on gel filtration is optimal (Fig. 7, lower panel), the 6.2 kilodalton peak is immediately preceded by two components of 8 and 10 kilodaltons. The second peak to elute from the column corresponds to a material of 3.5 kilodaltons. The last peak is compatible with a peptide of 1.2 to 1.4 kilodaltons (1.4K preproSS(25-33)-LI peptide). If the N-terminally directed antibody (SMo5) recognizes the various molecular forms observed after gel filtration on an equimolar basis, the 6.2K peptide then represents the most abundant prosomatostatin derived peptide in brain extracts after somatostatin-14 and somatostatin-28(1-12).

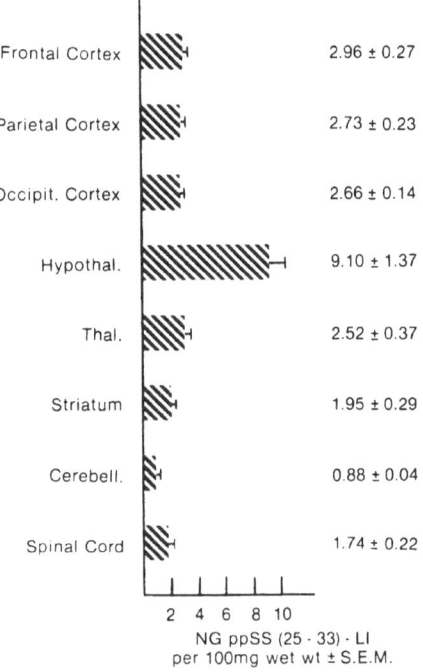

CENTRAL NERVOUS SYSTEM

Frontal Cortex	2.96 ± 0.27
Parietal Cortex	2.73 ± 0.23
Occipit. Cortex	2.66 ± 0.14
Hypothal.	9.10 ± 1.37
Thal.	2.52 ± 0.37
Striatum	1.95 ± 0.29
Cerebell.	0.88 ± 0.04
Spinal Cord	1.74 ± 0.22

2 4 6 8 10
NG ppSS (25 - 33) - LI
per 100mg wet wt ± S.E.M.

Fig. 6. Distribution of preprosomatostatin(25-33)-like immunoreactive material in various regions of the rat central nervous system.

Further purification of each immunoreactive component from gel filtration can be achieved by reverse-phase high pressure liquid chromatography (HPLC) using octadecylsilylsilica (C_{18}) as the solid phase and acetonitrile with trifluoroacetic acid (TFA) as the mobile phase.

10K preproSS(25-33)-LI peptide. The 10K material (Fig. 7, lower panel) detected with antibodies directed against the N-terminus of prosomatostatin elutes as a single peak on HPLC (Fig. 8). If every fraction from the HPLC is also monitored for its content in somatostatin-14-like immunoreactivity using an antibody population directed against the central region of SS14, the same fraction that contained preproSS(25-33)-LI material also contains SS14. This strongly suggests that the 10K preproSS(25-33)-LI peptide represents the whole prosomatostatin molecule. Quantitation of prosomatostatin using the N-terminally directed antibody (SMo5) leads to an underestimation when compared to values obtained with the C-terminally directed antibody (SS_9). This could mean that the N-terminus of prosomatostatin is less exposed than the C-terminus and thus less available for antibody recognition.

8K preproSS(25-33)-LI peptide. Pooled fractions from the 8K component observed after gel filtration have also been chromatographed on C_{18} columns. The column effluent was again monitored by RIA using two antibodies, SMo5 and S320. The former recognizes the N-terminus of prosomatostatin and the latter recognizes somatostatin-28(1-12). Virtually all the preproSS(25-33)-like material eluted in one fraction which also

41

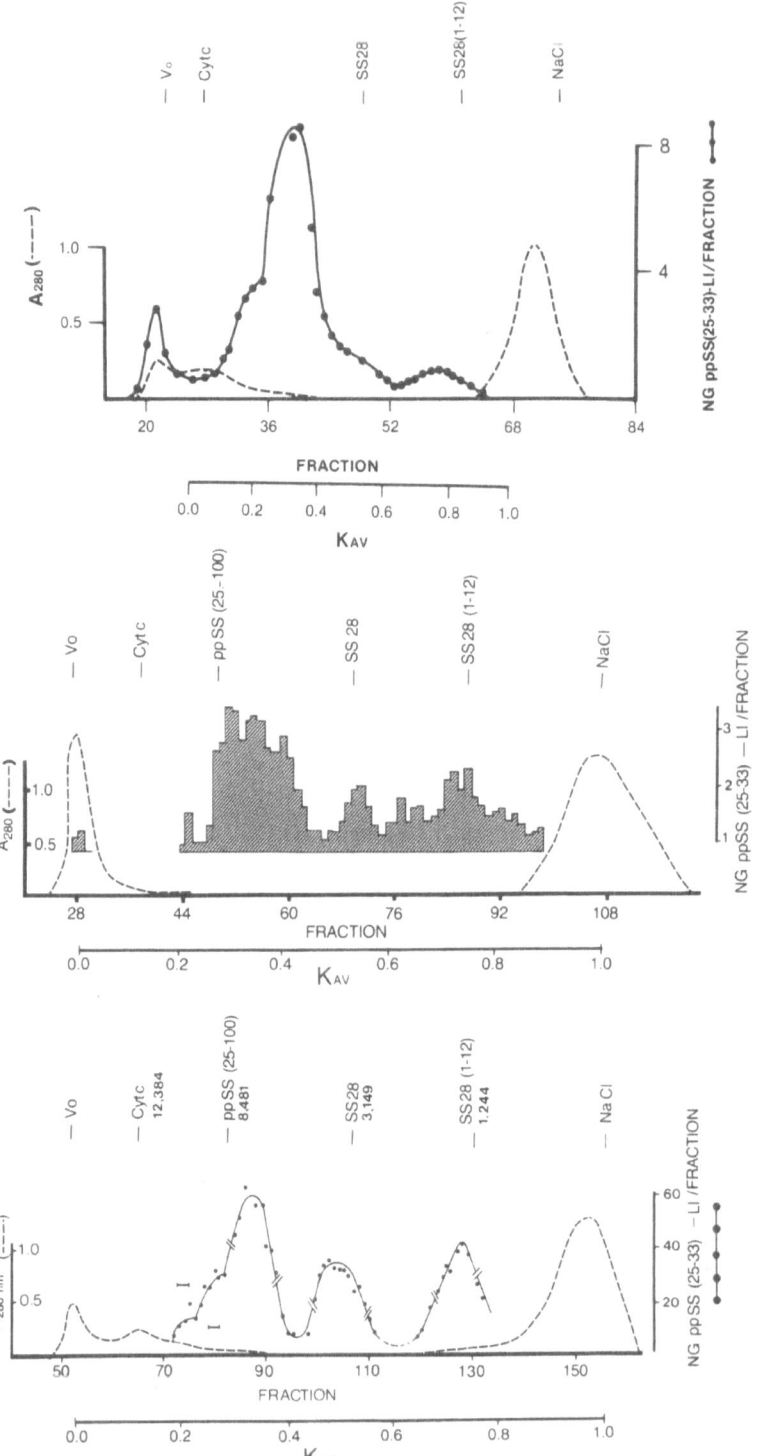

contained all the somatostatin-28(1-12)-like material eluted from the column (results not shown). We conclude from this data that the 8K peptide represents preproSS(25-100), a peptide already characterized in brain (13) and which contains somatostatin-28(1-12) at its C-terminus.

6.2K preproSS(25-33)-LI peptide. We have been unable using gel permeation chromatography to separate completely preproSS(25-100) from the 6.2K preproSS(25-33)-like immunoreactive peptide. Further purification has been achieved on HPLC using shallow acetonitrile gradients (Fig. 9). In these conditions, the 6.2K preproSS(25-33)-like immunoreactive material elutes in 4 consecutive fractions. The last 2 fractions which also contain somatostatin-28(1-12)-like immunoreactivity presumably represent the residual preproSS(25-100) remaining in the 6.2K cuts after gel filtration. The first two fractions contain a peptide with the N-terminus of prosomatostatin and without SS28(1-12) at its C-terminus. The structure of this molecule is unknown as well as its exact content in somatostatin-containing tissue. Several additional purification steps on HPLC will be required in order to isolate this peptide. It may represent preproSS(25-88) or a closely related molecule.

3.5K preproSS(25-33)-LI material. The 3.5K zone is heterogeneous when fractionated on HPLC (results not shown). It contains at least three components eluting between 35 and 60% acetonitrile. This heterogeneity as well as the rather low levels found in brain does not suggest a biological role for the 3.5K N-terminal peptide in nervous tissue. This molecular form probably corresponds to the 4K N-terminal peptide described by Aron et al. in the rat medullary thyroid carcinoma cell line CA77 (47). The presence of the 3.5K N-terminal peptide in tissue extracts supports the hypothesis that cleavage occurs at the Leu-Leu bond present at position 56-57 of preprosomatostatin.

Fig. 7 (opposite page). Upper panel. Gel permeation chromatography (Sephadex G-75) of an extract of 3 adult rat brains (males, Sprague-Dawley, 300 g). After rapid dissection, the brains were heated for 15 min and homogenized (polytron) in 30 ml 2 M acetic acid containing pepstatin 20 mg/L, PMSF 20 mg/L and bacitracin 50 mg/L. The homogenate was centrifuged at 2°C during 20 min at 40,000 x g and the supernatant lyophilized. The dried material was dissolved in 7 ml 30% acetic acid and loaded onto a Sephadex G-75 column (2.5 x 100 cm). Elution was done at 4°C with 30% acetic acid. The first peak of immunoreactive material eluted with the void volume probably represents interfering substances in the RIA. Vo = 154 ml; flow rate 13 ml/hr; fraction size 7 ml.
Middle panel. Gel permeation chromatography of an extract of 9 rat brains. Conditions as described under upper panel except that tissue was frozen in liquid nitrogen and lyophilized after dissection. In addition, heating of tissue was done in 50 mM sodium phosphate pH 7.7 without enzyme inhibitor.
Lower panel. Gel permeation chromatography (Sephadex G-75) of an extract of 35 rat brains (Sprague-Dawley, 33 to 334 g). The tissue had been frozen in liquid nitrogen immediately after dissection, stored at -20°C for 10 months, lyophilized, homogenized in 2 M acetic acid (2°C) containing pepstatin 30 mg/L, PMSF 30 mg/L and bacitracin 250 mg/L. The supernatant was lyophilized, the dry material was dissolved in 29 ml cold 30% degassed acetic acid and centrifuged at 50,000 x g for 45 min at 4°C. The supernatant was loaded onto a Sephadex C-75 column (125 x 5.5 cm). Vo = 872 ml; V NaCl = 2.92 L; fraction size 20 ml.

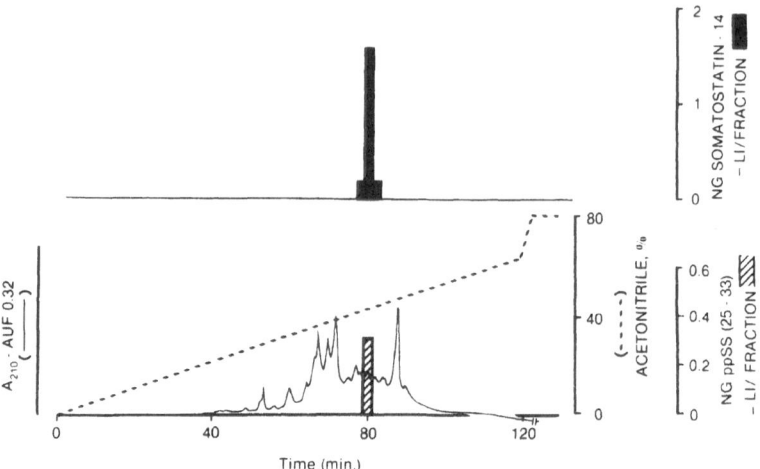

Fig. 8. Reverse-phase HPLC of 10 kilodalton preproSS(25-33)-LI
material from Sephadex G-75 gel permeation of brain extracts
(Fig. 7, lower panel, fractions 73-75). One mg of material
dissolved in 1 ml 0.1% trifluoroacetic acid (TFA) is loaded onto
a C_{18} analytical column (ALTEX ultrasphere, 4.6 x 150 mm, 5 μm
particle size). The mobile phase is 0.1% TFA with an acetonitrile gradient generated with a model 420 liquid chromatograph
from Beckman, Berkeley, CA. The preproSS(25-33)-like immunoreactive material is eluted at 80 min (lower panel). Monitoring
of HPLC fractions with a somatostatin-14 RIA, using SS9, shows
that virtually all the SS-14-like material is eluted also at 80
min (upper panel). The 10 kilodalton polypeptide from brain
contains both the amino-terminus and the carboxy-terminus of
prosomatostatin. Flow-rate 0.8 ml/min; fraction size 1.6 ml.

1.4K preproSS(25-33)-LI material. HPLC performed on pooled fractions
from the 1.4K zone reveals one major and two minor immunoreactive peaks
(Fig. 10). All these immunoreactive components are more hydrophobic than
a synthetic preproSS(25-33)-TYR standard. The levels of 1.4K peptide
appear rather low in brain when compared to those contained in the stomach
(see below).

Studies Performed in the Rat Digestive System

In the digestive system, the stomach contains the highest concentra-
tion of preproSS(25-33)-LI material, e.g., 6.2 ± 0.5 ng per 100 mg wet wt
± SEM. The lowest levels are seen in acid extracts of caecum and pancreas
(Fig. 11).

Sephadex G-75 chromatography of fresh rat stomach extract reveals a
preproSS(25-33)-like immunoreactivity profile similar to the one observed
after chromatography of brain extracts. The 6.2K immunoreactive peak
still predominates (Fig. 12) and is preceded by a shoulder representing
probably prosomatostatin and preproSS(25-100) which have not been resolved. A small amount of immunoreactive material elutes in the void
volume region. Its nature is unknown. A preproSS(25-33)-like peptide
elutes precisely at 0.51 Kav which is compatible with a molecule of 3.5
kilodaltons. This molecular form most probably corresponds to the peptide
recently isolated and characterized by Schmidt and co-workers from an

44

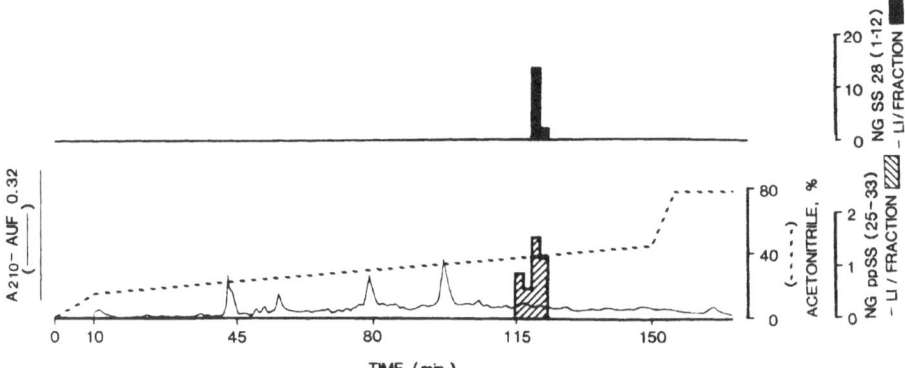

Fig. 9. <u>Lower panel</u>. Reverse-phase HPLC purification of the 6.2K preprosomatostatin(25-33)-like immunoreactive material from gel permeation of brain extracts (Fig. 7, <u>lower panel</u>, fractions 83-92). 1.2 mg of material dissolved in 0-8 ml 0.1% TFA is loaded onto a C_{18} analytical column (ALTEX ultrasphere, 4.6 x 150 mm, 5 μm particle size). The mobile phase is 0.1% TFA with an acetonitrile gradient. The immunoreactive material is eluted in 4 fractions. Monitoring of all HPLC fractions with a somatostatin-28(1-12) RIA using S320 (<u>upper panel</u>) reveals that the last two of the four fractions contain a somatostatin-28(1-12)-like peptide, most probably pre-proSS(25-100). The immunoreactive material eluted at 115 and 116 min does not contain the somatostatin-28(1-12) structure. Flow rate 0.8 ml/min, fraction size 1.6 ml.

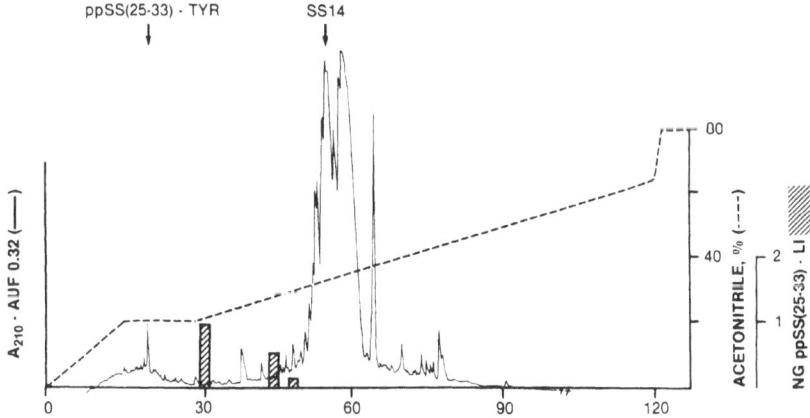

Fig. 10. Reverse-phase HPLC of the 1.4K preprosomatostatin(25-33)-like immunoreactive material from gel permeation of brain extracts (Fig. 7, <u>lower panel</u>, fractions 123-131). 1 mg of material dissolved in 0.8 ml 0.1% TFA is loaded onto a C_{18} analytical column. The mobile phase is 0.1% TFA with acetonitrile. The immunoreactive material elutes in one major peak and two minor ones. All immunoreactive components are eluted after synthetic preproSS(25-33)-TYR. Flow rate 0.8 ml/min, fraction size 1.6 ml.

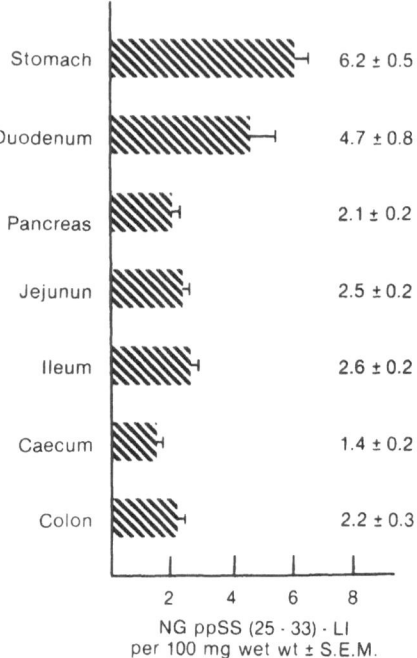

DIGESTIVE SYSTEM

Stomach	6.2 ± 0.5
Duodenum	4.7 ± 0.8
Pancreas	2.1 ± 0.2
Jejunun	2.5 ± 0.2
Ileum	2.6 ± 0.2
Caecum	1.4 ± 0.2
Colon	2.2 ± 0.3

NG ppSS (25 · 33) · LI
per 100 mg wet wt ± S.E.M.

Fig. 11. Distribution of preprosomatostatin-
(25-33)-like immunoreactive material in various regions of the rat digestive system.

upper porcine gut extract (49). The peptide identified by this group
represents the first 32 amino acids of prosomatostatin, e.g., proSS 1-32
or preproSS(25-56). The porcine peptide sequence (Fig. 4) is identical to
its human counterpart predicted by sequencing of the cDNA encoding human
preprosomatostatin (10) and it differs from the rat sequence (11,12) by
only one amino acid at residue 19 (ALA instead of THR). The existence of
such a peptide was postulated (13) but the molecule had not been isolated.
Preliminary quantitative data on rat brain and on rat stomach indicates
that the amount of 3.5K N-terminal peptide is low in these tissues. No
data are presently available on its content in porcine tissue. The work
of Schmidt et al. is important in that it provides solid data supporting
the Leu-Leu bond cleavage hypothesis, e.g., cleavage at position 56-57 of
preprosomatostatin during processing.

A preproSS(25-33)-like immunoreactive peptide of 1.2 to 1.4 kilodalton is also present in extracts of rat gastric tissue (Fig. 12). It is
virtually undetectable in pancreas and duodenum, while in the stomach it
accounts for up to one-third of the total preproSS(25-33)-LI material
present in that organ.

46

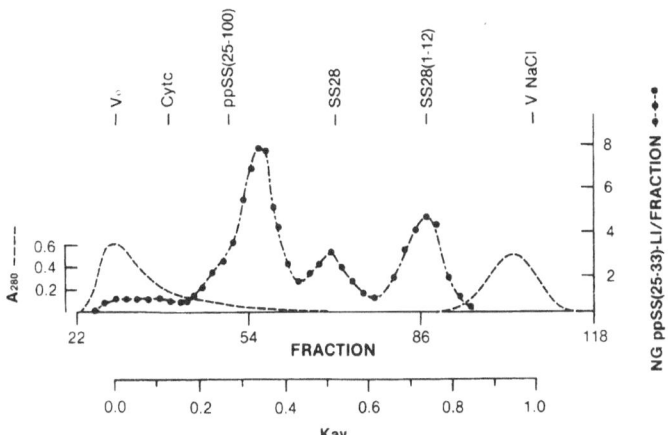

Fig. 12. Gel permeation chromatography (Sephadex G-75) of an extract of 2 adult rat stomachs (females, 280 g, fed ad libitum). The tissue was rapidly extracted in cold 2 M acetic acid without peptidase inhibitor. Otherwise, details of extraction and chromatography were as described in Fig. 7, <u>upper panel</u>. The immunoreactivity profile is essentially the same if peptidase inhibitors are used during extraction. The last immunoreactive peak (1.2 to 1.4 kilodalton) accounts for 1/3 of the total prepro-SS(25-33)-LI material eluted from the column.

ACKNOWLEDGMENTS

We are grateful to Dr. Nicholas Ling of the Salk Institute for providing us with the synthetic peptides used in these studies and to Miss Gina Gravel for technical assistance. We thank Dr. Maureen Kiely for her helpful suggestions and Miss Jean Walker for secretarial work. This research was supported by the Medical Research Council of Canada (Grant MA-9145), Fonds de Recherche en Sante du Quebec and by The Montreal General Hospital Research Institute.

REFERENCES

1. Brazeau P, Vale W, Burgus R, et al. Hypothalamic polypeptide that inhibits secretion of immunoreactive pituitary growth hormone. Science 1973; 179:77-9.
2. Reichlin S. Somatostatin. N Engl J Med 1983; 309:1495-501, 1556-63.
3. Pradayrol L, Jornvall H, Mutt V, Ribet A. N-terminally extended somatostatin: the primary structure of somatostatin-28. FEBS Lett 1980; 109:55-8.
4. Schally AV, Huang WY, Chang RCC, et al. Isolation and structure of prosomatostatin: a putative somatostatin precursor from pig hypothalamus. Proc Natl Acad Sci USA 1980; 77:4489-93.
5. Esch F, Bohlen P, Ling N, Benoit R, Brazeau P, Guillemin R. Primary structure of ovine hypothalamic somatostatin-28 and somatostatin-25. Proc Natl Acad Sci USA 1980; 77:6827-31.
6. Spiess J, Villarreal J, Vale W. Isolation and sequence analysis of a somatostatin-like polypeptide from ovine hypothalamus. Biochemistry

1981; 20:1982-8.

7. Benoit R, Ling N, Alford B, Guillemin R. Seven peptides derived from prosomatostatin in rat brain. Biochem Biophys Res Commun 1982; 107:944-50.

8. Patzelt C, Tager HS, Carroll RJ, Steiner DF. Identification of prosomatostatin in pancreatic islets. Proc Natl Acad Sci USA 1980; 77:2410-4.

9. Bohlen P, Brazeau P, Esch F, Ling N, Guillemin R. Isolation and chemical characterization of somatostatin-28 from rat hypothalamus. Regul Pept 1981; 2:359-69.

10. Shen L-P, Pictet RL, Rutter WJ. Human somatostatin I: sequence of the cDNA. Proc Natl Acad Sci USA 1982; 79:4575-9.

11. Goodman RH, Aron DC, Roos BA. Rat pre-prosomatostatin. Structure and processing by microsomal membranes. J Biol Chem 1983; 258:5570-3.

12. Funckes CL, Minth CD, Deschenes R, et al. Cloning and characterization of a mRNA encoding rat preprosomatostatin. J Biol Chem 1983; 258:8781-7.

13. Benoit R, Bohlen P, Esch F, Ling N. Neuropeptides derived from prosomatostatin that do not contain the somatostatin-14 sequence. Brain Res 1984; 311:23-9.

14. Spiess J, Vale W. Multiple forms of somatostatin-like activity in rat hypothalamus. Biochemistry 1980; 19:2861-6.

15. Patel YC, Zingg HH, Srikant CB. "Somatostatin-14 like immunoreactive forms in the rat: characterization, distribution and biosynthesis." In: Patel YC, Tannenbaum GS, eds. Somatostatin. New York: Plenum Press, 1985:71-87.

16. Morrison JH, Benoit R, Magistretti PJ, Bloom FE. Immunohistochemical distribution of prosomatostatin related peptides in cerebral cortex. Brain Res 1983; 262:344-51.

17. Ravazzola M, Benoit R, Guillemin R, Orci L. Immunocytochemical localization of prosomatostatin fragments in maturing and mature secretory granules of pancreatic and gastrointestinal D-cells. Proc Natl Acad Sci USA 1983; 80:215-8.

18. Marshak DW, Reeve JR, Shively JE, Hawke D, Takami MS, Yamada T. Structure of somatostatin isolated from bovine retina. J Neurochem 1983; 41:601-6.

19. Arakawa Y, Tachibana S. Somatostatin-20: a novel NH_2-terminally extended form of somatostatin isolated from porcine duodenum together with somatostatin-28 and somatostatin-25. Life Sci 1984; 35:2529-36.

20. Land H, Schutz G, Schmale H, Richter D. Nucleotide sequence of cloned cDNA encoding bovine arginine vasopressin-neurophysin II precursor. Nature 1982; 295:299-303.

21. Vinik AI, Gaginella TS, O'Dorisio TM, Shapiro B, Wagner L. The distribution and characterization of somatostatin-like immunoreactivity in epithelial cells, submucosa and muscle of the rat stomach and intestine. Endocrinology 1981; 109:1921-6.

22. Patel YC, Wheatley T, Ning C. Multiple forms of immunoreactive somatostatin: comparison of distribution in neural and non neural tissues and portal plasma of the rat. Endocrinology 1981; 109: 1943-9.

23. Trent DF, Weir GC. Heterogeneity of somatostatin-like peptides in rat brain, pancreas and gastrointestinal tract. Endocrinology 1981; 108:2033-8.

24. Baskin DG, Ensinck JW. Somatostatin in epithelial cells of intestinal mucosa is present primarily as somatostatin-28. Peptides 1984; 5:615-21.

25. Spira AW, Shimizu Y, Rorstad OP. Localization, chromatographic characterization and development of somatostatin-like immunoreactivity in the guinea pig retina. J Neurosci 1984; 4:3069-79.

26. Benoit R, Bohlen P, Ling N, et al. Presence of somatostatin-28(1-12)

in hypothalamus and pancreas. Proc Natl Acad Sci USA 1982; 79:917-21.

27. Spiess J, Villarreal J, Vale W. Isolation and sequence analysis of a somatostatin-like polypeptide from ovine hypothalamus. Biochemistry 1981; 20:1982-8.

28. Zingg HH, Patel YC. Processing of synthetic somatostatin-28 and a related endogenous rat hypothalamic somatostatin-like molecule to somatostatin-14 by hypothalamic enzymes. Life Sci 1982; 30:525-33.

29. Zingg HH, Patel YC. Biosynthesis of immunoreactive somatostatin by hypothalamic neurons in culture. J Clin Invest 1982; 70:1101-9.

30. Robbins RJ, Mothon S, Reichlin S. Somatostatin-28 is not the precursor of somatostatin-14 in cerebral cortical cells. Endocrinology 1983; 112:A18.

31. Van Itallie CM, Fernstrom JD. In vivo studies of somatostatin-14 and somatostatin-28 biosynthesis in rat hypothalamus. Endocrinology 1983; 113:1210-7.

32. Gluschankof P, Morel A, Gomez S, Nicolas P, Fahy C, Cohen P. Enzyme processing somatostatin precursors: an ARG-LYS esteropeptidase from the rat brain cortex converting somatostatin-28 into somatostatin-14. Proc Natl Acad Sci USA 1984; 81:6662-6.

33. Gluschankof P, Morel A, Benoit R, Cohen P. The somatostatin-28 convertase of rat brain cortex generates both somatostatin-14 and somatostatin-28(1-12). Biochem Biophys Res Commun 1985; 128:1051-7.

34. Harmar A, Ivell R, Keen P. The de novo biosynthesis of somatostatin and a related peptide in isolated rat dorsal root ganglia. Brain Res 1982; 242:365-8.

35. Ackland J, Ratter S, Bourne GL, Rees LH. Characterization of immunoreactive somatostatin in human fetal hypothalamic tissue. Regul Pept 1983; 5:95-101.

36. Low MJ, Hammer RE, Goodman RH, Habener JF, Palmiter RD, Brinster RL. Tissue-specific posttranslational processing of pre-prosomatostatin encoded by a metallothionein-somatostatin fusion gene in transgenic mice. Cell 1985; 41:211-9.

37. Conlon JM, McCarthy DM. Fragments of prosomatostatin isolated from a human pancreatic tumour. Mol Cell Endocrinol 1984; 38:81-6.

38. Bakhit C, Benoit R, Bloom FE. Release of somatostatin-28(1-12) from hypothalamus in vitro. Nature 1983; 301:524-6.

39. Sheward WJ, Benoit R, Fink G. Somatostatin-28(1-12)-like immunoreactive substance is secreted into hypophysial portal vessel blood in the rat. Neuroendocrinology 1984; 38:88-90.

40. Guy J, Benoit R, Pelletier G. Immunocytochemical localization of somatostatin-28(1-12) in the rat hypothalamus. Brain Res 1985; 330:283-9.

41. Campbell MJ, Lewis DA, Benoit R, Morrison JH. Regional heterogeneity in the distribution of somatostatin-28 and somatostatin-28(1-12)—immunoreactive profiles in monkey neocortex. J Neurosci 1986 (submitted).

42. Benoit R, Ling N, Bakhit C, Morrison JH, Alford B, Guillemin R. Somatostatin-28(1-12)-like immunoreactivity in the rat. Endocrinology 1982; 111:2149-51.

43. Benoit R, Bohlen P, Ling N, et al. Somatostatin-28(1-12)-like peptides. In: Patel YC, Tannenbaum GS, eds. Somatostatin. New York: Plenum Press, 1985:89-107.

44. Lechan RM, Goodman RH, Rosenblatt M, Reichlin S, Habener JF. Prosomatostatin-specific antigen in rat brain: localization by immunocytochemical staining with an antiserum to a synthetic sequence of pre-prosomatostatin. Proc Natl Acad Sci USA 1983; 80:2780-4.

45. Varndell IM, Sikri KL, Hennessy RJ, et al. Mammalian somatostatin-containing D cells exhibit rat somatostatin cryptic peptide (RSCP) immunoreactivity. An electron microscopical study. Cell Tissue Res 1986 (in press).

46. Low MJ, Lechan RM, Rosenblatt M, Goodman RH. Distribution and content of pro-somatostatin specific antigen in rat brain [Abstract]. Endocrinology 1982; 110:281.

47. Aron DC, Andrews PC, Dixon JE, Roos BA. Identification of cellular prosomatostatin and nonsomatostatin peptides derived from its amino terminus. Biochem Biophys Res Commun 1984; 124:450-6.

48. Aron DC, Roos BA. Nonsomatostatin secretory peptides derived from prosomatostatin's amino terminus in a rat medullary thyroid carcinoma cell line. Endocrinology 1986; 118:218-22.

49. Schmidt WE, Mutt V, Kratzin H, Carlquist M, Conlon JM, Creutzfeldt W. Isolation and characterization of proSS(1-32), a peptide derived from the N-terminal region of porcine preprosomatostatin. FEBS Lett 1985; 192:141-6

5

EXPRESSION OF PREPROSOMATOSTATIN IN FOREIGN CELLS: SECRETION OF MATURE SOMATOSTATIN BY YEAST (SACCHAROMYCES CEREVISIAE)

Dennis Shields,* Reza Green,* Michael Schaber,[2] and Richard Kramer[2]

*Departments of Anatomy and Developmental Biology and Cancer, Albert Einstein College of Medicine Bronx, New York 10461

[2]Department of Molecular Genetics, Roche Research Center Hoffman-LaRoche, New Jersey 07110

INTRODUCTION

Most small peptide hormones are synthesized as part of larger precursors which undergo proteolytic processing to generate the bioactive peptides (1). These precursors are excellent models to study protein trafficking within the secretory pathway since they are cotranslationally inserted into the lumen of the RER (1-3), transported through the Golgi apparatus and packaged into secretory vesicles (4). In the process, they undergo a variety of covalent modifications that serve as biochemical markers for intercompartmental transfer. At present it is unclear what structural information within peptide hormone precursors determines appropriate intracellular transit and secretion of the mature peptide product. In order to analyze putative sorting and processing domains, we are currently studying the biosynthesis of one of the simplest of these molecules, preprosomatostatin (preproSRIF).

Preprosomatostatin is a Mr 11,000 protein synthesized in the endocrine pancreas, intestine, central nervous system, and other tissues (5). In anglerfish, preprosomatostatin I consists of a 25 amino acid signal peptide which is cleaved cotranslationally to form proSRIF (3,6), an 82-residue pro region, and the biologically active moiety, SRIF, which comprises the carboxy-terminal 14 amino acids of the precursor (3,7,8). The SRIF sequence is flanked by a single pair of basic amino acids, typical of prohormone proteolytic processing sites (4). This Arg-Lys sequence is preceded by a highly conserved tetrapeptide (Ala-Pro-Arg-Glu) which may also play a role in proteolytic processing (7,8). ProSRIF migrates to the Golgi apparatus and co-localizes with a dibasic-specific protease that cleaves the mature hormone from its precursor (9). The absence of other paired basic residues (and, hence, other cryptic hormones) within the pro region implies that it functions to facilitate the biosynthesis and secretion of SRIF, including targeting the molecule to appropriate compartments. Our aim is to identify sorting and processing determinants within the pro region by studying the biosynthesis of predictively altered preproSRIF molecules. We have previously described the expression of preproSRIF in Cos 7 (monkey kidney) cells and demonstrated that these cells are able to correctly process proSRIF and secrete the mature hormone, suggesting that heterologous cells can recognize processing domains within proSRIF (10).

Genetic and biochemical evidence suggests that yeast have a secretory pathway that is similar if not identical to that found in higher cells (11). Of particular relevance is that yeast contain the necessary machinery to process, package and secrete peptide hormones. Yeast of the alpha mating type synthesize and secrete alpha factor (αF), a 13 amino acid mating pheromone (12). αF is synthesized as part of a precursor consisting of four tandem repeats of the peptide, preceded by a pro region of 89 amino acids that contains three potential glycosylation sites. The mature αF sequence is flanked by a processing site consisting of a Lys Arg pair and a spacer sequence of several Glu-Ala and Asp-Ala pairs. The extreme amino terminus of proαF resembles a signal sequence; however, there is no direct evidence for cotranslational cleavage in vivo or in vitro (13). Consequently, it remains to be determined which part of proαF mediates RER translocation. αF is processed from this precursor in the Golgi apparatus by the action of at least two membrane-bound enzymes: a paired-basic-specific protease (product of the KEX2 gene) which cleaves on the carboxyl side of Arg residues (14,15) and a dipeptide aminopeptidase (product of the STE13 gene) which trims the Glu-Ala and Asp-Ala pairs (16). ProαF follows a similar intracellular route in yeast to that taken by proSRIF in higher cells, as shown by its transport in yeast secretory pathway mutants (13). Therefore, it is likely that the pro region of proαF has a function similar to that of the pro region of proSRIF in insuring appropriate processing and secretion of the αF peptide.

Here we describe the construction of proαF-SRIF hybrid molecules and examine the secretion of SRIF from yeast. A similar approach has been used to express several heterologous proteins in yeast, including interferon (17,18), epidermal growth factor (19), and endorphin (17). These studies suggested that the ability of yeast to correctly process αF-hybrids and secrete foreign peptide products varied considerably, depending on the particular construction employed; in contrast, our data reveal accurate processing and efficient secretion of SRIF from yeast.

RESULTS

Construction of αFactor—SRIF Hybrid Genes

The initial aim of these studies was to determine if the yeast S. cerevisiae could package and secrete mature SRIF. For this purpose, we utilized the pro region of proαF to provide signals for intercompartmental transfer and proteolytic processing of the 14 amino acid sequence of SRIF. We constructed recombinant DNA molecules (Fig. 1) which included the DNA encoding the entire αF pro region (residues 1-89) terminating with the processing sequence Lys-Arg-Glu-Ala-Glu-Ala-Glu-Ala fused in frame to the DNA coding for the SRIF sequence. These plasmids were designated p82-1 and p82-5. These fusion were constructed to determine if yeast processing enzymes could excise mature SRIF from the chimeric precursor. The chimeric DNA molecules were inserted into a yeast expression vector (containing a TRP1 selectable marker) under the control of either the native αF promoter region (p82-5) or the inducible yeast PHO5 (acid phosphatase) promoter (p82-1). Transcription directed by the latter promoter can be induced by depletion of inorganic phosphate (P_i) and thus afforded the opportunity to modulate the expression of the hybrid protein under experimental conditions.

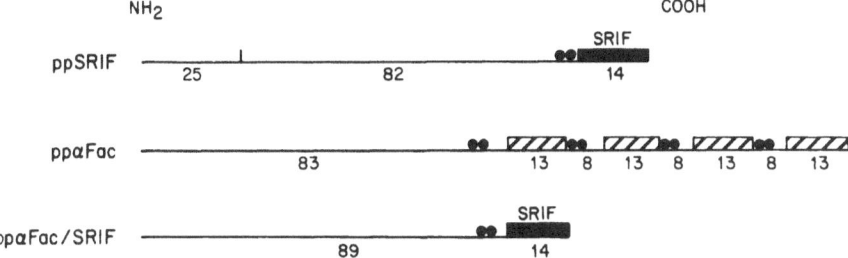

Fig. 1. Structure of αFactor-SRIF hybrid precursor. The structures of anglerfish preproSRIF (8) and yeast pro αFactor, ppαFac (12) and the ppαFac/SRIF hybrid, designated p82-1 are diagrammed schematically. The 25 amino acid signal peptide of preproSRIF is indicated by a vertical line; the proregions of preproSRIF and proαFac (82 and 83 amino acids, respectively) are also indicated. The black box represents the 14-amino acid sequence of mature SRIF; the 13-amino acid sequence of mature αFactor is shown by hatched boxes. The spacer regions flanking the αFactor peptide in the native precursor are shown by numbered boxes. The filled-in circles represent pairs of basic amino acids at the proteolytic processing site for mature SRIF (Arg-Lys) and αFactor (Lys-Arg); the processing site and spacer region in the proαFact/SRIF hybrid is: Lys-Arg-Glu-Ala-Glu-Ala-SRIF. Construction of the DNA encoding p82-1 (ppαFac/SRIF) and its insertion into the high copy number yeast expression vector pYE7, is described in detail elsewhere (35). It should be noted that this construction was placed under the control of either the acid phosphatase promoter (PHO5) (designated p82-1) or under the control of the αFactor promoter (p82-5). In the former case, expression was regulated by the absence or presence of phosphate, whereas in the latter case, expression was independent of the presence of phosphate.

Secretion of SRIF

Transformants carrying the plasmids p82-1 and p82-5 were screened for SRIF production by radioimmunoassay of culture media utilizing a rabbit antibody raised against synthetic SRIF. Exponentially growing cells were transferred to fresh medium in the presence (hi-P_i) or absence (no-P_i) of phosphate and incubated for various times, after which immunoreactive SRIF and cell number were determined. Yeast harboring the PHO5 construction (p82-1) secreted low but detectable levels of SRIF in hi-P_i medium. In contrast, a parallel incubation of cells in no-P_i medium resulted in the secretion of up to 200 ng/ml SRIF (Fig. 2). Normalization of data for the slower cell growth under phosphate-depleted conditions revealed a 70-fold induction of SRIF accumulation. As expected from previous studies (26), this induction was due to increased transcription of the chimeric gene under the control of the PHO5 promoter. This was shown by Northern blot analysis comparing uninduced and induced hybrid mRNAs using a SRIF-specific probe (data not shown). Yeast transformed with the αF promoter construct (p82-5) were shown to secrete SRIF constitutively at a level equivalent to that induced by no-P_i medium; however, this secretion was independent of the presence of phosphate (Fig. 2). In both cases, the rate of secretion of SRIF remained constant (approximately 1-3 ng/10^7 cells/hour) for the 30-hour duration of the experiment. It is noteworthy that the constitutive and induced secretion of SRIF were equivalent, suggesting that this represents a maximal level.

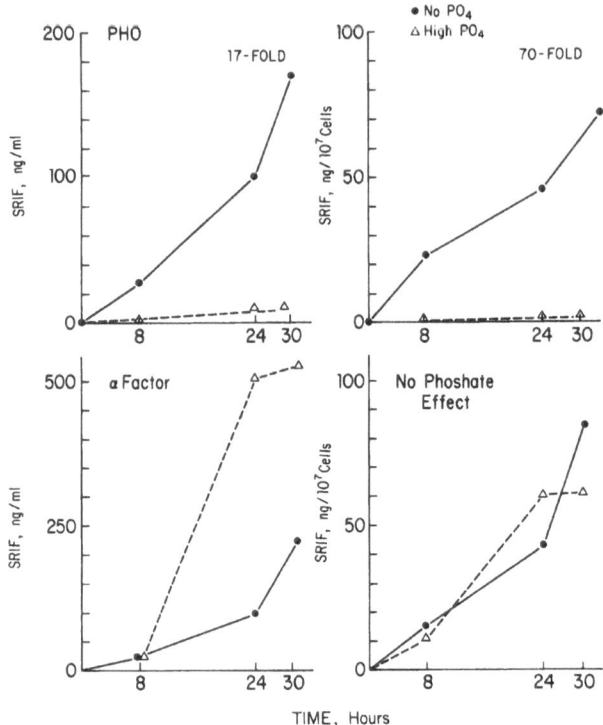

Fig. 2. Detection of SRIF immunoreactive material secreted into the growth medium. Yeast transformed with
plasmids p82-1 or p82-5 (Fig. 1) were grown in either
hi-P_i medium (open symbols) or no-P_i medium (closed
symbols), and incubation continued at 30°C for the
indicated times. At each time point, cell density was
determined spectrophotometrically and the SRIF present
in 100 μl of culture medium determined by radioimmunoassay. Due to differential growth in hi-P_i vs. no-P_i
medium, results are expressed as ng/10^7 cells, as well
as ng/ml secreted into the medium.

Characterization of Secreted SRIF-Immunoreactive Material

It was of primary interest to determine the biochemical nature of the
secreted immunoreactive material. This was particularly important in
light of earlier studies in which β endorphin was expressed in yeast as a
similar fusion protein, and the only secreted immunoreactive products were
proteolytic fragments generated by trypsin-like cleavages at internal
basic amino acids (17). Since there are two lysine residues in the 14
amino acids of SRIF, we wished to explore whether yeast would also nonspecifically degrade this peptide. Furthermore, previous studies indicated that cleavage at the Lys-Arg processing site was efficient with a
variety of proαF hybrids, irrespective of the downstream sequences;
however, subsequent trimming of the Glu-Ala pairs from the excised heterologous peptides occurred with highly variable efficiency (17,18,19).
Therefore, a second aim of these experiments was to determine the precise
amino terminus of the secreted molecule(s).

Yeast transformed with p82-1 were induced in no-P$_1$ medium for four hours, and then metabolically labeled for 2.5 hours with ^{35}S cysteine, an amino acid present only in SRIF and not in proαF (8,12). At the end of the incubation, media and cell lysates were treated with the RSS1 anti-SRIF antibody, which has been shown to immunoprecipitate preproSRIF and proSRIF as well as the mature hormone (6). Immune precipitates were supplemented with unlabeled SRIF, exhaustively reduced and carboxy-methylated, and analyzed by reverse phase HPLC using conditions which resolve native and carboxymethylated SRIF (Fig. 3).

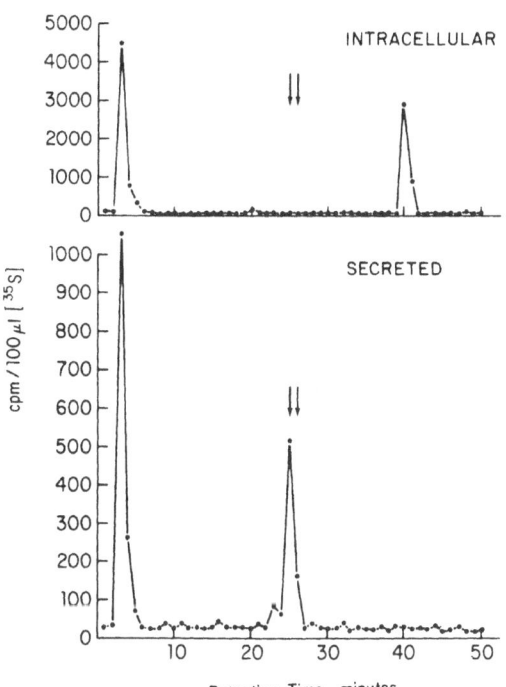

Fig. 3. Analysis of SRIF-immunoreactive material by HPLC. Yeast harboring p82-1 were induced no-P$_1$ for 4 hours, then resuspended in medium containing 100 μCi/ml ^{35}S Cysteine. After a further 2.5-hour incubation, cells and media were separated by centrifugation and cells lysed (35). Media and cell lysates were incubated with 20 μl of rabbit anti-SRIF antiserum; immune complexes were then isolated by adsorption to Protein A Sepharose beads. After washing, 3 μg unlabeled SRIF were added and samples exhaustively reduced and carboxymethylated. Radio-labeled SRIF was eluted from the Sepharose beads (35). The supernatants were applied directly to a Vydac C$_{18}$ reverse phase HPLC column and eluted with a 15-50% gradient of acetonitrile in 0.1% TFA. A 100 μl aliquot of each fraction was dried and radioactivity determined by liquid scintillation counting. Upper panel: intracellular SRIF-immunoreactive material. Lower panel: secreted SRIF-immunoreactive material. Arrows indicate the elution positions of native SRIF (fraction 26) and reduced and carboxymethylated SRIF (fraction 25).

The intracellular SRIF-immunoreactive material retention time 40 min, was found to correspond to unprocessed proαFactor-SRIF hybrid (Green and Shields, submitted). The medium samples from the transformants showed a major peak of radioactivity with the same retention time as unlabeled SRIF. Furthermore, labeled material that had not been subjected to reduction and carboxymethylation eluted one minute later, as did native SRIF. The identity of retention times and similarity of behavior following reduction and carboxymethylation strongly suggested that the yeast paired-basic protease and dipeptide aminopeptidase were able to correctly process this hybrid molecule and secrete mature disulfide-bonded SRIF. To test this directly, we then sequenced the HPLC purified material from p82-1 by automated Edman degradation. Major peaks of radiolabeled cysteine appeared at cycles 3 and 14 of Edman degradation (Fig. 4), exactly corresponding to the positions of this amino acid in mature SRIF.

The HPLC profile also showed a small amount of immunoreactive material that eluted 1-2 fractions earlier than reduced and carboxymethylated SRIF. We consistently observed this small peak and hypothesized that it might represent incorrectly processed peptide. Consequently, we also determined its amino acid sequence to establish its relationship to SRIF (Fig. 4). This material was identical to the major labeled peak in possessing cysteine residues at positions 3 and 14. Thus, it does not represent a processing intermediate, but most probably is mature SRIF that subsequently undergoes some additional modification, e.g., partial oxidation.

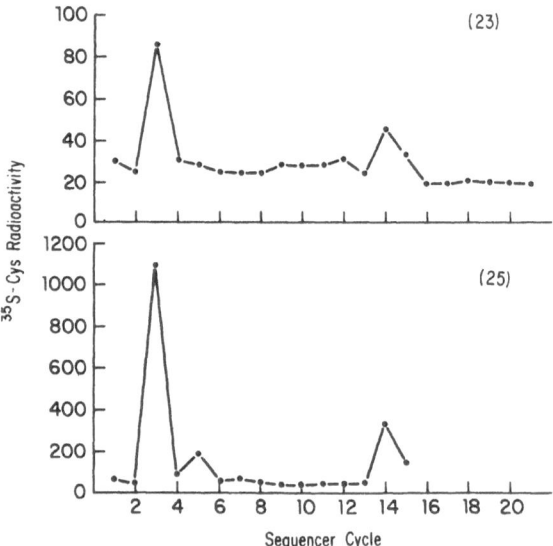

Fig. 4. Amino acid sequence determination of secreted SRIF-immunoreactive material. Yeast transformed with p82-1 were induced in no-P$_4$ medium and labeled with ^{35}S cysteine. SRIF-immunoreactive material was reduced, carboxymethylated, and purified by HPLC. The purified material eluting at 23 min (upper panel) and 25 min (lower panel) (see Fig. 3) was subjected to automated Edman degradation. The total ^{35}S radioactivity from each sequencer cycle was determined by liquid scintillation counting.

DISCUSSION

There is increasing evidence that proteins contain topogenic sequences which target them to different destinations within the cell (32,33). The best studied example is the signal peptide, which generally constitutes the amino-terminal 20-25 amino acids of secretory and membrane proteins and mediates their cotranslational insertion into the RER. Studies employing chimeric and predictively mutated proteins have supported the idea that the transient presence of such a signal sequence is both necessary and sufficient to direct a protein to the RER (33,34). However, the precise mechanisms by which proteins cross the lipid bilayer, including structural requirements other than the signal, remain unclear. Furthermore, it is proving more difficult to identify analogous topogenic determinants that subsequently localize these proteins to ER, Golgi, or plasma membrane. Such domains, in contrast with signal sequences (and the nuclear and mitochondrial targeting sequences that have been identified), may be derived from the interactions of noncontiguous amino acids and are thus likely to be permanent features of these proteins. Therefore, good models for identifying these epitopes would be secretory proteins of relatively simple structure and obvious functional domains.

The precursors to the small peptide hormones SRIF and αF fulfill these criteria and, as such, can be used to address several fundamental aspects of the secretory process: (1) Is there a minimum size (postulated to be 60-70 amino acids) required for successful translocation across the ER membrane, i.e., does the pro region of these precursors function primarily as a spacer? (2) Can a small peptide hormone contain information for intracellular sorting as well as for biological activity, or alternatively, does such information reside in the pro region? (3) What determines the specificity of proteolytic processing and appropriate packaging of the small peptide product? Our approach is to express native and recombinant preproSRIF and proαF molecules in heterologous cells. Their domain structure allows one to retain the biologically active moiety while altering or replacing parts of the precursor that may function in sorting and processing.

The experiments reported here describe the expression in yeast of a novel chimeric protein consisting of the pro region of yeast proαF, fused to the 14 amino acids of mature SRIF. Our results indicate that the pro region of proαF, can direct the intracellular transport and processing of SRIF. The final precursors are considerably shorter than native proαF (103 amino acids vs. 165) but can be translocated across the ER membrane in vivo and in vitro. Subsequently, these molecules are correctly compartmentalized with the paired-basic-specific protease and dipeptide aminopeptidase that process intact proαF. There was no detectable intracellular accumulation of mature SRIF and conversely, no secretion of the uncleaved precursors; similar results were observed with proαF (13). In contrast to studies in which β endorphin was expressed as a similar hybrid protein in yeast (17), we found no evidence for cleavage of the SRIF peptide itself. The only immunoreactive species secreted was native, disulfide-bonded SRIF as shown by elution behavior on HPLC and amino acid sequencing. These data support our hypothesis that the pro region, rather than the mature hormone sequence, mediates intracellular transport, since yeast cells do not distinguish between F and SRIF at the level of processing and secretion.

ACKNOWLEDGMENTS

We thank Mr. M. Brenner for expert technical assistance, and Ms. Rita Romita for typing the manuscript. This work was supported, in part, by

NIH grant AM-21860. D.S. is the recipient of a Research Career Development Award AM01208 and an Irma T. Hirschl Salary Award. R.G. was supported by NIH training grant 5T32CA09060.

REFERENCES

1. Douglass J, Civelli O, Herbert E. Annu Rev Biochem 1984; 53:665-715.
2. Shields D, Blobel G. Proc Natl Acad Sci USA 1977; 74:2059-63.
3. Shields D. Proc Natl Acad Sci USA 1980; 77:4074-8.
4. Steiner DF, Quinn PS, Chan SJ, Makh J, Tager HS. Ann NY Acad Sci 1980; 343:1-39.
5. Reichlin S. N Engl J Med 1983; 309:1495-1501.
6. Warren TG, Shields D. Biochemistry 1984; 23:2684-90.
7. Goodman RH, Aron DC, Roos BA. J Biol Chem 1983; 258:5570-3.
8. Hobart P, Crawford R, LuPing S, Raymond P, Rutter WJ. Nature 1980; 288:137-41.
9. Noe BD, Debo G, Spiess J. J Cell Biol 1984; 99:578-87.
10. Warren TG, Shields D. Cell 1984; 39:547-55.
11. Novick P, Field C, Schekman R. Cell 1980; 21:205-15.
12. Kurjan J, Herzkowitz I. Cell 1982; 30:933-43.
13. Julius D, Schekman R, Thorner J. Cell 1984; 36:309-18.
14. Julius D, Brake A, Blair L, Kunisawa R, Thorner J. Cell 1984; 37:1075-89.
15. Achstetter T, Wolf DH. EMBO J 1984; 4:173-7.
16. Julius D, Blair L, Brake A, Sprague G, Thorner J. Cell 1983; 32:839-52.
17. Bitter GA, Chen KK, Banks AR, Lai P-H. Proc Natl Acad Sci USA 1984; 81:5330-4.
18. Singh A, Lugovoy JM, Kohn WJ, Perry LJ. Nucleic Acids Res 1984; 12:8927-38.
19. Brake A, Merryweather JP, Coit DG, et al. Proc Natl Acad Sci USA 1984; 81:4642-6.
20. Kramer RA, Anderson N. Proc Natl Acad Sci USA 1980; 7:6541-5.
21. Andersen N, Thill GP, Kramer RA. Mol Cell Biol 1983; 3:562-9.
22. Schaber MD, DeChiara TM, Kramer RH. Methods Enzymol 1986; 119:417-23.
23. Hinnen A, Hicks JB, Fink GR. Proc Natl Acad Sci USA 1978; 75:1929-33.
24. Jones E. Genetics 1977; 85:23-33.
25. Morinaga Y, Franceschini T, Inouye S, Inouye M. Biotechnol 1984; 2:636-9.
26. Kramer RH, DeChiara TM, Schaber MD, Hilliker S. Proc Natl Acad Sci USA 1984; 81:367-70.
27. Speiss J, Villarreal J, Vale W. Biochemistry 1981; 20:1982-8.
28. Green R, Shields D. Endocrinology 1984; 114:1990-4.
29. Sripati, Warner J. Methods Cell Biol 1978; 20:61.
30. Poruchynsky MS, Tyndall C, Both GW, Sato F, Bellamy R, Atkinson PH. J Cell Biol 1985; 101:2199-2209.
31. Tarentino AL, Maley F. J Biol Chem 1974; 249:811-7.
32. Blobel G. Proc Natl Acad Sci USA 1980; 77:1496-1500.
33. Sabatini DD, Kreibich G, Morimoto T, Adesnik M. J Cell Biol 1982; 92:1-22.
34. Lingappa VR, Chaidez J, Yost CS, Hedgpeth J. Proc Natl Acad Sci USA 1984; 81:456-60.
35. Green R, Schaber M, Shields D, Kramer R. J Biol Chem 1986 (in press).

6

COTRANSLATIONAL AND POSTTRANSLATIONAL PROTEOLYTIC PROCESSING OF PREPROSOMATOSTATIN-I AND PREPROSOMATOSTATIN-II IN INTACT ISLET TISSUE

Bryan D. Noe,* Robert B. Mackin,* John K. McDonald,* Philip C. Andrews,[2] Jack E. Dixon,[2] and Joachim Spiess[3]

*Department of Anatomy and Cell Biology, Emory University School of Medicine, Atlanta, GA 30322; [2]Department of Biochemistry, Purdue University, West Lafayette, IN 47907; [3]Clayton Foundation Laboratories for Peptide Biology, The Salk Institute, La Jolla, CA 92037

INTRODUCTION

Somatostatin-14 (SS-14) and somatostatin-28 (SS-28) are synthesized as part of a larger precursor, prosomatostatin. This has been demonstrated by results from experiments employing pulse-chase incubations or chemical characterization of products from intact tissue (1-9). In addition, use of recombinant DNA methodology has provided the deduced amino acid sequences for preprosomatostatins from a number of sources (10-17). Prosomatostatins or prosomatostatin cleavage products have been identified in pancreatic islets of anglerfish (1,2,10-12,18-20), catfish (13,14,21), and rats (4); in hypothalamus of mouse (22), rat (7,23-27), sheep (28,29) and pigs (30); gut of pigs (31); and from diverse sources such as a medullary thyroid carcinoma cell line (12,15,16,32-34) and a phaeochromocytoma (35). Both the human (36) and rat (37,38) genes which code for preprosomatostatins (PPSS) have been characterized. The evidence currently available indicates that mammalian SS-14 and SS-28 are cleaved by differential processing from the same precursor in each tissue in which the PPSS gene is expressed. However, in the anglerfish islet there are two separate cell types in which two different forms of PPSS are expressed (39). In one of these cell types PPSS-I is synthesized and in the other PPSS-II is synthesized. To facilitate comparisons, the basic structures and primary cleavage sites of the fish and human PPSS are shown in Figure 1. The primary cleavage product of PPSS-I is SS-14 (1,2,40,41), whereas the primary cleavage product of PPSS-II is a unique form of SS-28 (aSS-28) which has [Tyr^7,Gly^{10}] SS-14 as its C-terminus and is hydroxylated at Lys^{23} (42-46).

At the present time, the foregoing information regarding prosomatostatin (PSS) processing is fairly well established. What is less well understood regarding the posttranslational processing of various PSS forms is the frequency and significance of cleavages which release peptides other than the primary products. A multiplicity of prosomatostatin fragments of varying size have been isolated from diverse tissue sources (23-35,47-50). With the exception of SS-14, SS-28 and SS-28$_{1-12}$, it is not clear whether any of the other fragments of prosomatostatin are metabolic cleavage products with potential bioactivity. In most cases, the possibility that these peptides are random degradation products of the somatostatin precursor cannot be excluded. In order to ascertain whether any of these peptides are metabolic cleavage products, it is necessary to perform biosynthetic studies. We have developed procedures for performing such studies.

Recently, several fragments which are potential cleavage products of anglerfish islet prosomatostatin-I (aPSS-I) and prosomatostatin-II (aPSS-II), but do not contain SS-14 or SS-28, have been isolated and characterized by Andrews and Dixon (51,52). The availability of these peptides for use as markers in biosynthetic studies has made it possible to study their production in intact islet tissue. We report here the results of studies designed to quantitate the amounts of these peptides which are synthesized and stored in islets, along with information which confirms the cleavage sites for the signal peptides of PPSS-I and PPSS-II.

RESULTS AND DISCUSSION

Identification of the Signal Cleavage Site in PPSS-I in Intact Islets

Anglerfish islets were incubated in the presence of various combinations of radioactively labeled amino acids, extracted in 2M acetic acid, desalted on Bio-Gel P-2, then gel filtered on columns of Bio-Gel P-30 and the M_r 8,000 to 15,000 labeled peptides were subjected to reverse phase HPLC on Vydac C18 columns in 0.1% TFA, using acetonitrile gradients. The

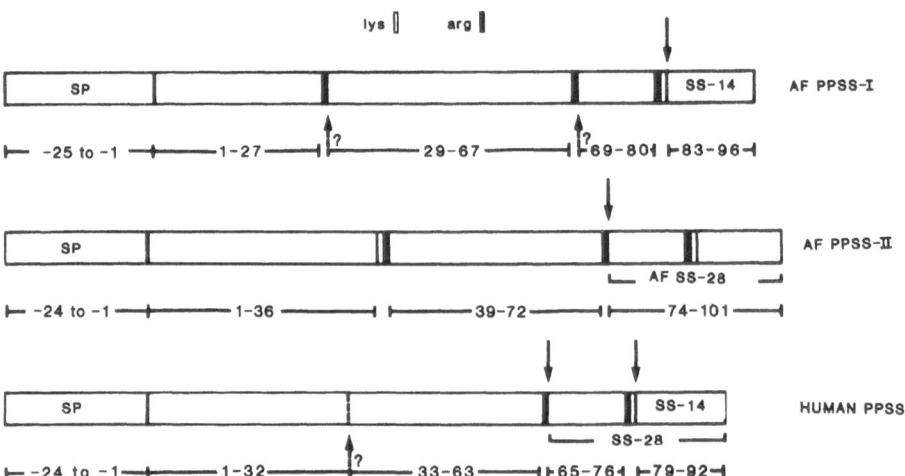

Fig. 1. Size and cleavage site comparisons between anglerfish and human preprosomatostatins. Numbering of residues assigns the N-terminal amino acid of prosomatostatin as +1; residues of signal peptides (SP) are assigned negative numbers. Known sites of posttranslational endopeptidase and exopeptidase cleavage are indicated by downward pointing solid arrows. Postulated sites of endopeptidase cleavage are indicated by upward pointing dashed arrows. Positions where arginine residues are located are indicated by solid rectangles; lysines are indicated by open rectangles.

elution positions of aPSS-I and aPSS-II were identified by their labeling patterns and radioimmunoassays. The portions of the HPLC eluates which contained aPSS-I and aPSS-II were pooled and the labeled material contained in them was further purified by additional HPLC chromatography. Confirmation that the suspected precursors were actually aPSS-I and aPSS-II was obtained by incubating each purified peptide in the presence of islet secretory granule lysates under conditions in which the islet prohormones are converted to products by enzymes in the granule lysate. After incubation, the products were subjected to HPLC and the HPLC eluates were monitored for the presence of the cleavage products of aPSS-I and aPSS-II. It was found that the major product of the precursor suspected to be aPSS-I was SS-14 and the major product of the precursor suspected to be aPSS-II was aSS-28 which verified the identity of each precursor.

In order to determine the position of signal peptide cleavage and the partial N-terminal structure of aPSS-I, aPSS-I previously labeled with [^{3}H]tryptophan and [^{14}C] leucine was purified by HPLC, reduced and S-carboxymethylated and subjected to sequential Edman degradation in an automated sequencer. Significant [^{14}C]Leu radioactivity was found in the products from cycles 10,12,13,14,19,31,34,35,36,39, and 40. No ^{3}H-labeling was observed through the first 44 sequencer cycles. The positions of each of the labeled leucine residues correspond precisely with the predicted positions of 11 leucine residues of PPSS-I as determined by Hobart et al. (10) and Goodman et al. (11,12). The observations that the peptide which was sequenced exhibited SS-like immunoreactivity, and that leucine residues were found in precise correspondence with the predicted sequence information, indicate that the peptide partially sequenced was aPSS-I. As it would be expected that signal sequences would be removed from any prohormones extracted from islet tissue, these results indicate that the N-terminal amino acid of aPSS-I is located 9 residues upstream from the first leucine residue observed. It follows that signal peptide cleavage occurs just N-terminal to this amino acid. According to the predicted sequence of aPSS-I (10-12), the signal cleavage site would thus be at a Cys-Ser bond, indicating a signal peptide 25 amino acids in length (Fig. 1). These results have been presented in more detail elsewhere (53).

This was the first identification of the amino terminus of aPSS-I extracted from islet tissue. These results confirm the previous findings of Warren and Shields (20) who demonstrated signal cleavage at this site by performing cell-free translation of PPSS-I mRNA in the presence of dog pancreatic microsomes. Our results are also consistent with the fact that one of the peptides isolated and characterized by Andrews and Dixon (51) was aPSS-I$_{1-27}$, a potential cleavage product of aPSS-I (see Fig. 1). Taken together, the results from all of these studies establish the signal cleavage site of PPSS I in anglerfish islets at the position following the 25th residue downstream from the initiator Met of PPSS-I (Fig. 1).

Identification and Quantification of Products of aPSS-I Processing Other Than SS-14

Several peptides which are potential cleavage products of aPSS-I have been isolated from anglerfish islets and characterized by Andrews and Dixon (51). These peptides are aPSS-I$_{1-27}$, aPSS-I$_{1-67}$, and aPSS-I$_{69-80}$. The peptide aPSS-I$_{29-67}$ was also prepared by tryptic digestion of the I-67 peptide. It could be predicted that each of these peptides may be a cleavage product of aPSS-I because each is flanked by basic amino acids in the precursor (Fig. 1). Moreover, the 1-27, 1-67 and 69-80 peptides isolated by Andrews and Dixon lacked the C-terminal basic residues by which they are extended in the precursor, suggesting the action of a carboxypeptidase in the final processing of these potential products.

We have developed procedures for performing biosynthetic studies to determine whether, and in what amounts, each of these peptides is produced during the processing of aPSS-I in intact islets. Extracts of tissue incubated 5 hours in the presence of a ^{3}H-amino acid mixture were subjected to gel filtration and peptides of varying molecular size were subsequently separated by reverse phase HPLC. The distribution of radioactivity incorporated was compared to the absorption profile of the eluted peptides by monitoring the eluate at 210 nm. The predominant peptide in the M_r 1,000-2,000 pool, both in terms of labeling and amount of peptide recovered, was SS-14. The elution positions of SS-14 and aPSS-I$_{69-80}$, the only other peptide of those available which was expected to be present in the M_r 1,000-2,000 pool, were established in separate standardization runs. Only small amounts of labeled aPSS-I$_{69-80}$ were recovered in extracts. The UV profiles confirmed that very little of this peptide was stored in the tissue. For the purpose of comparison, the peak areas from the computing integrator were used to calculate the amounts of each peptide found in a number of tissue extracts. The results, tabulated as nmol/gm islet tissue, are presented in Table 1. The tissue extracts contained 27 times more SS-14 than aPSS-I$_{69-80}$.

The other potential products of aPSS-I are significantly larger than SS-14 and aPSS-I$_{69-80}$. These were therefore found in the M_r 2,500-9,000 gel filtration pool. Quantitation of the amounts of aPSS-I$_{1-27}$, 1-67 and 29-67 which were labeled during the pulse incubation and quantities accumulated and stored in islets was accomplished by employing the procedures indicated above. When compared with the amounts of SS-14 recovered, the quantities of these peptides were extremely low (Table 1). No aPSS-I$_{29-67}$ was detected. The results from these studies are described in more detail in a separate communication (53). The data obtained indicate that SS-14 is by far the predominant cleavage product of aPSS-I with the other peptides being produced as only minor cleavage products of this precursor. A schematic diagram which depicts the structure of aPSS-I and its cleavage products is shown in Figure 2. The major product (SS-14) is cross hatched and the minor products are stippled.

Table 1. Comparison of the amounts of prosomatostatin cleavage products recovered from islet tissue extracts.

| | Prosomatostatin-I | |
Peptide	Nanomoles/gm Tissue*	Peptide as Percent of SS-14
SS-14	287.1 ± 20.1	100.0
aPSS-I$_{69-80}$	10.4 ± 3.5	3.6
aPSS-I$_{1-67}$	6.9 ± 1.5	2.4
aPSS-I$_{29-67}$	none detected	0.0
aPSS-I$_{1-27}$	16.0 ± 1.1	5.5

| | Prosomatostatin-II | |
Peptide	Nanomoles/gm Tissue**	Peptide as Percent of aSS-28
aSS-28	62.2 ± 3.8	100.0
aPSS-II$_{1-36}$	41.4 ± 2.8	66.5

*Mean ± SEM (n=5)
**Mean ± SEM (n=13)

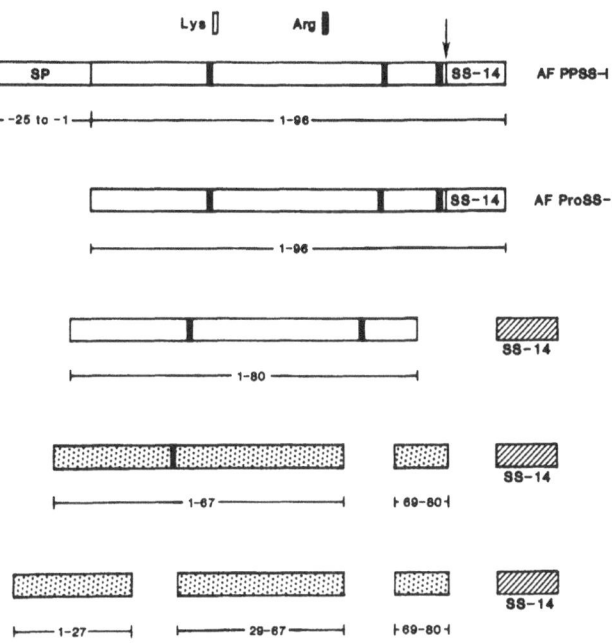

PROCESSING OF PREPROSOMATOSTATIN-I

Fig. 2. Diagram indicating several of the potential cleavage products of anglerfish preprosomatostatin-I which may be generated as products of proteolytic processing. Numbering of residues is the same as in Figure 1. The major product (SS-14) is cross hatched. Minor products are stippled.

The examination of a wide variety of tissue extracts from different species for peptides contained within the structure of mammalian prosomatostatin has led to the identification of a number of peptides in addition to SS-14 and SS-28 which may be cleavage products of this precursor. Prominent among these peptides derived from mammalian tissues are $SS-28_{1-12}$ (human PSS_{65-76} in Fig. 1) (23-26,48) and a 32 residue peptide, corresponding to human PSS_{1-32} (50) (Fig. 1). A peptide similar to PSS_{1-32} has been found in rat medullary thyroid carcinoma (34) and can be inferred to be present from work in which prosomatostatin cleavage products in rat brain were characterized (25). Other fragments of mammalian prosomatostatin have been described as well (47,48). However, just the fact that these peptides can be extracted from somatostatin-producing tissues is not sufficient to demonstrate that they are normal metabolic cleavage products of prosomatostatin. Whether a peptide is an actual processing product cleaved from prosomatostatin or an artifact of nonspecific proteolysis can be determined accurately only by quantitating the amount of each peptide produced in biosynthetic studies and by monitoring the amount of each of these peptides accumulated and stored in somatostatin-producing tissues. After comparing the amounts of the proposed product which are synthesized and stored with the quantity of SS-14 which is synthesized and stored in the same tissue, estimates can then be made regarding the relative abundance of other PSS cleavage products.

Our observation that relatively low levels of $aPSS-I_{1-27}$, $aPSS-I_{1-67}$, $aPSS-I_{69-80}$ and $aPSS-I_{29-67}$ are recovered, compared to amounts of $SS-14$, suggests that the major site of aPSS-I cleavage occurs at the basic dipeptide, Arg-Lys, which immediately precedes SS-14 in the precursor (Figs. 1 and 2). The results also indicate that secondary cleavages occur but appear to be minor, resulting in the production of the small amounts of the nonsomatostatin containing fragments which were recovered. That such small amounts of these minor products are generated suggests that none of these peptides is likely to be a bioactive cleavage product of aPSS-I. It is possible that these peptides are not normal metabolic cleavage products of aPSS-I at all. It cannot be excluded that each may be generated by random basic residue-specific endopeptidase activity combined with a carboxypeptidase B-like activity. It should be noted, however, that in the study of Andrews and Dixon (51) the relative proportions of each of these peptides recovered from separate islet tissue extracts differed to some extent from those obtained in the biosynthetic studies. These differences may relate to differential extraction and/or recovery of each of the peptides as a result of the procedures used in each laboratory. It is also possible that the larger peptides are not as readily extracted as the smaller peptides. However, the fact that in both laboratories the levels of the "propeptide" fragments recovered were found to be significantly lower than the amounts of SS-14 recovered is consistent with the argument that none are major cleavage products of aPSS-I.

In view of the data from both of these studies, a question remains regarding the nature of the major cleavage product(s) of aPSS-I other than SS-14. Considering the observation that $aPSS-I_{29-67}$ was not detected at all in tissue extracts in the present study, one possible cleavage product other than SS-14 is $aPSS-I_{29-80}$ (see Fig. 1). If $aPSS-I_{29-80}$ were a cleavage product, then the other major cleavage product would be aPSS-I_{1-27}. However, since the recovered levels of $aPSS-I_{1-27}$ were significantly lower than those of SS-14 (Table 1), this is considered unlikely. Thus, in accordance with the observation that recovery of $aPSS-I_{69-80}$ was also quite low (Table 1), it is proposed that the major cleavage product of aPSS-I other than SS-14 may be $aPSS-I_{1-80}$ (Fig. 2). This peptide has not yet been identified in extracts of anglerfish islets. It is possible that this is a result of poor recovery of the peptide during extraction or purification. Alternatively, the major sites of processing of the "propeptide" may be at positions other than at Arg^{28} or Arg^{68} resulting in cleavage products completely different from those identified to date.

Identification and Quantification of a Product of aPSS-II Other Than aSS-28

A peptide which corresponds to a specific sequence found near the N-terminus of PPSS-II has also been isolated from extracts of anglerfish islets and characterized by Andrews and Dixon (53). As discussed below, this peptide consists of 36 amino acids and appears to form the N-terminus of aPSS-II. It has therefore been designated $aPSS-II_{1-36}$ (see Fig. 1). As is the case for the nonsomatostatin containing products of aPSS-I already described, $aPSS-II_{1-36}$ could be a predicted cleavage product of aPSS-II because it is flanked in the precursor by a Lys-Arg sequence at its C-terminal end (Fig. 1). In order to determine whether this peptide is a normal cleavage product of aPSS-II, radiolabeled peptides from the M_r 2,500-8,000 region of gel filtration eluates were pooled, concentrated and subjected to HPLC analysis. Comparison of the elution patterns of labeled peptides with the elution position of the isolated peptide demonstrated that a labeled peptide eluted with an identical retention time. In differential labeling experiments, the peptide exhibited a labeling pattern consistent with the amino acid composition of $aPSS-II_{1-36}$ (10,52,54).

64

These results suggest that aPSS-II$_{1-36}$ is a normal metabolic cleavage product of aPSS-II. An additional observation which supports this hypothesis is the fact that the 1-36 peptide was found to lack the C-terminal Lys-Arg, both in the form isolated and characterized (52), and in the form demonstrated to be synthesized in islet tissue (54). This implies the participation of a carboxypeptidase to remove one or both C-terminal basic residues after endopeptidase cleavage. However, it is also possible that the 1-36 peptide is generated as the result of nonspecific degradation which occurs either within the tissue or during extraction and purification of islet peptides. In order to determine the amount of aPSS-II$_{1-36}$ relative to quantities of aSS-28 which are normally stored in islets, we performed HPLC analyses on a number of extracts and employed the peak area data from the computing integrater to calculate the nmol/gm of aPSS-II$_{1-36}$ and aSS-28 in the extracts. It was found that the amount of aPSS-II$_{1-36}$ present in islets was two-thirds the amount of aSS-28 (Table 1). This observation suggests that aPSS-II$_{1-36}$ is a significant cleavage product of aPSS-II in anglerfish islets. Because it is synthesized in in vitro incubations (54), because it is a prominent component of extracts from frozen islets (52), and because it is present in amounts similar to aSS-28 (Table 1 [53]), we hypothesize that aPSS-II$_{1-36}$ forms the N-terminus of aPSS-II. According to the predicted sequence of PPSS-II (10), signal cleavage would then occur at a Ser-Gln bond giving rise to a signal peptide of 24 amino acids (Fig. 1).

As they are located at the C-terminus of their precursors, the cleavage of both SS-14 and aSS-28 does not require the activity of an exopeptidase. Conversely, the production of the "propeptide" fragments of aPSS-I (discussed earlier) and aPSS-II$_{1-36}$ requires the action of a carboxypeptidase B (CPB)-like enzyme. Because significant amounts of aPSS-II$_{1-36}$ are normally synthesized in anglerfish islets, it was possible to perform experiments to determine whether this peptide serves as a substrate for the islet CPB which has recently been identified and characterized (55). Anglerfish proinsulin, aPSS-I and aPSS-II were purified by HPLC (54). Each of these prohormones was incubated with islet secretory granule lysate in the presence or absence of 1,10-phenanthroline (1,10-P), a chelator known to be an inhibitor of the islet CPB (55). The secretory granule lysates contain both the endoproteolytic and exoproteolytic enzymes which mediate islet prohormone processing. The processing of both insulin and aPSS-II$_{1-36}$ was altered in the presence of 1,10-P as indicated by a reduction in their retention time upon HPLC analyses. The processing of SS-14 and aSS-28 were not affected by 1,10-P (an expected result because the islet prohormone processing endopeptidases are not metalloproteinases [56,57]).

Although the reduction in retention time for the "incompletely converted" forms of insulin and aPSS-II$_{1-36}$ induced by 1,10-P is consistent with the C-terminal extension of these peptides by one or two basic amino acids, it was necessary to confirm this supposition. Therefore, the "incompletely converted" forms of insulin and aPSS-II$_{1-36}$ which were generated during in vitro conversion in the presence of 1,10-P were isolated by HPLC, concentrated, and reincubated in the presence or absence of purified porcine pancreatic CPB. Subsequent HPLC analysis demonstrated that treatment with the porcine CPB resulted in the generation of aPSS-II$_{1-36}$ and insulin having HPLC retention times identical to the natural product peptides which are produced in intact tissue or by in vitro incubation of the prohormones with secretory granule lysates in the absence of 1,10-P (54). As the porcine CPB could act only to remove one or more basic amino acids from the C-terminus of either substrate, we conclude that it mimics the action of the islet CPB. The results therefore demonstrate the physiologic relevance of the islet CPB in mediating final processing of both insulin and aPSS-II$_{1-36}$ after endopeptidase cleavage of their precursors. The results also provide further support for the argument that, because it is a normal cleavage product of aPSS-II and is produced in significant amounts, aPSS-II$_{1-36}$ may serve some important biologic function. The information available to date on aPSS-II processing is summarized diagrammatically in Figure 3.

The signal peptide of aPSS-II (-24 to -1) would be removed cotranslationally. The major posttranslational endoproteolytic cleavages occur at the C-terminus of Arg^{73} (to release aSS-28) and at the C-terminus of either the Arg at position 38 or the Lys at position 37 to release aPSS-II$_{1-36}$ extended by either one or two basic residues. C-terminal sequence analysis of the cleavage product generated during conversion in the presence of 1,10-phenanthroline would have to be performed to determine whether the endoproteolytic event occurs C-terminal to Arg^{38} or between Lys^{37} and Arg^{38}. Action of the islet carboxypeptidase removes the C-terminal basic residue(s), completing the processing of aPSS-II$_{1-36}$. Because the tissue produces 2/3 as much aPSS-II$_{1-36}$ as aSS-28, both peptides are indicated (cross hatched) as major products of aPSS-II processing in Figure 3.

The residual peptide from the precursor, aPSS-II$_{39-73}$ (or $_{38-72}$ depending on where the endopeptidase cleavage occurs in the Lys^{37}-Arg^{38} pair and whether carboxypeptidase activity removes Arg^{73}) is not indicated as a major product because this peptide has not yet been identified in

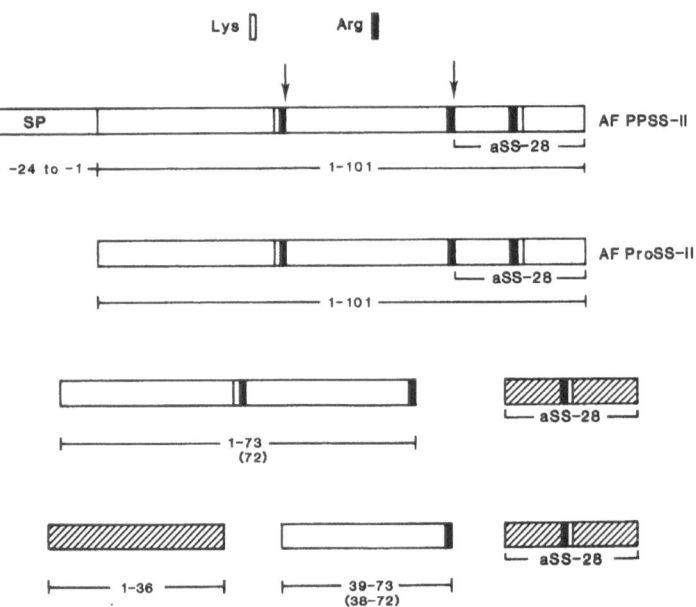

PROCESSING OF PREPROSOMATOSTATIN-II

Fig. 3. Diagram indicating the cleavage products of anglerfish preprosomatostatin-II which are generated as products of proteolytic processing. Numbering of residues is the same as in Figure 1. Both aSS-28 and aPSS-II$_{1-36}$ are major products (cross hatched). The exact structure of the residual peptide (residues 39-73 or 38-72) is as yet undetermined (see text).

tissue extracts (Fig. 3). However, since significant amounts of aPSS-II_{1-36}, are cleaved from aPSS-II, the residual peptide is presumably generated in quantities which are at least equimolar with those of aPSS-II_{1-36}.

The similarity in size of aPSS-I_{1-27} (Fig. 2) and aPSS-II_{1-36} Fig. 3) to potential cleavage products of prosomatostatins which have been isolated from several different mammalian tissues should be emphasized. Aron et al. have reported the presence of a M_r 4,000 peptide derived from the N-terminus of prosomatostatin synthesized in a rat medullary thyroid carcinoma cell line (33). However, this peptide is not secreted from its cells of origin in response to secretogogue challenge (34), suggesting that it may be a product of nonspecific degradation. Benoit et al. have examined peptides derived from rat brain prosomatostatin that do not contain SS-14 (25). It can be inferred from this work that one of the products is a peptide which consists of the first 32 residues of prosomatostatin. More recently, Schmidt et al. have isolated and sequenced a peptide found in extracts of porcine upper intestine (50). This peptide proved to have a sequence almost completely homologous (one amino acid substitution) with the first 32 residues of rat prosomatostatin (15,16). It is therefore possible that PSS_{1-32} may represent a normal cleavage product of mammalian prosomatostatin (see Fig. 1). However, it has not been demonstrated that this peptide is a normal metabolic cleavage product in biosynthetic studies. It is thus possible that it is generated by random degradation of prosomatostatin, or that it is normally produced in small amounts relative to quantities of SS-14 cleaved from the precursor. If PSS_{1-32} is a normal cleavage product, processing would occur at a Leu-Leu bond. Although it does not exclude the possibility that PSS_{1-32} is generated by in vivo processing, this difference in the nature of the cleavage site makes any comparisons between this peptide and aPSS-II_{1-27} or aPSS-II_{1-36} (Fig. 1) somewhat more tenuous. Clearly, further investigation is necessary.

Application of Methods Developed for Study of PSS Processing in Fish Islets to Examine PSS Processing in Mammalian Systems

Although the evidence available indicates that many similarities exist, it is clear that the characteristics of prosomatostatin processing in mammalian somatostatin-producing tissues cannot be completely deduced from the results of experiments performed with fish islets. In order to examine prosomatostatin processing in mammalian tissues more rigorously, the methodology employed with anglerfish islets could be applied. Application of these procedures would establish the amounts of the various putative cleavage products of prosomatostatin which are actually produced and stored in the tissue relative to those of the primary product, SS-14. This information, in turn, could then be used to facilitate the determination of whether any of the prosomatostatin fragments found in these tissues might possibly play a biologic role. Finally, it is possible that varying amounts of specific cleavage products may be produced in the same tissue under differing physiologic conditions as a result of differential cleavage. This is a possibility which can readily be tested in the anglerfish islet system and probably in mammalian systems as well.

ACKNOWLEDGMENTS

The authors express appreciation to Gail Debo, Julie Mackin and John Heil for excellent technical assistance and to Gail Morton for preparing the manuscript for publication. This work was supported by NIH grants AM 16921 (B.D.N.), AM 26378 (B.D.N. and J.S.), AM 18849 (J.E.D.), and AM 18024 (J.E.D.).

REFERENCES

1. Noe BD, Fletcher DJ, Bauer GE, Weir GC, Patel Y. Somatostatin biosynthesis occurs in pancreatic islets. Endocrinology 1978; 102:1675.
2. Noe BD, Fletcher DJ, Spiess J. Evidence for the existence of a biosynthetic precursor for somatostatin. Diabetes 1979; 28:724.
3. Zuhlke H, Ziegler M, Jahr H, Titze R, Schmidt S. Biosynthesis of somatostatin in pancreatic islets of Wistar rats. Acta Biol Med Germ 1978; 37:K15.
4. Patzelt C, Tager HS, Carroll RJ, Steiner DF. Identification of prosomatostatin in pancreatic islets. Proc Natl Acad Sci USA 1980; 77:2410.
5. Ensinck JW, Laschansky EC, Kanter RA, Fujimoto WY, Koerker DJ, Goodner CJ. Somatostatin biosynthesis and release in the hypothalamus and pancreas of the rat. Metabolism 1978; 27:1207.
6. Van Itallie CM, Fernstrom JD. In vivo studies of somatostatin-14 and somatostatin-28 biosynthesis in rat hypothalamus. Endocrinology 1983; 113:1210.
7. Zingg HH, Patel YC. Biosynthesis of immunoreactive somatostatin by hypothalamic neurons in culture. J Clin Invest 1982; 70:1101.
8. Yamada T, Basinger S. Biosynthesis of somatostatin-like immunoreactivity by frog retinas in vitro. J Neurochem 1982; 39:1539.
9. Robbins RJ, Reichlin S. Somatostatin biosynthesis by cerebral cortical cells in monolayer culture. Endocrinology 1983; 113:574.
10. Hobart P, Crawford R, Shen L-P, Pictet R, Rutter WJ. Cloning and sequence analysis of cDNAs encoding two distinct somatostatin precursors found in the endocrine pancreas of anglerfish. Nature 1980; 288:137.
11. Goodman RH, Jacobs JW, Chin WW, Lund PK, Dee PC, Habener JF. Nucleotide sequence of a cloned structural gene coding for a precursor of pancreatic somatostatin. Proc Natl Acad Sci USA 1980; 77:5869.
12. Goodman RH, Jacobs JW, Dee PC, Habener JF. Somatostatin-28 encoded in a cloned cDNA obtained from a rat medullary thyroid carcinoma. J Biol Chem 1982; 257:1156.
13. Minth CD, Taylor WL, Magazin M, Tavianini MA, Collier K, Weith HL, Dixon JE. The structure of cloned DNA complementary to catfish pancreatic somatostatin-14 messenger RNA. J Biol Chem 1982; 257: 10372.
14. Magazin M, Minth CD, Funckes CL, Deschenes R, Tavianini MA, Dixon JE. Sequence of a cDNA encoding pancreatic preprosomatostatin-22. Proc Natl Acad Sci USA 1982; 79:5152.
15. Goodman RH, Aron DC, Roos BA. Rat pre-prosomatostatin. Structure and processing by microsomal membranes. J Biol Chem 1983; 258:5570.
16. Funckes CL, Minth CD, Deschenes R, et al. Cloning and characterization of a mRNA-encoding rat preprosomatostatin. J Biol Chem 1983; 258:8781.
17. Shen LP, Pictet RL, Rutter WJ. Human somatostatin I: sequence of the cDNA. Proc Natl Acad Sci USA 1982; 79:4575.
18. Shields D. In vitro biosynthesis of fish islet preprosomatostatin: evidence of processing and segregation of a high molecular weight precursor. Proc Natl Acad Sci USA 1980; 77:4074.
19. Shields D. In vitro biosynthesis of somatostatin. Evidence for two distinct preprosomatostatin molecules. J Biol Chem 1980; 255:11625.
20. Warren TG, Shields D. Cell-free biosynthesis of multiple preprosomatostatins: characterization by hybrid selection and aminoterminal sequencing. Biochemistry 1984; 23:2684.
21. Andrews PC, Dixon JE. Isolation and structure of a peptide hormone predicted from a mRNA sequence--a second somatostatin from the catfish pancreas. J Biol Chem 1981; 256:8267.
22. Lauber M, Camier M, Cohen P. Higher molecular weight forms of

immunoreactive somatostatin in mouse hypothalamic extracts: evidence of processing in vitro. Proc Natl Acad Sci USA 1979; 76:6004.

23. Benoit R, Bohlen P, Ling N, et al. Presence of somatostatin-28(1-12) in hypothalamus and pancreas. Proc Natl Acad Sci USA 1982; 79:917.

24. Benoit R, Ling N, Bakhit C, Morrison JD, Alford B, Guillemin R. Somatostatin-28(1-12)-like immunoreactivity in the rat. Endocrinology 1982; 111:2149.

25. Benoit R, Bohlen P, Esch F, Ling N. Neuropeptides derived from prosomatostatin that do not contain the somatostatin-14 sequence. Brain Res 1984; 311:23.

26. Bakhit C, Benoit R, Bloom FE. Release of somatostatin-28(1-12) from rat hypothalamus in vitro. Nature 1983; 301:524.

27. Spiess J, Vale W. Multiple forms of somatostatin-like activity in rat hypothalamus. Biochem 1980; 19:2861.

28. Esch F, Bohlen P, Ling N, Benoit R, Brazeau P, Guillemin R. Primary structure of ovine hypothalamic somatostatin-28 and somatostatin-25. Proc Natl Acad Sci USA 1980; 77:6827.

29. Spiess J, Villarreal J, Vale W. Isolation and sequence analysis of a somatostatin-like polypeptide from ovine hypothalamus. Biochem 1981; 20:1982.

30. Schally AV, Huang W-Y, Chang RC, et al. Isolation and structure of pro-somatostatin: a putative somatostatin precursor from pig hypothalamus. Proc Natl Acad Sci USA 1980; 77:4489.

31. Pradayrol L, Jornvall H, Mutt V, Ribet A. N-terminally extended somatostatin: the primary structure of somatostatin-28. FEBS Lett 1980; 109:55.

32. Saito S, Saito H, Matsumura M, Ishimaru K, Sano T. Molecular heterogeneity and biological activity of immunoreactive somatostatin in medullary carcinoma of the thyroid. J Clin Endocrinol Metab 1981; 53:1117.

33. Aron DC, Andrews PC, Dixon JE, Roos BA. Identification of cellular prosomatostatin and nonsomatostatin peptides derived from its amino terminus. Biochem Biophys Res Commun; 124:450.

34. Aron DC, Roos BA. Nonsomatostatin secretory peptide(s) derived from prosomatostatin's amino terminus in a rat medullary thyroid carcinoma cell line. Endocrinology 1986; 118:218.

35. Wu P, Penman E, Coy DH, Rees LH. Evidence for direct production of somatostatin-14 from a larger precursor than somatostatin-28 in a phaeochromocytoma. Regul Pept 1983; 5:219.

36. Shen LP, Rutter WJ. Sequence of the human somatostatin I gene. Science 1984; 244:168.

37. Montminy MR, Goodman RH, Horovitch SJ, Habener JF. Primary structure of the gene encoding rat preprosomatostatin. Proc Natl Acad Sci USA 1984; 81:3337.

38. Tavianini MA, Hayes TE, Magazin MD, Minth CD, Dixon JD. Isolation, characterization and DNA sequence of the rat somatostatin gene. J Biol Chem 1984; 259:11798.

39. McDonald JK, Greiner F, Bauer GE, Elde RP, Noe BD. Separate cell types which express two forms of somatostatin in anglerfish islets can be differentiated immunohistochemically. J Histochem Cytochem [submitted 1986].

40. Noe BE, Spiess J, Rivier JE, Vale W. Isolation and characterization of somatostatin from anglerfish pancreatic islet. Endocrinology 1979; 105:1410.

41. Noe BD. Synthesis of one form of pancreatic islet somatostatin predominates. J Biol Chem 1981; 256:9397.

42. Noe BD, Spiess J. Evidence for biosynthesis and differential posttranslational proteolytic processing of different (pre)prosomatostatins in pancreatic islets. J Biol Chem 1983; 258:1121.

43. Noe BD, Spiess J. Identification and characterization of a primary cleavage product of (pre)prosomatostatin-II in pancreatic islets.

Abstracts 65th Annual Meeting of the Endocrine Society, 1983:85.

44. Morel A, Gluschankof P, Gomez S, Fefeur V, Cohen P. Characterization of a somatostatin-28 containing the (Tyr-7,Gly-10) derivative of somatostatin-14: a terminal active product of prosomatostatin II processing in anglerfish pancreatic islets. Proc Natl Acad Sci USA 1984; 81:7003.

45. Spiess J, Noe BD. Processing of an anglerfish somatostatin precursor to a hydroxylysine containing somatostatin-28. Proc Natl Acad Sci USA 1985; 82:277.

46. Andrews PC, Hawke D, Shively JE, Dixon JE. Anglerfish preprosomatostatin II is processed to somatostatin-28 and contains hydroxylysine at residue 23. J Biol Chem 1984; 259:15021.

47. Benoit R, Ling N, Alford B, Guillemin R. Seven peptides derived from pro-somatostatin in rat brain. Biochem Biophys Res Commun 1982; 107:944.

48. Conlon JM, McCarthy DM. Fragments of prosomatostatin isolated from a human pancreatic tumour. Mol Cell Endocrinol 1984; 38:81.

49. Patel YC, Wheatley T, Ning C. Multiple forms of immunoreactive somatostatin: comparison of distribution in neural and non-neural tissues and portal plasma of the rat. Endocrinology 1981; 109:1943.

50. Schmidt WE, Mutt V, Kratzin H, Carlquist M, Conlon JM, Creutzfeldt W. Isolation and characterization of proSS$_{1-32}$, a peptide derived from the N-terminal region of porcine preprosomatostatin. FEBS Lett 1985; 192:141

51. Andrews PC, Dixon JE. Isolation and characterization of prosomatostatin-I fragments from anglerfish islets: use of fast atom bombardment mass spectrometry as a tool for structure determination. J Biol Chem [submitted 1986].

52. Andrews PC, Dixon JD. Pancreatic preprosomatostatin processing: isolation and structure of intermediates and final products of processing. Conference on Peptide Sequencing Methodology, San Diego, November, 1985.

53. Noe BD, Andrews PC, Dixon JE, Spiess J. Cotranslational and post-translational proteolytic processing of preprosomatostatin-I in intact islet tissue [submitted 1986].

54. Mackin RB, Noe BD. The islet secretory granule carboxypeptidase B is involved in prohormone processing and exhibits functional homology with enkephalin convertase [submitted 1986].

55. Mackin RB, Noe BD. Characterization of a carboxypeptidase B-like enzyme in secretory granules and microsomes of pancreatic islets [submitted 1986].

56. Fletcher DJ, Noe BD, Bauer GE, Quigley JP. Characterization of the conversion of a somatostatin precursor to somatostatin by islet secretory granules. Diabetes 1980; 29:593.

57. Fletcher DJ, Quigley JP, Bauer GE, Noe BD. Characterization of proinsulin and proglucagon converting activities in isolated islet secretory granules. J Cell Biol 1981; 90:312.

70

7

ENVIRONMENTAL REGULATION OF NEUROTRANSMITTER PHENOTYPIC

EXPRESSION IN SYMPATHETIC NEURONS

John A. Kessler

Albert Einstein College of Medicine
1300 Morris Park Avenue
Bronx, New York 10461

The development of cellular specialization within the nervous system requires precise mechanisms for regulating expression of diverse neurotransmitter phenotypes. Neuronal choice of transmitter does not depend solely on intrinsic cellular information, but is influenced by neuronal interactions with the environment. Thus, it is now well established that neurons may alter the transmitters they synthesize and secrete (1-4) or their mode of synaptic communication (5,6) in response to alterations in the milieu. Moreover, this plasticity is not restricted to the conventional developmental period but extends into adult life; appropriate environmental stimuli alter transmitter phenotypic expression in mature as well as immature neurons (7,8). Indeed, emerging evidence suggests that continuing neuronal change is the rule, not the exception, and that transmitter mutability may be central to neuronal function (for review see reference 9).

The potential scope of such plasticity has been vastly expanded by the discovery that peptides may function as neurotransmitters, and that peptides and "conventional" transmitters, such as norepinephrine, may coexist in the same neuron. However, knowledge of the molecular mechanisms governing peptide development is limited. Do the well-defined mechanisms which influence development of conventional transmitter phenotypic characters similarly regulate peptide ontogeny? The study of sympathetic neuron development in culture provided a means of approaching this question, since autonomic neurons may express somatostatin (SO), substance P (SP), and other peptides (for review see 10), as well as norepinephrine and acetylcholine.

This chapter focuses on a series of experiments which compared mechanisms regulating expression of SO and SP in cultured rat sympathetic neurons with processes regulating noradrenergic and cholinergic development (11-13). These experiments addressed a number of specific issues. What molecular mechanisms foster SO and SP expression? Are transmitters which are colocalized in the same neurons also coregulated by the environment? Is there a fixed relationship between pairs of transmitters, or can the neuron express different combinations of transmitters, and in different proportions, in the appropriate milieu? Can we begin to formulate general rules that govern peptide development?

It has long been recognized that neuronal interactions with non-neuronal cells may influence neurotransmitter development. For example, sympathetic neurons which in vivo express predominantly noradrenergic characteristics become cholinergic when cultured in the presence of certain nonneuronal cells (1,2). Do similar interactions regulate peptide development in autonomic neurons? To approach this question, neonatal rat sympathetic neurons were cultured for varying periods of time in the presence and absence of ganglion nonneuronal elements (principally Schwann cells) and were examined for content of SO and SP (Fig. 1). Tyrosine hydroxylase (TH), the rate limiting enzyme in catecholamine biosynthesis, was also measured as an index of noradrenergic development, and the acetylcholine synthesizing enzyme, choline acetyltransferase (CAT), was utilized to monitor cholinergic development. In pure neuron cultures, levels of somatostatin increased approximately 12-fold during the first 2 weeks in culture. Coculture with nonneuronal cells, however, reduced this increase by more than 50% and slightly reduced levels of tyrosine hydroxylase. However, in the presence of nonneuronal cells, sympathetic neurons expressed significant levels of SP and CAT, and both traits increased continuously during the 4-week period of culture. By contrast, even after a month in vivo, pure neuron cultures contained virtually no SP and negligible levels of CAT activity. Thus, sympathetic ganglion non-neuronal cells inhibited somatostatin and noradrenergic development, but fostered SP and cholinergic expression.

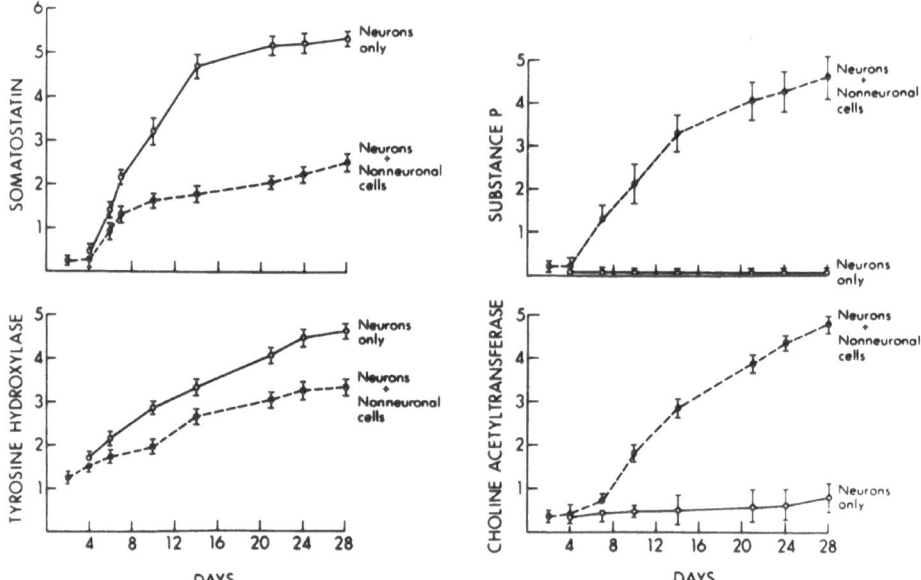

Fig. 1. Effects of nonneuronal cells on neurotransmitter expression. Dissociated sympathetic neurons were cultured in the presence and absence of ganglion nonneuronal cells and were examined after varying periods of time for content of somato-statin (mean fg/neuron ± SEM), tyrosine hydroxylase activity (mean fmole product/neuron/min ± SEM), substance P (mean fg/neuron ± SEM) and choline acetyltransferase activity (mean pmole product/neuron/min ± SEM). N=8 for each measurement.

NEURON-NEURON INTERACTIONS

Since neuronal interactions with nonneuronal cells influenced transmitter development, it seemed possible that neuron-neuron interactions might also be critical. To test this hypothesis, sympathetic neurons were cultured at different densities and were examined for content of SO, SP, TH, and CAT. Culture at high density resulted in clustering of neurons, whereas in low density cultures the neurons grew as singlets or doublets. Increasing neuron density significantly decreased somatostatin levels per neuron and marginally decreased TH activity per neuron (13). By contrast, increasing neuron density significantly increased both SP levels and CAT activity per neuron (13,14). The effects of increased neuron density were similar in pure neuronal cultures and in cultures containing nonneuronal cells. Thus, neuron-neuron interactions inhibited somatostatin development but stimulated SP and cholinergic expression.

PLASMA MEMBRANE REGULATION OF TRANSMITTER DEVELOPMENT

By what mechanisms did increased neuron density or coculture with nonneuronal cells influence transmitter development? Treatment of sympathetic neurons with culture medium conditioned by exposure to nonneuronal cells stimulated CAT activity (1) indicating that some of the effects of nonneuronal cells were mediated by soluble factors. However, treatment with medium conditioned by ganglion nonneuronal cells did not alter levels of SO or SP (13,15), suggesting that other factors mediated effects on peptide development. Moreover, treatment of low density cultures with medium conditioned by exposure to high density cultures also had no effect on levels of SO, SP, CAT, or TH (13,14), suggesting that soluble factors did not mediate the effects of increased density.

Were the effects of density or of coculture with nonneuronal cells mediated by direct cell-cell contact? To approach this question, neurons were exposed to purified plasma membranes isolated from cultured sympathetic neurons or from cultured ganglion nonneuronal cells (15) by sucrose density gradient centrifugation. Treatment of cultured sympathetic neurons with neuronal plasma membranes elevated CAT activity 12-fold and more than tripled SP. By contrast, somatostatin content was reduced by 30%. Treatment with membranes isolated from nonneuronal cells had an even larger effect; CAT activity was increased 25-fold and SP 16-fold, while somatostatin content was decreased by 35%. Thus, cell-surface molecules, which have been shown previously to influence neuronal morphogenesis and neurite elongation, may also help determine the transmitter phenotype of the neuron. This suggests that transmitter phenotype may be influenced, for example, by cell surface molecules encountered by migrating neural crest cells (the precursors of sympathetic ganglion neurons), or by the process of cell aggregation which leads to the formation of the ganglion.

SOLUBLE DIFFERENTIATING FACTORS

Neuronal interactions with target tissues are essential for both the development of immature neurons (16,17) and for the maintenance of adult phenotypic traits (18,19). At least some of the interactions between neurons and their targets appear to be mediated by chemical factors capable of supporting survival and development of responsive neurons (for review see 20). Is peptide development influenced by such soluble neuronotrophic factors? In early studies we found that the trophic protein, nerve growth factor (NGF), stimulated somatostatin and substance P development in dorsal root ganglion sensory neurons (21,22), and that target organ influences on peptidergic sensory neuron development were mediated by the trophic protein (21). Moreover, other investigators found that culture medium conditioned by certain nonneuronal cells stimulated somatostatin levels in sensory neurons without altering SP (23). These observations suggested that diffusible factors may influence peptide development, a conclusion supported by recent studies of somatostatin and substance P in sympathetic neurons.

Coculture of sympathetic neurons with pineal or salivary glands, which are target tissues in vivo for the sympathetic superior cervical ganglion (SCG), increased SP levels more than 9-fold without altering levels of SO (24). To determine whether these target influences on peptide expression were mediated by soluble factors, the effects of treatment with pineal conditioned medium (PCM) were examined (Fig. 2). PCM treatment of neurons cultured in the presence of ganglion nonneuronal cells significantly increased SP, reproducing the effects of the target tissue itself (11,12). Immunohistochemical examination of these cultures demonstrated SP-like immunoreactivity in neurons but not in nonneuronal cells, and the increase in peptide was directly proportional to the dose of PCM (Fig. 2). Under these conditions, levels of SO were unaffected by PCM treatment. However, elimination of ganglion nonneuronal cells decreased SP to negligible levels and abolished the stimulatory effects of PCM on SP. In these pure neuronal cultures, however, PCM treatment increased somatostatin in a dose-dependent manner (Fig. 2). Thus, PCM increased either SO or SP in sympathetic neurons depending upon whether nonneuronal cells were absent or present in the culture. This suggests that contact with nonneuronal cells determined which peptide would be preferentially expressed, and that PCM then quantitatively stimulated that peptide. It is apparent, therefore, that different environmental factors may interact in regulating transmitter development, and that the effects of a factor may be altered or abolished by other environmental influences.

EFFECTS OF MEMBRANE DEPOLARIZATION

Neuronal development and transmitter expression may be regulated transsynaptically by innervating neurons. For example, previous studies have indicated that nerve impulse activity in vivo (25,26) and membrane depolarization in culture (27) stimulate development of noradrenergic traits, such as TH, and increase catecholamine synthesis in sympathetic neurons. K^+-induced membrane depolarization of cultured sympathetic neurons increased the number of TH enzyme molecules by mechanisms apparently regulated at the transcriptional level (28). By contrast, nerve impulse activity in vivo decreased SP levels in the adult (21) and neonatal (4) SCG, and K^+- or veratridine-induced membrane depolarization decreased both SP and SO levels in cultured sympathetic neurons (Table 1). The decreased peptide levels could have resulted from increased release, decreased synthesis, or increased catabolism of the peptides, or a combination of these mechanisms. K^+ or veratridine treatment did, in fact, increase SO release in culture, but the amount released was small in comparison to the decrease in peptide levels in the neurons (13). Turnover studies indicated that the effects of membrane depolarization on peptide levels resulted primarily from decreased net synthesis of SO. Since TH levels increased in the same cultures in response to K^+-induced depolarization (Table 1), and since content of total protein was unchanged, the decrease in SO synthesis reflected a specific inhibition of peptide metabolism.

The decrease in net SO synthesis in response to membrane depolarization could have reflected alterations in transcriptional, translational, or posttranslational events. To help define the mechanisms regulating peptide metabolism, SO-mRNA and TH-mRNA levels were quantitated in sym-

74

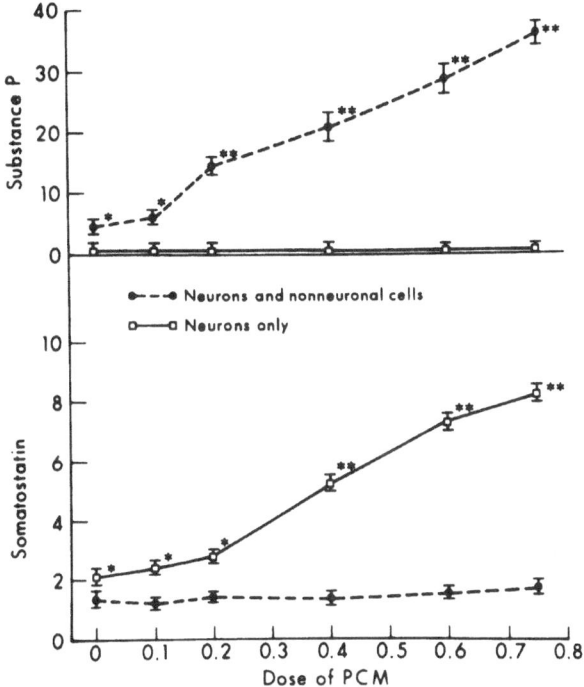

Fig. 2. Effects of pineal conditioned medium (PCM) on somatostatin and substance P in sympathetic neurons. Sympathetic
neurons cultured in the presence (circles) or absence (squares)
of ganglion nonneuronal cells were treated with PCM on the
second day of culture. After 7 days of treatment the cultures
were examined for content of somatostatin and substance P, which
are expressed as mean fg per neuron ± SEM. Neuron numbers did
not differ significantly among the groups. *Differs at $P < 0.05$.
**Differs at $P < 0.01$. Reprinted with permission (12).

pathetic neurons cultured under depolarizing conditions. Northern blot
analysis of mRNA levels demonstrated that potassium treatment greatly
reduced levels of SO-mRNA, in parallel with the decrease in neuronal SO
levels (30). Although alterations in mRNA stability have not been excluded, these observations suggest that membrane depolarization regulated
gene transcription of both SO and TH. Moreover, since SO and TH are
co-localized within the same neurons in culture (13), it is apparent that
membrane depolarization may simultaneously stimulate development of one
transmitter phenotype while inhibiting expression of another, thus altering the phenotype of the neuron.

EFFECTS OF CYCLIC NUCLEOTIDES

The intracellular signals regulating peptide metabolism in sympathetic neurons are unknown. Since cAMP was known to stimulate sympathetic
noradrenergic development (31), sympathetic neuron SO and SP were examined
after treatment with membrane-permeable cAMP analogs or with forskolin, a
stimulator of adenylate cyclase.

Treatment with forskolin or with any of several membrane-permeable cAMP analogs resulted in a 3-fold increase in TH activity (15). By contrast, none of these treatments increased somatostatin levels and dibutyryl cAMP treatment actually decreased somatostatin content more than 50%. Since treatment with butyrate also more than halved somatostatin levels, it seems likely that the butyryl moiety of the dibutyryl cAMP molecule was responsible for the diminished peptide content. Interestingly, butyrate also decreased TH activity by almost 50%, possibly by inhibiting histone deacetylation (32). These observations suggest that cAMP does not regulate somatostatin metabolism in sympathetic neurons. Similarly, treatment with guanosine 3',5'-phosphate (cGMP) analogs also failed to increase peptide levels.

EFFECTS OF CATECHOLAMINE DEPLETION

Since SO and SP were localized within noradrenergic sympathetic neurons, it was logical to ask whether depletion of norepinephrine (NE) would influence peptide development in SCG neurons. Cultures were treated with reserpine, guanethidine or tyramine—drugs which are known to deplete NE—and were examined for content of somatostatin, SP and norepinephrine. Neurons were treated both in the absence and presence of nonneuronal cells. In each instance treatment with these drugs decreased neuronal content of NE. However, in no instance did treatment alter levels of SP or somatostatin significantly. Consequently, it is possible to alter the ratio between levels of different transmitters in sympathetic neurons by manipulating regulatory processes (in this case uptake and storage) which are specific for one transmitter.

EFFECTS OF SERUM-FREE MEDIUM

Neurotransmitter phenotypic expression by sympathetic neurons cultured in defined (serum-free) and serum-containing medium differed in many

Table 1. Effects of membrane depolarization on somatostatin levels and on tyrosine hydroxylase activity.

	Somatostatin	Tyrosine Hydroxylase
Control	2.9 ± 0.24	2.7 ± 0.15
K^+ (55mM)	0.1 ± 0.01*	4.4 ± 0.31**
Veratridine (10^{-6} µM)	0.1 ± 0.02*	4.2 ± 0.27**
Veratridine + tetrodotoxin	3.0 ± 0.26	2.6 ± 0.33
Tetrodotoxin (10^{-7} µM)	3.1 ± 0.28	2.5 ± 0.17

Sympathetic neurons were treated with K^+ or drugs from day 2 of culture to day 14 when they were examined for content of somatostatin (mean fg/neuron ± SEM) and tyrosine hydroxylase activity (mean fmole product/ neuron/min ± SEM). N=8. *Differs from control at $P < 0.001$. **Differs from control at $P < 0.02$.

respects (5,33). For example, SCG neurons cultured in defined medium failed to develop normal levels of dopamine B-hydroxylase, expressed only low levels of CAT, and failed to develop cholinergic synapses (5,33). To determine whether peptide expression was also altered in the absence of serum, SP and somatostatin development in defined and serum-containing media were compared both in the presence and absence of nonneuronal cells. In each instance, neuronal peptide levels were substantially reduced compared to levels in cultures grown in serum-containing medium. By contrast, SP levels in dissociated dorsal root ganglion sensory neurons were greater in defined than in serum-containing medium (unpublished observation).

CO-REGULATION OF TRANSMITTER PHENOTYPES

Our observations regarding the expression and regulation of sympathetic transmitter traits suggest that there is no fixed relationship between any pair of the four phenotypes examined. (For summary see Table 2). For example, factors which stimulate noradrenergic development may decrease SP and somatostatin levels (membrane depolarization), increase them (NGF) or leave them unchanged (cAMP). Although TH and CAT development tend to be inversely related, their regulatory mechanisms were dissociated in neurons cultured in serum-free medium; under these conditions CAT diminished without any change in TH. Finally, cholinergic and SP development paralleled each other in most instances, but cAMP decreased CAT activity without altering SP levels. Consequently, each phenotype appears to be independently regulated in cultured sympathetic neurons. Nevertheless, the similarities between cholinergic and SP development on the one hand, and between noradrenergic and somatostatin development on the other, may indicate some as yet unclarified functional relationships. Taken all together, these observations suggest that neurotransmitter phenotypic expression is a complex process in which the environment regulates a balance among multiple transmitters. The intracellular mechanisms mediating effects of cell contact, soluble differentiating factors, and other aspects of the milieu remain to be clarified.

Table 2. Summary of environmental effects on neurotransmitter phenotypic expression.

	Somato-statin	Substance P	Tyrosine hydroxy-lase	Choline acetyl-transferase
Membrane depolarization	↓	↓	↑	↓
cAMP	→	→	↑	↓
Nonneuronal cells	↓	↑	↓	↑
PCM*	↑	→	↑	→
PCM* and non-neuronal cells	→	↑	↓	↑
Serum-free medium	↓	↓	→	↓
NGF	↑	↑	↑	↑
Neuron density	↓	↑	↓	↑

*Pineal gland conditioned medium[12].

REFERENCES

1. Patterson PH, Chun LLY. The induction of acetylcholine synthesis in primary cultures of dissociated sympathetic neurons. I. Effects of conditioned medium. Dev Biol 1977; 56:263.
2. Johnson M, Ross D, Myers M, Bunge R, Wakshull E, Burton H. Synaptic vesicle cytochemistry changes when cultured sympathetic neurons develop cholinergic interactions. Nature (London) 1976; 262:308.
3. LeDouarin NM, Teillet M, Ziller C, Smith J. Adrenergic differentiation of cells of the cholinergic ciliary and Remak ganglia in avian embryos after in vivo transplantation. Proc Natl Acad Sci USA 1978; 75:2030.
4. Kessler JA, Adler J, Bohn MC, Black IB. Substance P in principal sympathetic neurons: regulation by impulse activity. Science 1981; 214:335.
5. Higgins D, Burton H. Electrotonic synapses are formed by fetal rat sympathetic neurons maintained in a chemically defined culture medium. Neuroscience 1982; 7:2241.
6. Kessler JA, Spray DC, Saez JC, Bennett MVL. Determination of synaptic phenotype: insulin and cAMP independently initiate development of electrotonic coupling between cultured sympathetic neurons. Proc Natl Acad Sci USA 1984; 81:6325.
7. Hendry IA, Iversen LL, Black IB. A comparison of the neural regulation of tyrosine hydroxylase activity in sympathetic ganglia of adult mice and rats. J Neurochem 1973; 20:1683.
8. Thoenen H, Mueller RA, Axelrod J. Trans-synaptic induction of adrenal tyrosine hydroxylase. J Pharmacol Exp Ther 1969; 169:249.
9. Black IB. Stages of neurotransmitter development in autonomic neurons. Science 1982; 215:1198.
10. Kessler JA, Black IB. Mechanisms governing peptidergic phenotypic expression and development. In: Krieger DT, et al., eds. Brain peptides. New York: Wiley, 1983.
11. Kessler JA. Environmental co-regulation of substance P, somatostatin, and neurotransmitter synthesizing enzyme in cultured sympathetic neurons. Brain Res 1984; 321:155.
12. Kessler JA. Non-neuronal cell conditioned medium stimulates peptidergic expression in sympathetic and sensory neurons in vitro. Dev Biol 1984; 106:61.
13. Kessler JA. Differential regulation of peptide and catecholamine characters in cultured sympathetic neurons. Neuroscience 1985; 15:827.
14. Adler J, Black IB. Sympathetic neuron density differentially regulates transmitter phenotypic expression in culture. Proc Natl Acad Sci USA 1985; 82:4296.
15. Kessler JA, Conn G, and Hatcher VB. Isolated plasma membranes regulate neurotransmitter expression and facilitate effects of a soluble brain cholinergic factor. Proc Natl Acad Sci USA (in press).
16. Hamburger V. The effects of wing bud extirpation on the development of the central nervous system in chick embryos. J Exp Zool 1934; 68:448.
17. Prestige MC. The control of cell number in the lumbar spinal ganglia during the development of Xenopus laeuis tadpoles. J Embryol Exp Morphol 1967; 17:453.
18. Olson L, Malmfors T. Growth characteristics of adrenergic nerves in the adult rat. Acta Physiol Scand 1970; 348(suppl):1.
19. Hendry IA, Iversen LL. Changes of enzyme pattern in the sympathetic nervous system of adult mice after submaxillary gland removal: response to exogenous nerve growth factor. J Neurochem 1974; 22:999.
20. Berg DK. New neuronal growth factors. Annu Rev Neurosci 1984; 7:149.
21. Kessler JA, Black IB. Nerve growth factor stimulates the development

of substance P in sensory ganglia. Proc Natl Acad Sci USA 1980; 77:649.

22. Kessler JA, Black IB. Similarities in development of substance P and somatostatin in peripherial sensory neurons: effects of capsaicin and nerve growth factor. Proc Natl Acad Sci USA 1981; 78:4644.

23. Mudge AW. Effects of chemical environment on levels of substance P and somatostatin in cultured sensory neurons. Nature (London) 1981; 292:764.

24. Kessler JA, Adler J, Jonakait GM, Black IB. Target organ regulation of substance P in sympathetic neurons in culture. Dev Biol 1984; 103:71.

25. Black IB, Geen SL. Trans-synaptic regulation of adrenergic neuron development. Inhibition by ganglionic blockade. Brain Res 1973; 63:291.

26. Thoenen H. Trans-synaptic enzyme induction. Life Sci 1974; 14:223.

27. Walicke P, Campenot R, Patterson P. Determination of transmitter function by neuronal activity. Proc Natl Acad Sci USA 1977; 74:5767.

28. Hefti F, Gnahn H, Schwab ME, Thoenen H. Induction of tyrosine hydroxylase by nerve growth factor and by elevated K+ concentrations in culture, of dissociated sympathetic neurons. J Neurosci 1982; 2:1554.

29. Kessler JA, Black IB. Regulation of substance P in adult rat sympathetic ganglia. Brain Res 1982; 234:182.

30. Spiegel K, Kessler JA. Environmental regulation of neurotransmitter gene transcription (Abstract). Soc Neurosci 1985; 11:669.

31. Mackay A, Iversen L. Increased tyrosine hydroxylase activity of sympathetic ganglia cultured in the presence of dibutyryl cyclic AMP. Brain Res 1972; 48:424.

32. Candido E, Reeves R, Davie J. Sodium butyrate inhibits histone deacetylation in cultured cells. Cell 1978; 14:105.

33. Iacovetti L, Johnson M, Joh T, Bunge R. Biochemical and morphological characterization of sympathetic neurons grown in a chemically defined medium. Neuroscience 1982; 7:2225.

II. MECHANISMS OF ACTION

8

SIDE CHAIN CONFORMATIONS OF SOMATOSTATIN ANALOGS

WHEN BOUND TO RECEPTORS

Ruth F. Nutt, C. Dylion Colton, Richard Saperstein and
Daniel F. Veber

Merck Sharp & Dohme Research Laboratories
West Point, Pennsylvania 19486

Conformationally based design has resulted in greatly simplified constrained analogs of somatostatin which show a high degree of metabolic stability and improved duration of action. In our laboratory, these studies have resulted in the highly potent analog, MK-0678 (I) (1). Small, cyclic somatostatin analogs such as II, III, and IV have been developed at other laboratories and some have also been evaluated in clinical studies in humans. All of these analogs, which are shown in Figure 1, represent significant advances over somatostatin for therapeutic application but show, at best, only low oral availability. Should the present clinical studies, using such analogs, show useful therapeutic properties, improved analogs will be required. Physical studies of MK-0678 and related structures have given us an opportunity to develop a uniquely detailed picture of the features of somatostatin which are required for biological activity. These studies should form the basis for future analog design.

The structure of somatostatin and analogs can be viewed at two levels of detail. One level relates to the peptide backbone conformation and the way this presents the general spatial relationships of the individual amino acid side chains. Models of both the cyclic hexapeptides and somatostatin were developed on the basis of such data and the two structures have been compared (5). A second level of detail involves the specific spatial relationships of the side chains as defined by the rotational angle between the α and β carbons, the so-called χ_1 angle.

The important conformation to be defined is that at the receptor. Such definition can only be done by indirect means since direct observations of receptor bound hormones has not yet been accomplished using current technology. Observations of structural features in solution of partially restricted analogs can be used only to infer probable features at the receptor. On the other hand, observations of bioactivity in covalently constrained analogs gives positive information about the receptor bound conformation. Somatostatin conformation is a uniquely detailed example of a peptide where observations of solution structural features have been related to the receptor bound conformation through synthesis of covalently constrained bioactive analogs. We describe here three new cyclic hexapeptide somatostatin analogs having constraints on the two phenylalanine side chains and which help define the χ_1 angles at the receptor and relate them to NMR chemical shift data in solution.

```
        NMe-Ala-Tyr-D-Trp
          |         |              I¹ (MK-0678)
        Phe-Val    Lys


        H-D-Phe-Cys-Phe-D-Trp
               |        |          II² (SMS-201-995)
        Thr(ol)-Cys-Thr——Lys


         H-Cys-Phe-Phe-D-Trp
            |            |         III³
        HO-Cys-Phe-Thr  Lys


         Asn-Phe-Phe-D-Trp
           |           |           IV⁴ (CGP-15425)
        GABA-Phe-Thr——Lys
```

Fig. 1. Some key classes of small ring analogs
of somatostatin (GABA is α-aminobutyric acid).

Specific side chain relationships are recognized in cyclic hexapeptide analogs of somatostatin through upfield shifts caused by the three
aromatic rings in the molecule. The aromatic ring of tryptophan is close
to the aliphatic chain of lysine as seen in larger ring analogs (6). The
aromatic ring of phenylalanine-11 is recognized as close to one face of
the proline ring at the α and β carbons. In analogs such as VIII, it is
recognized as close to the α-methyl group of N-methyl alanine (7).

In analog V, the aromatic ring of phenylalanine-7 is seen as being
close to both the CH_2 group of tryptophan and to one face of the proline
at the γ-position. These two proximities cannot occur at the same time
and must reflect a significant occurrence in solution of at least two
rotamers involving rotation about the α-β carbon-carbon bond of phenylal-
anine-7. Only one of these two rotamers is likely to be involved in
receptor binding.

In order to establish the receptor binding rotamer for phenylalanine-
7, a bulky group (acetoxy) was introduced into the γ-position of proline
as both the cis and trans isomer relative to the carboxamide of proline.
Synthesis of VI and VII were accomplished via the transhydroxyproline
analog having the lysine ε-amino group protected by the 2-chloroCBZ. The
protected cyclic peptide was prepared using standard methodology previously reported from these laboratories (8). The transacetoxy analog VI was
then prepared by acetylation of the hydroxyl followed by HF removal of the
2-chloroCBZ group. Preparation of the cis isomer requires tosylation of
the hydroxyl followed by displacement of tosyl with inversion using cesium
acetate in DMF. Removal of the 2-chloroCBZ in liquid HF gave VII.

The isomer having the trans relationship (VI) has the acetoxy group
away from the aromatic ring of phenylalanine-7 and it should therefore
have no influence on the phenylalanine rotamer population. This lack of
effect is confirmed by the lack of change in chemical shift of the CH_2 of
tryptophan in compound VI (2.9 ppm) compared to the proline unsubstituted
analog V (2.95 ppm). The observed retention of equivalent bioactivity
(Fig. 2) in VI compared to V is therefore expected in view of a similar
rotamer population.

84

	Rel. Pot. for Inhibition of Release of:		
	INS	GLU	GH
V	5	8	1.7
VI	11	22	~3
VII	95	84	~5

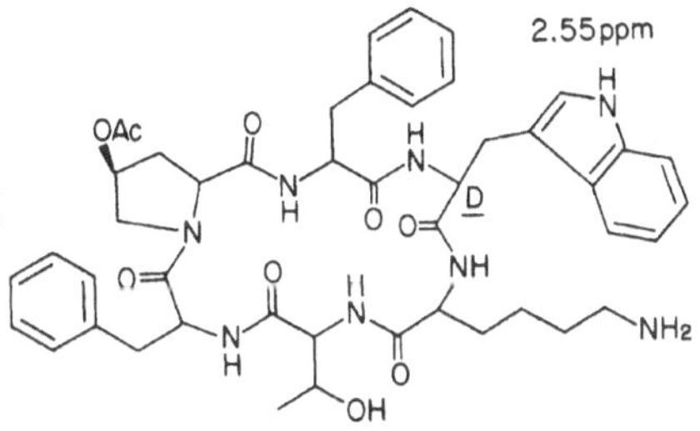

Fig. 2. The parent cyclic hexapeptide V has the β protons on D-tryptophan and the cis proton of the γ-position of proline 6 shifted upfield in the PMR spectrum. The trans-acetoxy proline analog, VI, has the same chemical shift for the β-CH$_2$ of D-Trp, about 0.4 ppm, upfield from the normal position for these protons. The large effect of the acetoxy substitution on the γ-position of proline limits the evaluation of its chemical shift. The cis acetoxy proline has the CH$_2$ of D-Trp shifted upfield a further 0.35 ppm. Analog potency relative to somatostatin (1.0) is given for inhibition of insulin (INS) and glucagon (GLU) release in rats as well as inhibition of growth hormone (GH) from dispersed rat pituitary cells (9).

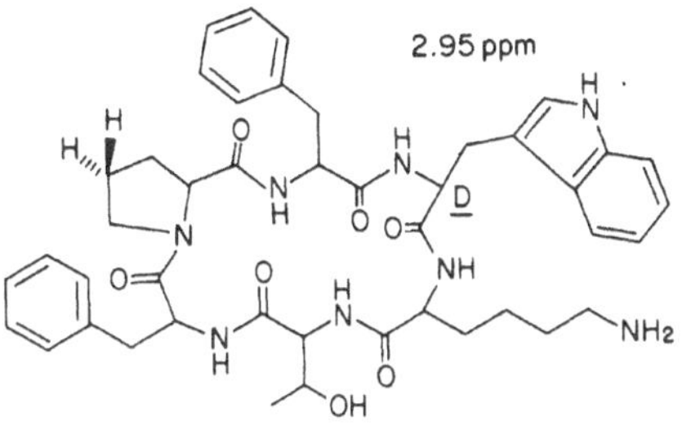

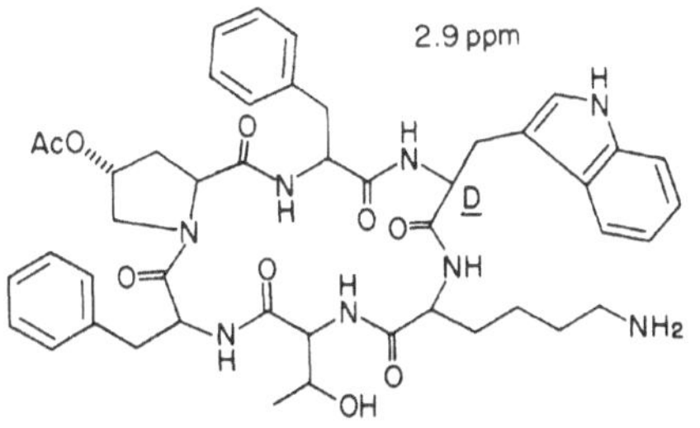

In contrast, the isomer with a cis proline configuration has the acetoxy group directed toward the side chain of phenylalanine-7 and does not allow the rotamer having the aromatic ring close to the proline. Thus, in this compound (VII) we see a much enhanced upfield shift of the CH_2 of tryptophan (2.55 ppm) compared to the other analogs (V and VI) indicating a greatly increased population of the rotamer having the phenyl group directed toward the tryptophan. The retention of high activity in this analog argues against any receptor role for the rotamer having the phenyl group close to proline. Indeed, the apparent higher potency of VII for inhibition of insulin and glucagon release is consistent with a receptor bound conformation having the phenyl group close to the CH_2 of tryptophan. It is important to recognize that this conformation is quite compatible with tryptophan rotamers which have the indole ring close to lysine side chain as we have previously proposed (6). It is not compatible with the stacking of the phenyl and indole groups as proposed by Momany (8) since this conformation precludes the upfield shift of the CH_2 group on tryptophan.

A direct test of the rotamer of phenylalanine-11 responsible for biological activity has been accomplished through synthesis of the isomeric pair of peptides VIII and IX. The highly potent N-methyl alanine containing cyclic peptide (VIII) shows an exceptional upfield shift of the c-methyl group of N-methyl alanine. The phenyl of phenylalanine-11 which is responsible for this upfield shift is known to contribute greatly to the potency as analogs lacking this group show only about 0.05 the potency (10). To test the biological significance of the proximity of the phenyl to the methyl of N-methyl alanine, the isomer IX (Fig. 3) was prepared using methods as described in reference 8. This analog has the phenyl now covalently attached at the β-carbon of the N-methyl amino acid and the attachment to the 11-position amino acid has been broken. We see from the NMR spectrum in solution that in spite of the lack of a bond to the 11-position amino acid, the phenyl ring is still close to the remaining methyl group. This methyl group is now shifted upfield to 0.15 ppm, a position comparable to the methyl group in the isomer VIII. It must be concluded that the spatial position of the phenyl ring is basically the same in analogs VIII and IX even though the point of covalent attachment has been moved six atoms away from the original one. The high biological activity of IX for inhibition of insulin and glucagon release suggests that the common spatial position of this phenyl ring seen in solution is retained on receptor binding. The apparent lower potency for GH release may reflect a receptor selectivity. We do not believe this to be a general phenomenon, however, as the selectivity did not translate into a series of closely related analogs of IX.

The various studies in our laboratories of cyclic hexapeptide somatostatin analogs have shown that all of the binding energy of somatostatin can be accounted for by contributions from phenylalanine-11 (8), phenylalanine-7 (10), tryptophan-8 (10), and lysine-9 (11). There is apparently no contribution of the amide backbone since highly active retro-cyclo isomeric analogs can be prepared (13). Specific rotational relationships have also been defined for the lysine side chain (14) and the tryptophan side chain (15). The proximity of these two side chains is inferred by NMR studies and it is inferred that this proximity must exist for biological activity (6). The studies reported here establish rotational relationships for the two phenylalanine side chains and complete the picture of the relationships of all of the groups required for receptor binding. It is hoped that such a detailed picture of somatostatin analogs will allow the design of even further simplified analogs which meet all of the expected criteria of useful drugs relating to duration of action and oral bioavailability.

IX

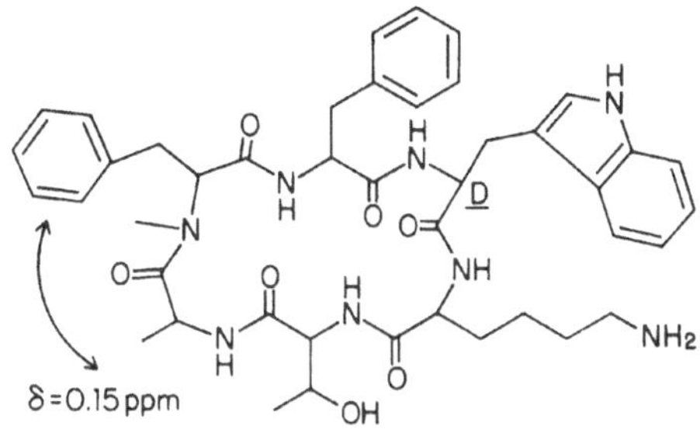

δ=0.15ppm

| Insulin | Glucagon | GH (in vitro) |
| 49(23,104) | 59(9,218) | 0.3(.08,.7) |

VIII

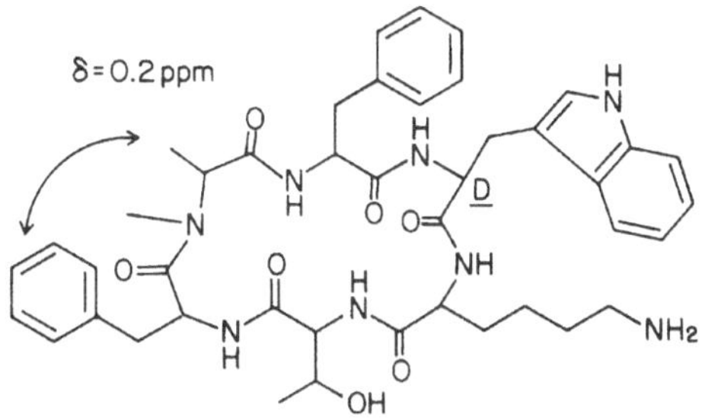

δ=0.2ppm

| Insulin | Glucagon | GH (in vitro) |
| 6(4,11) | 8(1,60) | 3(2,5) |

Fig. 3. Inhibition of the release of insulin and glucagon in rats and growth hormone from dispersed rat pituitary cells (9) for 2 isomeric cyclic hexapeptide somatostatin analogs. The chemical shift of the methyl group of alanine in compound IX in D_2O is 0.2 ppm and for the c-methyl group of the N-methylalanine in VIII is 0.15 ppm.

REFERENCES

1. Veber DF, Saperstein R, Nutt RF, et al. A super active cyclic hexapeptide analog of somatostatin. Life Sci 1984; 34:1371.
2. Bauer W, Briner U, Doepfner W, et al. SMS 201-995: a very potent and selective octapeptide analogue of somatostatin with prolonged action. Life Sci 1982; 31:1133.
3. Vale W, Rivier J, Ling N, Brown M. Metabolism 1978; 27(suppl 1): 1391.
4. Cyclo(Asn-Phe-Phe-D-Trp-Lys-Thr-Phe-Gaba) CGP-15425.
5. Veber DF. Design of a highly active cyclic hexapeptide analog of somatostatin. In: Rich DH, Gross E, eds. Peptides: synthesis—structure—function. Proceedings of the 7th American Peptide Symposium, 1981:685.
6. Arison BH, Hirschmann R, Veber DF. Inferences about the conformation

of somatostatin at a biologic receptor based on NMR studies. Bioorganic Chem 1978; 7:447.

7. Freidinger RM, Perlow DS, Randall WC, Saperstein R, Arison BH, Veber DF. Conformational modification of cyclic hexapeptide somatostatin analogs. Int J Pept Protein Res 1984; 23:142.

8. Momany FA, Bowers CY, Reynolds GA, Chang D, Hong A, Newlander K. Design, synthesis, and biological activity of peptides which release growth hormone in vitro. Endocrinology 1981; 108:31.

9. Veber DF, Holly FW, Paleveda WJ Jr, et al. Conformationally restricted bicyclic analogs of somatostatin. Proc Natl Acad Sci USA 1978; 75:2636-40.

10. Veber DF, Freidinger RM, Perlow DP, et al. A potent cyclic hexapeptide analog of somatostatin. Nature 1981; 292:55.

11. Veber DF, Randall WC, Nutt RF, et al. Circular dichroism aids interpretation of structure-activity relationships of somatostatin analogs. In: Blaha K, Malon P, eds. Proceedings of the 17th European Peptide Symposium, Peptides 1982, 1982:789.

12. Nutt RF, Veber DF, Curley PE, Saperstein R, Hirschmann R. Somatostatin analogs which define the role of the lysine-9 amino group. Int J Pept Protein Res 1983; 21:66.

13. Freidinger RM, Veber DF. Design of novel cyclic hexapeptide somatostatin analogs from a model of the bioactive conformation. In: Conformationally directed drug design. ACS Symposium Series 251, Am Chem Soc, Washington, DC, 1984.

14. Nutt RF, Saperstein R, Veber DF. Structural and conformational studies regarding tryptophan in a cyclic hexapeptide somatostatin analog. In: Hruby V, Rich D, eds. Peptides: structure and function. Proceedings of the 8th American Peptide Symposium, 1983.

15. Nutt RF, Curley PE, Pitzenberger SM, Freidinger RM, Saperstein R, Veber DF. Novel conformationally constrained amino acids as lysine-9 substitutions in somatostatin analogs. Proc 9th American Pept Symp 1985; 44.

9

SOMATOSTATIN RECEPTOR: EVIDENCE FOR FUNCTIONAL AND STRUCTURAL HETEROGENEITY

Coimbatore B. Srikant and Yogesh C. Patel

Fraser Laboratories, McGill University, Departments of
Medicine, and Neurology and Neurosurgery, Royal Victoria
Hospital and Montreal Neurological Institute, Montreal
Quebec H3A 1A1, Canada

INTRODUCTION

Somatostatin, like many other peptide systems, is a multigene family
with two principal bioactive forms corresponding to somatostatin-14 (S-14)
and somatostatin-28 (S-28) (1). The S-14 structure is totally conserved
in all vertebrate species whereas S-28 has undergone a great deal of
structural and perhaps functional evolution from fish to mammals (1-3).
Major differences exist in the expression of fish and mammalian somatostatin genes. There are two somatostatin genes in the catfish and anglerfish (2,4). These genes give rise to two separate precursors and two
separate products which appear to be expressed in two separate populations
of somatostatin cells (2,5). By contrast, the single mammalian somatostatin gene encodes for a single precursor which is differentially processed to two products, S-14 and S-28, which appear to be localized in the
same cell (1,6-8). Mammalian somatostatin cells consist typically of
neurons or endocrine-like cells (D-cells) found in many parts of the body
where they regulate a variety of physiological processes, acting both
locally as neurotransmitters, neuromodulators, paracrine regulators or
"lumones," and systemically as true hormones (9). The relative proportions of S-14:S-28 vary considerably in different tissues. S-14 is the
predominant form in the brain, pancreas, upper gut and enteric neurons
whereas S-28 is an important constituent of brain somatostatin and the
predominant molecular form in intestinal mucosa (1).

It is now well established that both S-14 and S-28 have a common
active site located in the ring segment which is responsible for both
receptor binding and biological activity. The actions of the two peptides
are, however, qualitatively similar but quantitatively different (Table
1). S-28 tends to be selective for inhibition of hypothalamic CRF release
and of GH, TSH, insulin, and pancreatic exocrine secretion, whereas S-14
appears to act preferentially on glucagon, gastric exocrine secretion, and
nonsecretory digestive events (10-16). Most of the tissue-selective
actions of the two peptides can be accounted for by different potencies
for interaction with somatostatin receptors. As in the case of the
biological actions, the binding affinity of S-14 and S-28 for tissue S-14
receptors is qualitatively similar but quantitatively different (17).
Such tissue selectivity clearly points to functional heterogeneity of the
somatostatin receptor and raised the possibility that S-14 and S-28

specific binding domains exist. Although pharmacological and biochemical studies with radioligands prepared from tyrosinated analogs of S-14 have now provided solid evidence for functional as well as structural heterogeneity of the S-14 binding region, the same approaches using tyrosinated S-28 agonists have so far failed to distinguish a separate S-28 receptor. On the other hand, recent in vivo and in vitro autoradiographic studies with these ligands strongly suggest that S-14 and S-28 specific binding sites exist in brain and pancreatic islets. In this chapter we provide a comparative evaluation of the interactions of these peptides with somatostatin receptors in different tissues of the rat and review evidence supportive of the differential receptor binding of these peptides.

DISTRIBUTION OF SOMATOSTATIN RECEPTORS

Somatostatin receptors on plasma membranes have been identified and characterized in a number of laboratories using as agonists three principal radioiodinated tyrosine analogs: $[^{125}I\text{-}Tyr^{11}]$ S-14, $[^{125}I\text{-}Tyr^{1}]$ S-14 or $[^{125}I\text{-}Tyr]$ S-14. Binding sites identified with such radioligands ("S-14 receptor") were originally found on GH_4C_1 rat pituitary cells (18). S-14 receptors in normal tissues were first characterized in rat brain membranes in our laboratory (19). Subsequently, we and others have described membrane receptors for S-14 in the rat pituitary, the adrenal cortex, the exocrine pancreas, guinea pig pancreatic acinar cells, and monkey and human brain (20-29). A number of studies have documented the presence of these receptors in several kinds of tumor cells, including AtT-20 mouse pituitary cells (30,31), rat insulinoma (32), hamster insulinoma (33), human somatotrophic tumors (34,35), and human meningioma (36). Structure-activity relationship studies have revealed that the cyclic

Table 1. Comparison of reported relative potencies of S-14 and
S-28 for inhibition of hypothalamic CRF release and of
pituitary, islet and digestive functions
(schematic depiction).

Biological Activity	S-14	S-28
CRF	−	+
GH	+	++
TSH	+	++
Insulin	+	+++
Glucagon	++	+
Gastric acid	++	+
Pepsin	++	+
Pancreatic secretion	+	++
Splanchnic blood flow	+	−
Intestinal motility	+	−
Receptor Binding Activity		
Cerebral cortex	++	+
Median eminence	−	++
Pituitary	+	++
Adrenal cortex	+	+
Exocrine pancreas	++	+

structure of S-14 is essential and that residues 7-11 constitute the
ligand recognition site for S-14 receptor binding. Membrane S-14 receptors in normal rat tissues exhibit high affinity (Kd = 0.5 - 1.7 nM)
(19,20,25,26). The highest receptor concentrations are found in the
cerebral cortex, anterior pituitary, adrenal cortex and exocrine pancreas
(250-400 fmol/mg protein) (Fig. 1). These receptors are localized in all
major brain regions with the highest concentration in the cerebral cortex
(Fig. 1). Thalamus, whole hypothalamus, striatum, amygdala, and hippocampus contain intermediate receptor densities whereas midbrain, medulla-
pons, cerebellum, and spinal cord exhibit low binding. The regional brain
concentration of S-14 receptors in general parallels the distribution of
somatostatin neuronal cell bodies in the CNS in keeping with the postulated interneuronal role of the majority of brain somatostatin neurons
(37). By ultrastructural in vivo autoradiography, somatostatin receptors
have been localized in the normal rat pituitary on somatotrophs, thyro-
trophs, and lactotrophs, the three known targets for normal somatostatin
action in the pituitary (38). Adrenal somatostatin receptors are localized virtually exclusively to the zona glomerulosa of the cortex as
determined by direct binding studies and by in vivo autoradiography
(21,39). A lower density of S-14 receptors occurs in the adrenal medulla
as visualized by in vitro autoradiography (40). By EM autoradiography,
islet S-14 receptors have been found on B, A, and D cells (41). The
presence of intracellular receptors for somatostatin has been suggested by
a number of reports which, however, need verification. The most compel-
ling evidence comes from studies which have demonstrated a rich concentration of receptors on secretory granule membranes of pituitary and islet
cells by direct binding and by in vivo autoradiography (38,42). Significant labeling of the nucleus of pituitary target cells following the
intravenous administration of labeled S-28 has raised the possibility of
nuclear binding sites for somatostatin (38). Although the occurrence of
cytoplasmic S-14 receptors in tissues such as the gut, pancreas and kidney
has been claimed (43-47), such binding sites are of low affinity and thus
of doubtful physiological significance.

HETEROGENEITY OF S-14 RECEPTORS

Differences in Tissue Binding of S-14 and Related Analogs

The properties of binding sites identified using $[^{125}I\text{-}Tyr^{11}]$ S-14 as
radioligand show sufficient variation between tissues to suggest that the
S-14 receptor itself is heterogeneous. First, there is a 2- to 3-fold
difference in the binding affinity of S-14 for S-14 receptors on pancreatic exocrine cells (Kd = 0.5 nM) compared to those in the cerebral
cortex, pituitary, and adrenal cortex (Kd = 1.7, 1.1, and 1.1 nM respectively) (17). Second, the addition of Ca^{++} (0.1 mM) increases the specific binding of S-14 receptors in the exocrine pancreas but not in the other
tissues (26). Third, the binding affinities of a number of structural
analogs of S-14 differ between tissues (17,20,25,26,48). For instance,
$[D\text{-}Br_5Trp^8]$ S-14 binds to S-14 receptors in the pituitary with an affinity
3 times greater than in brain and adrenal cortex while $[L\text{-}Br_5\text{-}Trp^8]$ S-14
exhibits a 3-fold greater affinity for S-14 receptors in the brain and
pituitary than for those in the adrenal cortex (Table 2). $[L\text{-}F_5\text{-}Trp^8]$
S-14 interacts with S-14 receptors with greater affinity in the adrenal
cortex and pituitary compared to exocrine pancreas and brain. Modified
phenylalanine substitution of the position 4 residue lysine (which is
removed from the active site) also results in tissue-specific binding as
evidenced by the 15-fold greater affinity of $[p\text{-}NH_2\text{-}Phe^4]$ S-14 compared to
S-14 in the exocrine pancreas. Two cyclic analogs of somatostatin, SMS
201-995 and cyclo-[Aha-Cys-Phe-D-Trp-Lys-Thr-Cys] show biphasic displacement of binding to S-14 receptors in the brain due to interaction with a

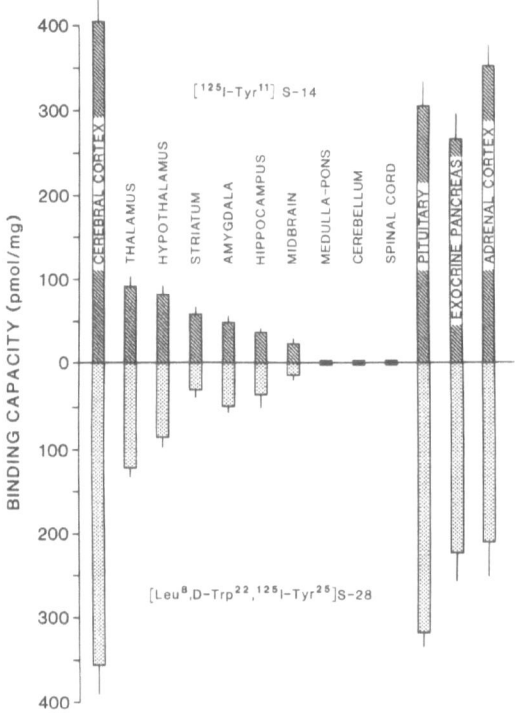

Fig. 1. Distribution of somatostatin receptors quantitated using [^{125}I-Tyr^{11}] S-14 (top panel) and [Leu^8, D-Trp^{22}, ^{125}I-Tyr^{25}] S-28 (bottom panel) in rat tissues.

high and a low affinity form of the S-14 receptor (49,50). The two receptor subtypes can only be differentiated through the biphasic interaction of these cyclic analogs with binding sites labeled with either [^{125}I-Tyr^{11}] S-14 or [^{125}I-Leu^8, D-Trp^{22}, Tyr^{25}] S-28 ([^{125}I-LTT] S-28 (see below); labeled tyrosinated analogs of SMS 201-995 react with only the high affinity form (51). The two receptor subpopulations are characterized by differential ionic requirements for binding and variable tissue distribution. The high affinity binding sites are increased by Mg^{2+} and decreased by Na$^+$ whereas the low affinity sites are increased by Na$^+$ and unaffected by Mg^{2+} (52). Both receptor subtypes have been identified in the brain where their relative amounts exhibit regional variation. On the other hand, peripheral tissues such as the pituitary and pancreas contain only the higher affinity form of the S-14 receptor (49,50).

Cross-Linking Studies

Recent cross-linking studies from our laboratory have provided evidence of molecular heterogeneity of the S-14 receptor. Chemical cross-linking of receptor-bound [^{125}I-Tyr^{11}] S-14 with disuccinimidyl suberate (DSS) has revealed the presence of a specifically labeled 200,000 dalton receptor protein in rat exocrine pancreas and adrenal cortex (Figures 2 and 3) (26,53). The S-14 receptor protein in adrenal cortex appears to be larger than that in the exocrine pancreas since its presence

Table 2. Relative affinities of S-14 analogs
for binding to S-14 receptors.

Peptide	Tissue			
	Adrenal Cortex	Cerebral Cortex	Exocrine Pancreas	Pituitary
S-14	1	1	1	1
D-Trp^8 S-14	2	5	3	10
D-F$_5$-Trp^8 S-14	46	32	32	31
L-F$_5$-Trp^8 S-14	18	6	1.2	14
D-Br$_5$-Trp^8 S-14	4	4	3	10
L-Br$_5$-Trp^8 S-14	22	7	2	7
Phe^4 S-14	2	2	1	4
p-NH$_2$-Phe^4 S-14	3	6	15	4

can be detected only under reducing conditions. Preliminary studies in our laboratory indicate the specific labeling of a 200,000 dalton receptor protein in rat brain and pituitary also (C. B. Srikant, unpublished results). In addition to the 200,000 dalton protein found in all tissues examined so far, two other specifically labeled bands of Mr = 80,000 and 70,000 have been observed in pancreatic acinar cells only (26). The structural uniqueness of the pancreatic acinar cell S-14 receptors compared to those in other tissues is interesting in view of the higher affinity and calcium sensitivity of S-14 binding for this receptor compared to S-14 receptors in other tissues. Our estimate of the molecular size of the S14 receptor differs from the value of 92,000 daltons reported for rat pancreatic acinar cell S-14 receptors cross-linked with [^{125}I-Tyr^1] S-14 and 4-hydroxysuccinimidyl-4-azidobenzoate (28). Whether these disparate estimates could be due to the use of different ligands and cross-linking reagents remains to be established.

S-14 Receptor Regulation

S-14 receptors appear to be reciprocally regulated by changes in somatostatin levels. Preincubation of AtT-20 cells with either S-14 or S-28 led to a marked reduction in the S-14 receptor binding capacity (31). S-28, which binds to these receptors with greater affinity than S-14, also caused a greater down-regulation of the receptors. Similar regulation of S-14 receptors has been shown to occur in vivo. One week after streptozotocin induced diabetes in rats, the resulting hypersomatostatinemia was found to be associated with a reduction in S-14 receptor concentration in pancreatic acinar cells (26). Conversely, depletion of endogenous brain somatostatin by cysteamine administration in rats led to up-regulation of cerebrocortical S-14 receptors (54). The relative potencies of S-14 and S-28 to down-regulate S-14 receptors have been assessed only in AtT-20 cells where S-28 is twice as effective as S-14. It remains to be established whether the abilities of these peptides to regulate S-14 receptors in other systems parallel their relative binding affinities.

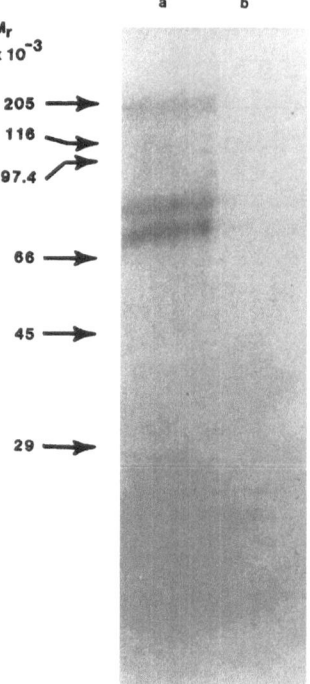

Fig. 2. Autoradiogram of $[^{125}\text{I-Tyr}^{11}]$ S-14 cross-linked to S-14 receptors in rat pancreatic acinar cell membranes. The receptor was cross-linked to bound radioligand using DSS and subjected to polyacrylamide gel electrophoresis. Three labeled protein bands corresponding to Mr = 200,000, 80,000, and 70,000 were detected by autoradiography (lane a). When excess S-14 was present at the time of binding, labeling of these proteins was inhibited (lane b).

Receptor Binding of Somatostatin-28

Tissue specific binding of S-28. While impressive pharmacological and biochemical evidence has been marshalled in support of the heterogeneity of the S-14 receptor unit, data favoring the existence of a distinct S-28 receptor are less firm. The separate phylogenetic origins of the two peptides argue strongly in favor of independent functions perhaps mediated through separate receptors. S-14 receptors in all tissues interact with both S-14 and S-28 but with notable differences in their relative affinities. As illustrated in Table 3, S-14 receptors in the pituitary bind S-28 with greater affinity than S-14 whereas those in the brain and exocrine pancreas bind S-14 with greater avidity than S-28 (26,55). The two peptides interact with adrenocortical S-14 receptors with comparable affinity (25). Such differences in binding affinities of S-14 and S-28 have also been observed in tumor cell models. The S-14 receptors in AtT-20 cells bind S-28 with greater affinity than S-14 (31) while in GH_4C_1 cells the binding affinity of S-28 is less than that of S-14 (56).

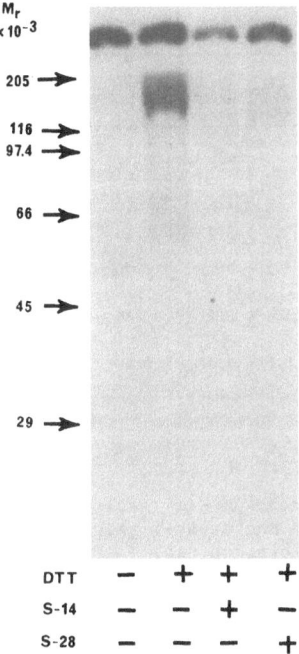

DTT	−	+	+	+
S-14	−	−	+	−
S-28	−	−	−	+

Fig. 3. Autoradiogram of cross-linked receptor bound [^{125}I-Tyr^{11}] S-14 in rat adrenocortical membranes. Cross-linking was carried out using DSS and solubilized under reducing and non-reducing conditions. Specific labeling of a 200,000 dalton protein subunit was observed under reducing conditions only.

Identification of [^{125}I-LTT] S-28 Binding Sites

Attempts to identify S-28 specific binding sites ("S-28 receptor") were first made by Reubi et al. with the labeled analog [^{125}I-LTT] S-28 (57). Somatostatin-28 was reported to interact with higher affinity than S-14 for rat brain membrane binding sites labeled by this radioligand. A detailed comparison of the inhibitory potency of S-14 and S-28 for binding to [^{125}I-LTT] S-28 sites in rat brain in our laboratory, however, failed to confirm this (Table 3). Indeed, as shown in Figure 1 and Table 3, the receptor concentration and binding parameters including the relative affinities of S-28 and S-14 calculated using [^{125}I-LTT] S-28 were virtually identical to those obtained with [^{125}I-Tyr^{11}] S-14 in the brain, pituitary, adrenal cortex and exocrine pancreas (17). Likewise, in limited studies of the binding of structural analogs of S-28, no differences could be elicited in the interactive potency of these peptides for [^{125}I-LTT] S-28 and [^{125}I-Tyr^{11}] S-14 sites (17). Similar results have been observed in AtT-20 cells also (31).

The failure of standard membrane binding assays to discriminate between [^{125}I-Tyr^{11}] S-14 and [^{125}I-LTT] S-28 binding sites, prompted additional lines of investigation, viz., pharmacological studies exploit-

Table 3. Comparison of $[^{125}I\text{-}Tyr^{11}]$ S-14 and $[^{125}I\text{-}LTT]$ S-28
binding sites in normal rat tissues.

Tissue	$[^{125}I\text{-}Tyr^{11}]$ S-14 Binding Sites			$[^{125}I\text{-}LTT]$ S-28 Binding Sites		
	B_{max} (fmol/mg)	Kd [nM]	Relative affinity of S-28*	B_{max} (fmol/mg)	Kd [nM]	Relative affinity of S-28*
Brain	410 ± 40	1.7 ± 0.2	0.20	360 ± 34	1.5 ± 0.11	0.23
Pituitary	305 ± 45	1.1 ± 0.09	3.20	320 ± 28	1.1 ± 0.07	2.78
Adrenal cortex	350 ± 40	1.1 ± 0.11	0.79	210 ± 30	1.2 ± 0.02	0.85
Exocrine pancreas	266 ± 22	0.5 ± 0.07	0.46	222 ± 24	1.2 ± 0.16	0.54

*Relative affinity of S-28 is expressed relative to that of S-14 taken as 1.

ing the differential effects of nucleotides and ions on radioligand binding, autoradiography and cross-linking studies to resolve the question of separate S-14 and S-28 receptors.

Effects of Nucleotides on $[^{125}I\text{-}Tyr^{11}]$ S-14 and $[^{125}I\text{-}LTT]$ S-28 Binding

Receptors coupled to adenylate cyclase are converted by guanine nucleotides from a high affinity to a low affinity state (58). Addition-ally, guanine nucleotides have been reported to inhibit binding in several peptide hormone receptor systems (59,60). We thus undertook a detailed evaluation of the influence of nucleotides on the binding of both $[^{125}I\text{-}Tyr^{11}]$ S-14 and $[^{125}I\text{-}LTT]$ S-28 to rat brain membranes. Both adenine and guanine nucleotides inhibited the binding of each radioligand by decreas-ing the receptor number without altering the affinity (61). The binding of $[^{125}I\text{-}Tyr^{11}]$ S-14 was inhibited by adenine nucleotides to a greater extent than guanine nucleotides as illustrated in Figure 4 (left panel) by the effects of ATP and GTP. By contrast, GTP had a greater effect than ATP on $[^{125}I\text{-}LTT]$ S-28 binding sites (Fig. 4, right panel). We have determined that the number of binding sites for the two radioligands is altered to different degrees by nucleotides. Among adenine nucleotides, ATP is more potent than cAMP and ADP in decreasing $[^{125}I\text{-}Tyr^{11}]$ S-14 binding whereas the potencies of these nucleotides for inhibiting LTT S-28 binding are comparable. For guanine nucleotides the rank order potency for inhibiting $[^{125}I\text{-}Tyr^{11}]$ S-14 binding is GTP > GMP-PNP GMP > GTP > cGMP. In the case of $[^{125}I\text{-}LTT]$ S-28 binding, maximum inhibition is observed with cGMP followed by GTP, GMP, GDP and GMP-PNP. In previously reported studies, guanine but not adenine nucleotides was found to inhibit the binding of a slightly different S-14 radioligand. In rat brain and pituitary, $[^{125}I\text{-}Tyr^{11}]$ S-14 binding sites were decreased by guanine nucleotides (62) whereas in GH_4C_1 cells the nucleotides altered the affinity of S-14 receptors without affecting their concentration (63). The effect of guanine nucleotides in inhibiting S-14 receptor binding appears to involve the inhibitory component of guanine nucleotide binding protein, N_1. Pretreatment of GH_4C_1 cells with pertussis toxin which ADP ribosylates N_1 and thereby blocks the inhibitory actions of S-14 also inhibits S-14 receptor binding almost completely (64). However, whether the effect of toxin was due to reduction in number or affinity, S-14 receptor could not be established. In rat pancreatic acini we have shown that guanine, but not adenine, nucleotides decreased the binding of [^{125}I-Tyr[11]] S-14 (26). The mechanism by which nucleotides decrease the number and/or affinity of somatostatin receptors is not precisely known but may depend on the modulation of the equilibrium between active/inactive and/or high/low affinity conformations.

Modulation of Binding By Ca[++]

Previous studies have reported that Ca[++] regulates the binding of [^{125}I-Tyr[11]] S-14 to intact cells and membranes from guinea pig pancreatic acini as well as to brain membranes (65). Binding in both systems was potentiated by Ca[++] concentrations up to ~0.1 mM; higher Ca[++] concentrations inhibited binding. We have extended these observations to a detailed comparison of the Ca[++] dependency of both [^{125}I-Tyr[11]] S-14 and [^{125}I-LTT] S-28 binding to rat brain membranes. Our studies show that Ca[++] progressively augments the binding of both [^{125}I-Tyr[11]] S-14 and [^{125}I-LTT] S-28 but that at high Ca[++] concentrations (> 15 mM) the binding of [^{125}I-LTT] S-28 but not that of [^{125}I-Tyr[11]] S-14 is inhibited. Competitive inhibition of [^{125}I-LTT] S-28 binding by S-28 and S-14 at high Ca[++] concentrations showed a 4-fold increase in the affinity of S-14 compared to that for S-28 (C. B. Srikant and A. Dahan, unpublished data). Thus, the normal ability of S-14 to interact more avidly than S-28 for [^{125}I-LTT] binding sites in rat brain at low (0.1 mM) Ca[++] concentrations (Table 3) is accentuated by high Ca[++] suggesting the presence of Ca[++]-dependent high and low affinity forms of [[125]I -LTT] S-28 binding sites. These data further highlight the heterogeneity of the somatostatin receptor. Unfortunately, the inability of pharmacological manipulations such as alterations in Ca[++] concentration to modify the affinity of [^{125}I-LTT] S-28 binding sites in favor of S-28 (rather than in favor of S-14) fail to provide definitive proof of separate S-14 and S-28 binding sites, at least in brain membranes. Additional studies exploiting such ionic effects on receptors in other tissues, as well as the use of more selective S-28 agonists, may further clarify this issue.

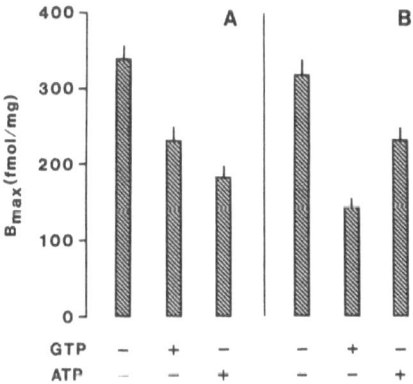

Fig. 4. Differential inhibition by GTP and ATP of the binding of [^{125}I-Tyr[11]] S-14 (panel A) and [Leu[8], D-TrP[22], ^{125}I-Tyr[25]] S-28 (panel B) in rat brain. The concentration of receptor sites (B_{max}) interacting with the radioligands was determined in the absence or presence of 10^{-4} M GTP or ATP as indicated.

Autoradiographic Characterization of $[^{125}I\text{-Tyr}^{11}]$ S-14 and $[^{125}I\text{-LTT}]$ S-28 Binding Sites

In recent years the techniques of in vivo and in vitro autoradiography have been extensively employed for visualizing somatostatin receptors in fixed tissue preparations. This approach has proved to be particularly promising for distinguishing separate populations of binding sites labeled with $[^{125}I\text{-Tyr}^{11}]$ S-14 and $[^{125}I\text{-LTT}]$ S-28. For instance, quantitative in vivo autoradiography has revealed a striking difference in the pattern of labeling of the circumventricular organs of the brain by intravenously administered $[^{125}I\text{-Tyr}^{11}]$ S-14 and $[^{125}I\text{-LTT}]$ S-28 (39). In particular, the median eminence labels preferentially with $[^{125}I\text{-LTT}]$ S-28 and shows virtually no specific $[^{125}I\text{-Tyr}^{11}]$ S-14 binding sites. Similarly, by in vitro autoradiography performed on slide-mounted frozen brain sections, selective labeling with $[^{125}I\text{-LTT}]$ S-28 has been demonstrated in cerebellar nuclei, in the nuclei of the solitary tract, the vagus nerve, the cochlear and vestibular nerves, in the lateral geniculate body and in the substantia nigra (66). Perhaps the most convincing demonstration of tissue selective labeling with these two radioligands comes from recent quantitative electron microscopic autoradiographic studies of binding sites on individual islet cells in monolayer culture. $[^{125}I\text{-Tyr}^{11}]$ S-14 preferentially associates with the glucagon-producing A cells whereas $[^{125}I\text{-LTT}]$ S-28 selectively labels the insulin-producing B cells (67). These observations strongly suggest the existence of separate binding sites for S-14 and S-28 on A and B cells respectively which mediate the A cell selective inhibitory effect of S-14 and the B cell selective action of S-28.

Cross-Linking Studies

Chemical cross-linking of $[^{125}I\text{-LTT}]$ S-28 has revealed a 200,000 dalton receptor protein detectable under reducing conditions in rat adrenal cortex (53). Additionally, in exocrine pancreas, brain, and pituitary, we have detected specific labeling with $[^{125}I\text{-LTT}]$ S-28 of a 200,000 dalton receptor protein identical to that observed with cross-linked $[^{125}I\text{-Tyr}^{11}]$ S-14 in these tissues (C. B. Srikant, unpublished data). In the case of the pancreatic acinar cells, the two additional protein bands of Mr = 80,000 and 70,000 are labeled by both radioligands (unpublished observations). Excess S-14 and S-28 completely inhibit the labeling of receptor proteins with both radioligands indicating a complete cross-reactivity of the respective binding sites. These data suggest that the differential receptor binding affinity of S-28 and S-14 is not dependent on separate receptor subunits.

Do Separate S-14 and S-28 Receptors Exist?

There is considerable direct pharmacological and biochemical evidence to suggest functional and structural diversity of the S-14 binding region. This evidence is based on (i) differential tissue binding affinities of S-14; (ii) tissue specific receptor interaction of S-14 analogs; (iii) identification of two receptor subpopulations interacting with cyclic analogs such as SMS 201-995; (iv) tissue-selective receptor modulation by Ca^{++}; (v) tissue-related structural differences in the receptor unit as revealed by chemical cross-linking.

Somatostatin-28 clearly binds to somatostatin-14 receptors. It does so with widely differing affinities in different tissues. While it is tantalizing to propose an S-28 specific receptor subpopulation, the only substantive evidence in support of this comes from autoradiography which has demonstrated sites either uniquely (brain) or preferentially (B cells) labeled with $[^{125}I\text{-LTT}]$ S-28 (38,66,67). However, even in these instances, crossover experiments to compare the inhibitory potencies of S-14 for interaction with [^{125}I-LTT] S-28 sites and of S-28 for interaction with [^{125}I-Tyr^{11}] S-14 sites have not been carried out and will be required for final confirmation of separate receptor sites for the two peptides. Were it not for the autoradiographic data, one could reconcile existing membrane and related binding data with the concept of a heterogeneous somatostatin receptor containing subclasses of S-14 specific (but not S-28 specific) binding domains. The different reactivity of S-28 could then be explained on the basis of the interaction of this peptide with different conformations of the S-14 binding region in different tissues. On the other hand, it is conceivable that the existence of an S-28 specific binding site has so far defied detection because of the use of [^{125}I-LTT] S-28 as radioligand. This analog is the sole S-28 agonist that has been used experimentally to identify S-28 receptors but its structure is altered sufficiently from the parent molecule to potentially mask S-28 specific binding. This applies particularly to the D-Trp^{22} modification which is theoretically capable of enhancing S-14 like activity (17). Perhaps with other S-28 radioligands more representative of S-28 activity, it may be possible with pharmacological and biochemical means to disclose an S-28 specific receptor or receptor subtype. Finally, since S-14 and S-28 exert qualitatively similar but quantitatively different effects, the possibility that these differences are due in part to differential modulation of receptor-linked membrane signaling pathways (adenyl cyclase, Ca^{++} mobilization) known to be activated by somatostatin has to be entertained. Some evidence for differential effects on post-receptor events has been obtained in the case of AtT-20 tumor cells where S-28 is more potent than S-14 for S-14 receptor down-regulation and for inhibition of stimulated but not basal ACTH secretion and cAMP concentration (31). The possibility of similar selective effects of S-14 and S-28 on cAMP-dependent and -independent actions of the two peptides in normal target tissues remains to be explored.

ACKNOWLEDGMENTS

We are grateful to Mrs. M. Correia for secretarial help in the preparation of this manuscript. This work was supported by grants from the Canadian Medical Research Council (MT 6832, MA 6196) and the USPHS (AM 21373).

REFERENCES

1. Patel YC, Zingg HH, Srikant CB. Somatostatin-14 like immunoreactive forms in the rat: characterization, distribution and biosynthesis. In: Patel YC, Tannenbaum GS, eds. Somatostatin. New York: Plenum Press, 1985.

2. Dixon JE, Andrews PC. Somatostatins of the channel catfish. In: Patel YC, Tannenbaum GS, eds. Somatostatin. New York: Plenum Press, 1985.

3. Spiess J, Noe BD. Processing of an anglerfish somatostatin precursor to a hydroxylysine containing somatostatin-28. Proc Natl Acad Sci USA 1985; 82:277.

4. Hobart P, Crawford R, Shen LP, Raymond P, Rutter WJ. Cloning and sequence analysis of cDNAs encoding two distinct somatostatin precursors found in the endocrine pancreas of anglerfish. Nature 1980; 288:137.

5. Noe BD, Debo G, Spiess J. Comparison of prohormone-processing activities in islet microsomes and secretory granules: evidence for distinct converting enzymes for separate islet prosomatostatins. J Cell Biol 1984; 99:578.

6. Montminy MR, Goodman RH, Horovitch SJ, Habener JF. Primary structure of the gene encoding rat preprosomatostatin. Proc Natl Acad Sci USA 1984; 81:3337.

7. Tavianini MA, Hayes TE, Magazin MD, Minth CD, Dixon JE. Isolation, characterization, and DNA sequence of the rat somatostatin gene. J Biol Chem 1984; 259:11798.

8. Ravazzola M, Benoit R, Ling N, Guillemin R, Orci L. Immunocytochemical localization of prosomatostatin fragments in maturing and mature secretory granules of pancreatic and gastrointestinal D cells. Proc Natl Acad Sci USA 1983; 80:215.

9. Reichlin S. Somatostatin. N Engl J Med 1983; 309:1495.

10. Brown MR, Rivier C, Vale W. Central nervous system regulation of adrenocorticotropin secretion: role of somatostatins. Endocrinology 1984; 114:1546.

11. Brazeau P, Ling N, Esch F, Bohlen P, Benoit R, Guillemin R. High biological activity of the synthetic replicates of somatostatin-28 and somatostatin-25. Regul Pept 1981; 1:255.

12. Klaff LJ, Barron JL, Levitt NS, Ling N, Millar RP. Somatostatin-28 inhibits thyroid-stimulating hormone release in man. S Afr Med J 1982; 62:929.

13. Konturek SJ, Tasler J, Jaworek J, et al. Gastrointestinal secretory, motor, circulatory, and metabolic effects of prosomatostatin. Proc Natl Acad Sci USA 1981; 78:1967.

14. Mandarino L, Stenner D, Blanchard W, et al. Selective effects of somatostatin-14, -25 and -28 on in vitro insulin and glucagon secretion. Nature 1981; 291:76.

15. Seal A, Yamada T, Debas H, et al. Somatostatin-14 and -28: clearance and potency on gastric function in dogs. Am J Physiol 1982; 243:G97.

16. Susini C, Esteve JP, Vaysse N, Pradayrol L, Ribet A. Somatostatin-28: effects on exocrine pancreatic secretion in conscious dogs. Gastroenterology 1979; 79:720.

17. Srikant CB, Patel YC. Somatostatin receptors. In: Patel YC, Tannenbaum GS, eds. Somatostatin. New York: Plenum Press, 1985.

18. Schonbrunn A, Tashjian A Jr. Characterization of functional receptors for somatostatin in rat pituitary cells in culture. J Biol Chem 1978; 253:6473.

19. Srikant CB, Patel YC. Identification and characterization of somatostatin receptors in rat brain synaptosomal membranes. Proc Natl Acad Sci USA 1981; 78:3930.

20. Srikant CB, Patel YC. Characterization of pituitary membrane receptors for somatostatin in the rat. Endocrinology 1982; 110:2138.

21. Aguilera G, Parker DS, Catt KJ. Characterization of somatostatin receptors in the rat adrenal glomerulosa zone. Endocrinology 1982; 111:1376.

22. Reubi J-C, Perrin M, Rivier J, Vale W. High affinity binding sites for somatostatin to rat pituitary. Biochem Biophys Res Commun 1982; 105:1538.

23. Enjalbert A, Tapia-Arancibia L, Rieutort M, Brazeau P, Kordon C, Epelbaum J. Somatostatin receptors in rat anterior pituitary membranes. Endocrinology 1982; 110:1634.

24. Aguilera G, Parker DS. Pituitary somatostatin receptors: characterization by binding with a non-degradable peptide analogue. J Biol Chem 1982; 257:1134.

25. Srikant CB, Patel YC. Somatostatin receptors in rat adrenal cortex: characterization and comparison with brain and pituitary receptors. Endocrinology 1985; 116:1717.

26. Srikant CB, Patel YC. Somatostatin receptors on rat pancreatic acinar cells: pharmacological and structural characterization and demonstration of down-regulation in streptozotocin diabetes. J Biol Chem 1986; 261:7690.

27. Esteve JP, Susini C, Vaysse N, et al. Binding of somatostatin to pancreatic acinar cells. Am J Physiol 1984; 247:G62.

28. Sakamoto C, Goldfine ID, Williams JA. The somatostatin receptor on isolated pancreatic acinar cell plasma membranes: identification of subunit structure and direct regulation by cholecystokinin. J Biol Chem 1984; 259:9623.

29. Beal MF, Tran VT, Mazurek MF, Chaltha G, Martin JB. Somatostatin binding sites in human and monkey brain: localization and characterization. J Neurochem 1986; 46:359.

30. Richardson UI, Schonbrunn A. Inhibition of adrenocorticotropin secretion by somatostatin in pituitary cells in culture. Endocrinology 1981; 108:281.

31. Srikant CB, Heisler S. Relationship between receptor binding and biopotency of somatostatin-14 and somatostatin-28 in mouse pituitary tumor cells. Endocrinology 1985; 117:271.

32. Bhathena SJ, Oie HK, Gazdar AF, Voyler NR, Wilkins SD, Recant L. Insulin, glucagon and somatostatin receptors in cultured cells and clones from rat islet cell tumor. Diabetes 1982; 31:521.

33. Reubi J-C, Rivier J, Perrin M, Brown M, Vale W. Specific high affinity binding sites for somatostatin-28 on pancreatic B-cells: differences with brain somatostatin receptors. Endocrinology 1982; 110:1049.

34. Reubi J-C, Landolt AM. High density of somatostatin receptors in pituitary tumors from acromegalic patients. J Clin Endocrinol Metab 1984; 59:1148.

35. Moyse E, Le Dafniet M, Epelbaum J, et al. Somatostatin receptors in human growth hormone and prolactin-secreting pituitary adenomas. J Clin Endocrinol Metab 1985; 61:98.

36. Reubi J-C, Maurer R, Klijin JGM, et al. High incidence of somatostatin receptors in human meningioma: biochemical characterization. J Clin Endocrinol Metab 1986; 63:433.

37. Elde R, Johansson O, Hokfelt T. Immunocytochemical studies of somatostatin neurons in brain. In: Patel YC, Tannenbaum GS, eds. Somatostatin. New York: Plenum Press, 1985.

38. Morel G, Mesguich P, Dubois MP, Dubois PM. Ultrastructural autoradiographic localization of somatostatin-28 in the rat pituitary gland. Endocrinology 1985; 116:1615.

39. Patel YC, Baquiran G, Srikant CB, Posner BI. Quantitative in vivo autoradiographic localization of [^{125}I-Tyr^{11}] somatostatin-14 and [Leu^8, D-Trp^{22}, ^{125}I-Tyr^{25}] somatostatin-28 binding sites in rat brain. Endocrinology 1986; 119:2262.

40. Maurer R, Reubi J-C. Distribution and coregulation of three peptide receptors in adrenals. Eur J Pharmacol 1986; 125:241.

41. Patel YC, Amherdt M, Orci L. Quantitative electron microscopic radiography of insulin, glucagon and somatostatin binding sites on islets. Science 1982; 217:1155.

42. Draznin B, Leitner JW, Sussman KE. Kinetics of somatostatin receptor migration in isolated pancreatic islets. Diabetes 1982; 31:467.

43. Reyl FJ, Lewin MJM. Intracellular receptor for somatostatin in gastric mucosal cells: decomposition and reconstitution of somatostatin-stimulated phosphoprotein phosphate. Proc Natl Acad Sci USA 1982; 79:978.

44. Reyl FJ, Lewin MJM. Evidence for an intracellular somatostatin receptor in pancreas: a comparative study with reference to gastric mucosa. Biochem Biophys Res Commun 1982; 109:1324.

45. Arilla E, Lopez-Ruiz MP, Guijarro LG, Prieto JC, Gomez-Pan A, Hirst B. Characterization of somatostatin binding sites in cytosolic fraction of rat intestinal mucosa. Biochim Biophys Acta 1984; 802:203.

46. Guijarro LG, Arilla E, Lopez-Ruiz MP, Prieto JC, Whitford C, Hirst BH. Somatostatin binding sites in cytosolic fraction isolated from

rabbit antral and fundic gastric mucosa. Regul Pept 1985; 10:207.

47. Arilla E, Colas B, Prieto JC. Specific somatostatin-binding to cytosol of bovine gallbladder mucosa. Biosci Rep 1986; 6:283.

48. Srikant CB, Patel YC. Somatostatin analogs: dissociation of brain receptor binding affinities and pituitary actions in the rat. Endocrinology 1981; 108:341.

49. Reubi J-C. Evidence for two somatostatin-14 receptor types in rat brain cortex. Neurosci Lett 1984; 49:259.

50. Tran V, Beal MF, Martin JB. Two types of somatostatin receptors differentiated by cyclic somatostatin analogs. Science 1985; 228:492.

51. Reubi J-C. Novel selective radioligand for one population of rat cortex somatostatin receptors. Life Sci 1985; 36:1829.

52. Reubi J-C, Maurer R. Different ionic requirements for somatostatin receptor subpopulations in the brain. Regul Pept 1986; 14:301.

53. Srikant CB, Patel YC. Chemical cross-linking of somatostatin receptors in rat adrenal cortex. Biochem Biophys Res Commun 1986; 139:757.

54. Srikant CB, Patel YC. Cysteamine-induced depletion of brain somatostatin is associated with up-regulation of cerebrocortical somatostatin receptors. Endocrinology 1984; 115:990.

55. Srikant CB, Patel YC. Receptor binding of somatostatin-28 is tissue specific. Nature 1981; 294:259.

56. Schonbrunn A, Rorstad OP, Westendrog JM, Martin JM. Somatostatin analogs: correlation between receptor binding affinity and biological potency in GH pituitary cells. Endocrinology 1983; 113:1559.

57. Reubi J-C, Rivier J, Perrin M, Brown M, Vale W. High affinity binding sites for a somatostatin-28 analog in rat brain. Life Sci 1981; 28:2191.

58. Rodbell M, Krans HM, Pohl SL, Birnhaumer L. The glucagon-sensitive adenylcyclase system in plasma membranes of rat liver: effects of guanyl nucleotides on binding of ^{125}I-glucagon. J Biol Chem 1971; 246:1872.

59. Kent RS, De Lean A, Lefkowitz RJ. A quantitative analysis of beta-adrenergic receptor interactions: resolution of high and low affinity states of the receptor by computer modelling of ligand binding data. Mol Pharmacol 1980; 17:14.

60. Smith KE, Hoss WP. Guanine nucleotides regulate ^{3}H-substance P binding in rat small intestine. Regul Pept 1985; 11:275.

61. Dahan A, Srikant CB. Differential effects of guanine and adenine nucleotides on [^{125}I-Tyr^{11}] S-14 and [Leu^8, D-Trp^{22}, ^{125}I-Tyr^{25}] S-28 binding sites in rat brain [Abstract]. International Conference on Somatostatin, Washington, DC, 1986.

62. Enjalbert A, Rasolonjanahary R, Moyse E, Kordon C, Epelbaum J. Guanine nucleotide sensitivity of [^{125}I] iodo N-Tyr somatostatin binding in rat adenohypophysis and cerebral cortex. Endocrinology 1983; 113:822.

63. Koch BD, Schonbrunn A. The somatostatin receptor is directly coupled to adenylate cyclase in GH$_4$C$_1$ pituitary cell membranes. Endocrinology 1984; 114:1784.

64. Koch BD, Dorflinger LJ, Schonbrunn A. Pertussis toxin blocks both cyclic AMP-mediated and cyclic AMP-independent actions of somatostatin. J Biol Chem 1985; 260:13138.

65. Susini C, Esteve JP, Vaysse N, Ribet A. Calcium-dependence of somatostatin binding to receptors. Peptides 1985; 6:831.

66. Leroux P, Quirion R, Pelletier G. Localization and characterization of brain somatostatin receptors studied with somatostatin-14 and somatostatin-28 receptor radioautography. Brain Res 1985; 347:74.

67. Amherdt M, Patel YC, Orci L. Selective binding of somatostatin-14 and somatostatin-28 to islet cells revealed by quantitative electron microscopic autoradiography. Science 1986 (submitted).

10

STRUCTURAL ANALYSIS OF SOMATOSTATIN RECEPTORS

John A. Williams and Christiane Susini

Cell Biology Laboratory, Mount Zion Hospital and
Medical Center and the Department of Physiology,
The University of California, San Francisco, CA

Somatostatin receptors have been characterized by ligand binding studies using intact cells or cell lines and membrane fractions from various tissues including brain (1,2), anterior pituitary (3-5), adrenal cortex (6,7), and both exocrine (8-10) and endocrine (11) pancreas. In general these studies indicate that somatostatin receptors in different tissues have similar affinity (Kd = 0.25 to 1.0 nM) although minor inter-tissue differences have been reported in specificity for somatostatin 14 and somatostatin 28 (11). Tissue-specific differences in receptor regulation by other peptides are also known. For example, cholecystokinin regulates somatostatin binding in pancreatic membranes but not those of the cerebral cortex (9).

Because ligand binding data provide only inferential information about the structure of the receptor, we have begun a program to label, isolate and sequence the somatostatin receptor. These studies reported here deal with the covalent labeling of the receptor by crosslinking bound ^{125}I-somatostatin to its receptor. Initial studies have been carried out using plasma membranes from pancreatic acinar cells as this provides a relatively easy source of homogenous membranes enriched in somatostatin receptors. We report here that the somatostatin receptor has an apparent molecular weight of 90,000 daltons and that labeled receptor can be solubilized under nondenaturing conditions.

METHODS

Pancreatic plasma membranes were prepared from isolated rat pancreatic acini as previously described (9). Cyclic somatostatin, [Tyr[1]]somatostatin 14 and [Tyr[11]]somatostatin 14 were obtained from Bachem Biochemicals, Inc., Torrance, CA. Both Tyr analogs were labeled with ^{125}I by chloramine-T iodination according to the procedure of Patel and Reichlin (12). ^{125}I-[Tyr[1]]somatostatin was also obtained from New England Nuclear. All crosslinking reagents were obtained from Pierce Chemical Company.

Binding and crosslinking studies using ^{125}I-[Tyr[1]]somatostatin 14 were carried out as described (9). In studies with ^{125}I-[Tyr[11]]somatostatin 14, binding was performed in buffer containing 50 mM Tris Cl, pH 7.5, 0.2 mM $CaCl_2$, 0.5 mM benzamidine, 1 mg/ml of bovine serum albumin and 0.2 mg/ml soybean trypsin inhibitor. The presence of Ca^{2+} has been shown to enhance binding of $[Tyr^{11}]$- but not $[Tyr^1]$somatostatin (8). Binding was carried out for 90 min at 24° with 100 µg/ml plasma membrane. To determine nonspecific binding, studies were also carried out with un-labeled cyclic somatostatin added at 1 µM. Binding was terminated by centrifugation of a 150 µl aliquot at 10,000 x g for 1 min in a micro-centrifuge.

For crosslinking, 1 ml aliquots were incubated as above with 100 pM to 1 nM ^{125}I-somatostatin. Incubation was terminated by centrifugation at 30,000 x g for 15 min at 4°, and the resulting pellet was washed and resuspended in phosphate buffered saline, pH 7.4. Heterobifunctional crosslinking agents were dissolved in DMSO just before use and added at a final concentration of 100 µM. After 4 min in darkness the suspension was exposed to UV light from a GE 275 watt sunlamp for 14 min at a distance of 12 cm. All operations were carried out at 4°. Excess 50 mM Tris Cl buffer containing 2 mM EDTA was then added to quench any remaining hydrox-ysuccinimide groups, the membranes centrifuged and the pellets either directly solubilized in sodium dodecyl sulfate (SDS) for gel electrophore-sis or taken up in specified nondenaturing detergent in 50 mM Tris Cl with 0.5 mM benzamidine. In the latter case, membranes were incubated with mixing for 2 hours followed by centrifugation at 100,000 x g for 1 hour all at 4°. The pellet and supernatant were then prepared in SDS buffer for gel electrophoresis. When indicated, samples were reduced with 50 mM dithiothreitol. Electrophoresis was performed according to Laemmli (13) using 1.5 mm thick slab gels containing 7.5% acrylamide. Autoradiograms were obtained from the dried gels after exposure for 3-10 days to Kodak X-omat AR film using Dupont Cronex Lightning plus screen at -70°C.

RESULTS AND DISCUSSION

In previous studies carried out with ^{125}I-$[Tyr^1]$somatostatin 14 and the heterobifunctional crosslinker n-hydroxysuccinimidyl-4-azidobenzoate (HSAB), we were able to label a single protein band centered at Mr = 92,000 which was not affected by reduction with DTT (9). Neither the homobifunctional reagent disuccinimidyl suberate (DSS) or UV light alone were effective in crosslinking somatostatin. Clearly the optimal cross-linking protocol is influenced by the structure of both the ligand and its receptor. DSS has been used for a number of receptors following the work of Czech on insulin receptors (14,15). We were led to try HSAB, however, since glucagon receptors are crosslinked by HSAB but not DSS (16).

Subsequently it became apparent that ^{125}I-$[Tyr^{11}]$somatostatin was probably a better ligand for receptor studies as it is less susceptible to degradation by aminopeptidases. We therefore carried out receptor binding using conditions found to be optimal for this ligand (8). Initial cross-linking studies (not shown) revealed a similar labeling pattern using three different heterobifunctional reagents HSAB, n-succinimidyl6-(4'azido-2' nitrophenylamino) hexanoate (SANAH) and n-5-azido-2-nitro-benzoyloxy-succinimide (ANB-NOS). Most efficient crosslinking was ob-served with ANB-NOS which is chemically similar to HSAB but which contains a nitro group on the aromatic ring which shifts the absorbance optimum from 260 to 350 nm. Optimal results were obtained with 50-100 µM cross-linker. Using this protocol, a broad Mr = 92,000 band was labeled which was unaffected by sulfhydryl reduction (Fig. 1). When excess somatostatin was present during binding, both binding of the ^{125}I-ligand and the appearance of the crosslinked band were essentially abolished. CCK is known to act via the CCK receptor to reduce the binding of somatostatin to its receptor. This resulted in a parallel reduction in ^{125}I-$[Tyr^{11}]$ somatostatin binding and reduction in the density of the crosslinked band (Fig. 1). In other studies (to be published) increasing concentrations of somatostatin and guanine nucleotides gave parallel inhibition of binding and the density of the crosslinked protein band. Thus there is a good correlation indicating that whatever ^{125}I-somatostatin (molecular weight about 2000) is bound, it can be proportionately crosslinked to a 90,000 dalton protein. Two caveats must of course be kept in mind that apply to all crosslinking studies of this type. First, the efficiency of cross-linking is low as is true for other ligand-receptor pairs. Second, the labeled protein could be merely adjacent to the receptor. The short distance between the two reactive groups (about 5 Å) and the lack of labeling even when nonspecific binding is increased (see below), however, make this unlikely and the Mr = 92,000 labeled band will therefore be tentatively referred to as the somatostatin receptor. Further support is provided by the observation of a similar crosslinked species using rat pituitary membranes (L. D. Lewis and J. A. Williams, to be published).

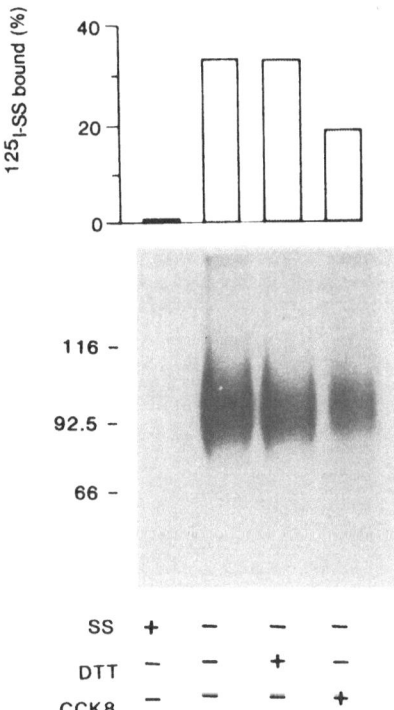

Fig. 1. Binding and crosslinking of [125]I-[Tyr[11]]somatostatin 14 to its receptors on rat pancreatic plasma membranes. Following binding of 250 pM ^{125}I-ligand for 90 min at 24° with 1 μM somatostatin or 10 nM CCK added as specified, aliquots were removed and centrifuged to determine % bound (upper panel). The remainder of each was cross-linked with 50 μM ANB-NOS in conjunction with UV light and subjected to gel electrophoresis with or without prior reduction by 50 mM DTT followed by autoradiography (lower panel). The position of molecular weight markers is indicated on the left side.

To increase the amount of labeled somatostatin receptor as starting material for further characterization, we investigated the effect of the ligand concentration on the appearance of the labeled band. Since nonspecific labeling increases linearly with ligand concentration, the ratio of specific to nonspecific binding decreases at ligand concentrations higher than the receptor Kd. As shown in Figure 2, however, this did not lead to the appearance of nonspecifically crosslinked proteins. Apparently nonspecifically bound hormone is not in close enough apposition to protein to result in crosslinking. This has been observed previously in studies of electron microscopic autoradiography of ^{125}I-insulin and ^{125}I-CCK where nonspecifically bound ligand did not fix with glutaraldehyde (crosslink) to the cells (17). The practical result is that to obtain maximal labeled receptor one can use saturating concentrations (1.0 nM ^{125}I-somatostatin) as well as scaling up the size of the binding reactions.

To study the nature of the receptor it is necessary for it to be solubilized under nondenaturing conditions. We therefore crosslinked ^{125}I-somatostatin to several mg of pancreatic membranes and incubated aliquots in the absence or presence of various nondenaturing detergents. After 2 hours at 4° the mixture was centrifuged and the pellet taken up in a volume equal to the supernatant so that the degree of solubilization could be readily determined. As expected, in the absence of detergent all crosslinked protein remained unsolubilized (Fig. 3). Complete solubilization was observed with Zwittergent 3-12 and Zwittergent 3-14. Partial solubilization was observed with CHAPS, octylglucopyranoside, and Triton X-100 and essentially none with digitonin and Zwittergent 3-08. Basically similar results were observed using 0.5, 1 and 2% detergent; in all cases membrane protein concentration was 1 mg/ml. Many of the detergents did not appear to solubilize membranes as effectively as when crosslinking had

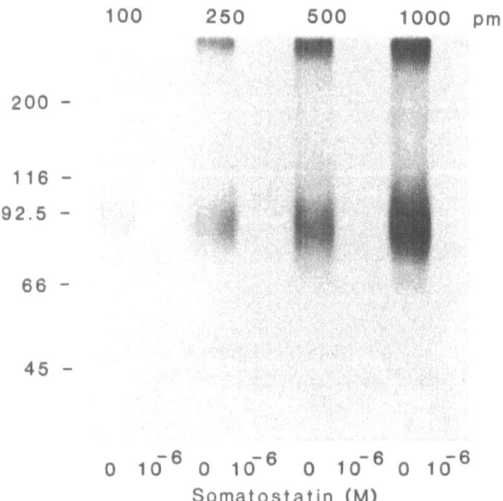

Fig. 2. Crosslinking of ^{125}I-[Tyr^{11}]somatostatin 14 following incubation of pancreatic membranes with various concentrations of ^{125}I-ligand in the presence or absence of 1 μM unlabeled cyclic somatostatin.

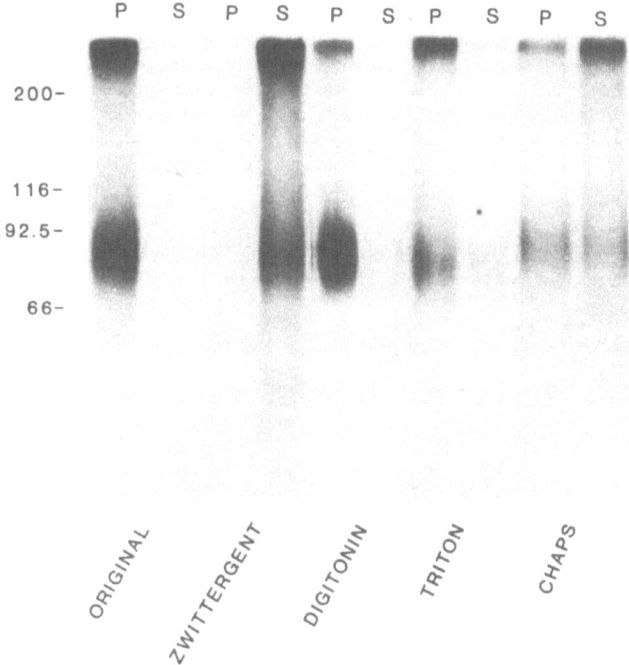

Fig. 3. Presence in pellet (P) or supernatant (S) following detergent extraction of ^{125}I-[Tyr^{11}]somato-statin crosslinked to pancreatic plasma membranes.

not been carried out. While conditions could be optimized for other detergents, we routinely use Zwittergent 3-12 and are able to store aliquots of solubilized labeled receptors in the freezer for several weeks.

Studies are currently in progress subjecting this material to gel exclusion chromatography, density gradient equilibrium and lectin chromatography (18). Preliminary studies have revealed that solubilized somatostatin receptor can be absorbed to specific lectins and eluted with appropriate sugar. Best results have been obtained with wheat germ agglutinin agarose and elution with N, N', N''-triacetylchitotriose (19). This indicates that the somatostatin receptor is a glycoprotein and provides an initial step in purification of the receptor.

For further study of the receptor it is also desirable to solubilize the receptor without prior crosslinking with retention of binding ability and follow its purification by ligand binding. To date we have been unsuccessful in this utilizing Zwittergent 3-12 or any of the other detergents. When conditions are developed permitting this, it will then be possible to purify the receptor by lectin and ligand affinity chromatography as has been carried out for the insulin and other receptors. Besides providing further structural information, the purified receptor can also be used to generate antireceptor antibodies.

Finally, the structural studies to date are not conclusive as to the existence of different subtypes of somatostatin receptors. Different somatostatin ligands including somatostatin 28 analogs (data not shown) all produce similar crosslinking patterns in pancreas membranes. The best evidence for receptor subtypes has been obtained in brain with a cyclic octapeptide somatostatin analog (20). To date, however, we have been unsuccessful at crosslinking brain somatostatin receptors. Further structural studies and purification of somatostatin receptors from various tissues will be necessary to fully characterize somatostatin receptors.

ACKNOWLEDGMENTS

This work was supported by NIH grant AM32994. The expert technical assistance of A. Bailey and D. McChesney is gratefully acknowledged.

REFERENCES

1. Srikant CB, Patel YC. Somatostatin receptors: identification and characterization in rat brain membranes. Proc Natl Acad Sci USA 1981; 78:3930.
2. Czernik AJ, Petrack B. Somatostatin receptor binding in rat cerebral cortex: characterization using a nonreducible somatostatin analog. J Biol Chem 1983; 258:5525.
3. Schonbrunn A, Tashjian AH Jr. Characterization of functional receptors for somatostatin in rat pituitary cells in culture. J Biol Chem 1978; 253:6473.
4. Srikant CB, Patel YC. Characterization of pituitary membrane receptors for somatostatin in the rat. Endocrinology 1982; 110:2138.
5. Reubi J-C, Perrin M, Rivier J, Vale W. High affinity binding sites for somatostatin to rat pituitary. Biochem Biophys Res Commun 1982; 105:1538.
6. Aguilera G, Parker DS, Catt KT. Characterization of somatostatin receptors in the rat adrenal glomerulosa zone. Endocrinology 1982; 111:1376.
7. Srikant CB, Patel YC. Somatostatin receptors in the rat adrenal cortex: characterization and comparison with brain and pituitary receptors. Endocrinology 1985; 116:1717.
8. Taparel D, Esteve JP, Susini C, et al. Binding of somatostatin to guinea-pig pancreatic membranes: regulation by ions. Biochem Biophys Res Commun 1983; 115:827.
9. Sakamoto C, Goldfine ID, Williams JA. The somatostatin receptor on isolated pancreatic acinar cell plasma membranes: identification of subunit structure and direct regulation by cholecystokinin. J Biol Chem 1984; 259:9623.
10. Esteve JP, Susini C, Vaysse N, et al. Binding of somatostatin to pancreatic acinar cells. Am J Physiol 1984; 247:G62.
11. Reubi J-C, Rivier J, Perrin M, Brown M, Vale W. Specific high affinity binding sites for somatostatin-28 on pancreatic β-cells: differences with brain somatostatin receptors. Endocrinology 1982; 110:1049.
12. Patel YC, Reichlin S. Somatostatin in hypothalamus, extrahypothalamic brain, and peripheral tissues of the rat. Endocrinology 1978; 102:523
13. Laemmli UK. Cleavage of structure proteins during the assembly of the head of bacteriophage T_4. Nature 1970; 227:680.
14. Pilch PF, Czech MP. The subunit structure of the high affinity insulin receptor. J Biol Chem 1980; 255:1722.
15. Massague J, Czech MP. The subunit structures of two distinct receptors for insulin-like growth factors I and II and their relationship to the insulin receptor. J Biol Chem 1982; 257:5038.
16. Johnson GL, MacAndrew VI Jr, Pilch PF. Identification of the glucagon receptor in rat liver membranes by photoaffinity crosslinking.

Proc Natl Acad Sci USA 1981; 78:875.

17. Goldfine ID, Williams JA. Receptors for insulin and CCK in the acinar pancreas: relationship to hormone action. Int Rev Cytol 1983; 85:1.

18. Hedo JA. Lectins as tools for the purification of membrane receptors. In: Venter JC, Harrison LC, eds. Receptor biochemistry and methodology, vol 2. New York: Alan R Liss, 1984.

19. Susini C, Bailey A, Szecowka J, Williams JA. Characterization of covalently crosslinked pancreatic somatostatin receptors [Abstract]. Gastroenterology 1986; 90:1653.

20. Reubi JC. New specific radioligand for one subpopulation of brain somatostatin receptors. Life Sci 1985; 36:1829.

11

MODE OF ACTION OF SOMATOSTATIN IN ISLET B-CELLS:
INFLUENCE ON GLUCOSE-, L-ISOLEUCINE- AND GLYBURIDE-
INDUCED ELECTRICAL ACTIVITY

Caroline S. Pace

University of Alabama at Birmingham
1808 7th Avenue South
Birmingham, Alabama 35294

INTRODUCTION

The widespread role of somatostatin (SRIF, somatotropin release inhibiting factor) as a modulator of neural activity as well as endocrine and exocrine secretion has stimulated interest in its mechanism of action. We have examined the mechanism of action of SRIF in the pancreatic islet B-cell and, in conjunction with results of other groups, have concluded that its primary effect resides in disrupting the transduction of receptor information at the level of the plasma membrane (1). SRIF inhibits the generation of cyclic AMP (1), decreases the membrane permeability to Ca^{++} (1), and disrupts the electrical activity associated with glucose-induced insulin secretion (1,2). The ability of SRIF to antagonize glucose activation of the electrical events in the B-cell plasma membrane may be due to a countermodulatory action of SRIF on K^+ permeability (P_k) (1,2). The evidence supporting this conclusion will be reviewed in this chapter.

Most of the evidence showing the involvement of cyclic AMP, Ca^{++} and K^+ permeabilities in the inhibitory action of SRIF have used glucose as the primary B-cell stimulant. However, SRIF has been found to inhibit insulin release provoked by leucine, arginine, tolbutamide, glucagon, secretin, and isoproterenol in man and/or baboon or dog (3-10). If SRIF also interacts with a membrane receptor, it is possible that it either alters receptor affinity for each of the above insulinotropic agents or binds to a specific receptor, the activation of which leads to cellular activity opposing that induced by a given stimulatory agent. Amino acids and hypoglycemic agents have been indicated to elicit electrical activity from B-cells by influencing P_k similar to glucose (11-13). We selected L-isoleucine and glyburide to determine if SRIF influences electrical activity elicited by these agents.

INFLUENCE OF SRIF ON GLUCOSE-INDUCED ELECTRICAL ACTIVITY

Depolarization of the B-cell membrane due to glucose appears to be primarily because of a reduction in P_k. This is supported by evidence that glucose inhibits efflux of $^{86}Rb^+$ (14,15) and $^{42}K^+$ (16-18) from islet cells. Furthermore, tetraethylammonium ion (TEA), a specific inhibitor of voltage-sensitive P_k in nerve and muscle membranes (19-21), was found to inhibit $^{86}Rb^+$ efflux, and potentiate the secretory and electrical responses to glucose (22,23). Quinine, an inhibitor of Ca^{++}-sensitive P_k in red blood cells (24), was found to augment glucose-induced electrical and secretory responses (25,26). The regulation of P_k has an important role in the maintenance of oscillatory pattern of electrical activity in the B-cell. This is characterized by a regular alteration of a depolarized phase, accompanied by the generation of spikes, with a silent repolarized phase. Prevention of an increase in P_k prevents repolarization producing continuous spike action; prevention of a decrease in P_k prevents depolarization producing a continuous silent phase. Gradations between continuous spike activity and silent phase can be quantitated by analyzing the percent of time occupied by the active phase fraction.

SRIF at 0.1 μg/ml has been found to elicit sustained hyperpolarization and inhibition of spike activity in cultured rat islet cells (1). This inhibition of glucose-induced electrical activity was almost completely antagonized by the addition of 20 mM TEA or 0.1 mM quinine (1). The sustained inhibitory influence of SRIF on cultured rat islet cells contrasts with the transient influence of SRIF on microdissected mouse islet cells (2). SRIF rapidly elicited a 2-fold increase in the duration of the silent phase, had no effect on the active phase, and provoked a hyperpolarization of about 5 mV. This effect was transient, lasting for about 3-4 min (Fig. 1, Cell 2), although the electrical activity was irregular until removal of SRIF. The different effect of SRIF on cultured and microdissected islet cells may be due to a greater sensitivity of the former to SRIF or to the alteration in the topography of the islet cells and, thereby, impairment of the paracrine influence of intraislet cell hormone release.

In other experiments with mouse islets TEA was used and was found to abolish the oscillatory pattern of electrical activity due to 11.1 mM

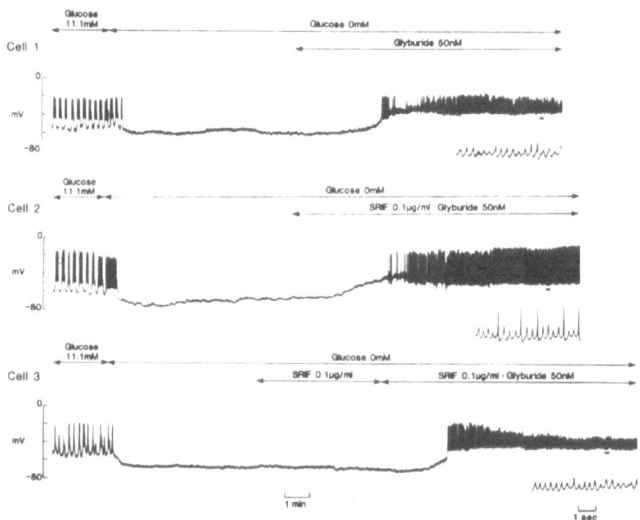

Fig. 1. Influence of SRIF on glyburide-induced electrical activity. Application of SRIF did not influence frequency of spike activity or time lag before onset of depolarization and spike activity.

glucose (2). Addition of 0.1 to 0.5 μg/ml SRIF did not revert the pattern of the electrical activity to oscillations. The effect of TEA and SRIF was reversible.

These results indicate that SRIF interrupts the mechanism leading to depolarization and maintenance of the pattern of oscillatory electrical activity, thereby suggesting that the hormone increases P_k. At first, any association with a Ca^{++}-sensitive P_k mechanism seems to be contradictory to the facts because an increase in P_k is associated with an increase in intracellular Ca^{++}, whereas SRIF inhibits Ca^{++} entry. However, this contradiction can be overcome by postulating that SRIF antagonizes the glucose-activated decrease in P_k. The absence of adequate depolarization, in turn, would prevent the activation of voltage-sensitive Ca^{++} gates. We tested this postulate by determining the influence of SRIF on the efflux of $^{86}Rb^+$ from islet cells.

INFLUENCE OF SRIF ON $^{86}Rb^+$ FLUXES IN ISLET CELLS

For these studies cultured rat islets were used (1). It was found that 0.1 μg/ml SRIF had no apparent influence on the uptake of $^{86}Rb^+$ into islet cells exposed to 16.7 mM glucose over a 30-min period compared with that obtained in the presence of glucose alone. These results indicate that SRIF may not hyperpolarize the plasma membrane via activation of a Na-K ATPase.

The addition of 0.1 μg/ml of SRIF to medium containing 16.7 mM glucose led to a 2-fold increase in the rate constant for $^{86}Rb^+$ efflux. The glucose-induced reduction of $^{86}Rb^+$ efflux was not further reduced by the addition of 20 mM TEA. However, the enhancement of the rate of $^{86}Rb^+$ efflux due to SRIF was reduced 80% by the simultaneous presence of TEA. In addition, 0.1 mM quinine partially reversed the SRIF-induced increase in the rate of $^{86}Rb^+$ efflux. It is clearly evident from the $^{86}Rb^+$ efflux studies that SRIF enhances P_k, thereby antagonizing the glucose-induced decrease in P_k. Either antagonist of P_k activation, TEA or quinine, effectively counteracted the SRIF-induced augmentation of $^{86}Rb^+$ efflux, lending further supporting evidence to a possible direct action of SRIF on P_k.

The definitive effects of SRIF on the inhibition of Ca^{++} uptake on the one hand (27), and the augmentation of $^{86}Rb^+$ efflux on the other (1,2), suggest that one or both of these phenomena prevent normal regulation of a Ca^{++}-sensitive P_k system. Accordingly, we determined the effects of an increase in extracellular Ca^{++} from 2.5 to 5.0 mM on the rate of $^{86}Rb^+$ efflux in the presence of 16.7 mM glucose with or without SRIF. The increase in Ca^{++} or addition of SRIF produced equal increases in the efflux rate when acting separately; when working together, there was about an additional 35% increase in $^{86}Rb^+$ efflux. These results are predictable assuming that the B-cell membrane possesses a Ca^{++}-sensitive P_k system.

The influence of excess Ca^{++} on $^{86}Rb^+$ efflux is consistent with electrophysiological studies that revealed the dynamic relationship between changes in Ca^{++} and K^+ permeabilities (25). These studies showed that an increase in the Ca^{++} level from 2.5 to 5.0 mM in the presence of 11.1 mM glucose elicited prolonged silent phases between bursts of spikes at a potential more negative than that obtained in the presence of 2.5 mM Ca^{++}. We have observed a similar effect of excess Ca^{++} on the membrane potential in previous studies in which cultured rat islet cells were used (1). Although excess Ca^{++} led to hyperpolarization and a decrease in the level of spike activity in the cultured islet cells, the addition of SRIF led to no further change in these parameters. The inability of excess Ca^{++} to reverse the influence of SRIF on either the membrane potential or the rate of $^{86}Rb^{+}$ efflux is probably due to activation of a Ca^{++}-sensitive P_k.

INFLUENCE OF SRIF ON GLUCOSE METABOLISM

In view of the hypothesis that a signal stemming from glucose metabolism serves as a trigger for both the membrane and the secretory events, it is important to determine if the action of SRIF could be mediated by inhibition of glucose metabolism. Our previously reported findings (1) are in agreement with other studies in which SRIF was found not to affect the metabolism of glucose through the glycolytic pathway (28), the Krebs cycle (29), or the pentose monophosphate shunt (28). In light of these results, it is apparent that SRIF can influence processes involved in the transduction of glucose activation without the mediating influence of glucose metabolism.

This conclusion does not rule out the possibility that SRIF may intercept or override the coupling between glucose metabolism and membrane-related processes.

INFLUENCE OF SRIF ON L-ISOLEUCINE AND GLYBURIDE-INDUCED ELECTRICAL ACTIVITY

SRIF has been clearly shown to inhibit glucose-induced electrical activity in microdissected mouse islets (2). Since both isoleucine and glyburide represent two primary stimulants of insulin secretion, it was of interest to determine if SRIF would inhibit the electrical response to these agents. The experiments were performed according to two different protocols: (1) Initially the cell was impaled in 11.1 mM glucose and then the solution was changed to one containing 20 mM isoleucine plus 5.6 mM glucose or 50 nM glyburide, after which 0.1 μg/ml SRIF was added. Subsequently SRIF was withdrawn. (2) After impaling the cell in glucose, glucose was withdrawn; after about 5 min SRIF was added. The cell was either preexposed to SRIF for 5 min before addition of isoleucine plus glucose or glyburide to the medium, or SRIF was added to the medium at the same time as the agents. The second protocol was used because it was found that addition of SRIF to a solution containing glyburide did not induce inhibition of electrical activity due to glyburide (Fig. 1). It was then decided to preexpose the cell to SRIF for 5 min before addition of the drug. This protocol also did not reveal any inhibitory influence of SRIF on glyburide-induced electrical activity (Fig. 1). The spike frequency was not altered (see expanded records). Furthermore, the time delay for onset of depolarization and onset of spike activity did not differ whether SRIF was present or not. The number of cells observed with glyburide alone was 7 and with SRIF preexposure was 5. The reason for this lack of inhibition is not known since SRIF has been found to inhibit insulin release due to another oral hypoglycemic agent, tolbutamide, in man (6,7), and the isolated perfused canine pancreas (10). It is conceivable that a higher concentration of SRIF was required, but 0.1 μg/ml was sufficient to inhibit electrical activity due to glucose (1,2) or isoleucine (Fig. 2).

Addition of SRIF to the medium containing glucose or isoleucine led to inhibition of the percent duration of the active phase, but did not influence the burst frequency (Fig. 2, Table 1). The electrical response was measured for 3.3 min after addition of SRIF. After 3 to 4 minutes, the inhibition of the electrical response was not as marked, but return to

114

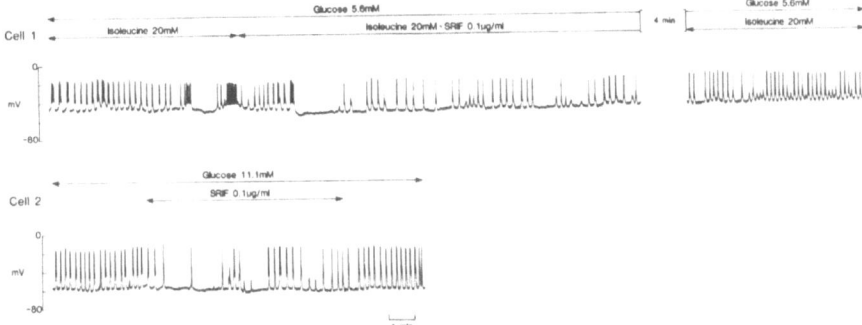

Fig. 2. Influence of SRIF on L-isoleucine- and glucose-induced electrical activity. Addition of SRIF resulted in a decrease in % duration of active phase (see Table 1).

control electrical activity did not occur until after withdrawal of SRIF (Fig. 2). Preexposure of the B-cell to SRIF before addition of isoleucine resulted in a delay of the onset of depolarization and spike activity, but did not significantly inhibit the percent duration of the active phase or burst frequency (Fig. 3). A total number of 4 cells with or without addition of SRIF was observed. In the presence of SRIF there was almost a 3-fold increase in the time necessary for onset of depolarization and a 2.5-fold increase in the time required for onset of spike activity after the addition of isoleucine (Fig. 4). It is not clear why addition of SRIF before addition of isoleucine does not inhibit the electrical activity, whereas addition of the hormone in the presence of isoleucine leads to inhibition. However, it is evident in the latter that the strongest inhibitory response occurs 3 to 4 min after addition of isoleucine. In view of this it is not surprising that when the cell is preexposed to SRIF there is about a 3-min delay before onset of the electrical response beyond that seen without SRIF.

Table 1. Effect of somatostatin on electrical response elicited by glucose or isoleucine plus glucose.

		n	%Duration Active Phase (M+SE)	P	Burst Frequency (M±SE)	P
A	Glucose, 11 mM	5	31 ± 4		4.3 ± 1.0	NS
	Glusoe, 11 mM +SRIF, 0.1 μg/ml	5	19 ± 3	<0.05	2.9 ± 1.2	
D	Isoleucine, 10 mM	4	44 ± 5		3.8 ± 1	NS
	Isoleucine, 10 mM +SRIF, 0.1 μg/ml	4	29 ± 2	<0.05	2.8 ± 2	

n - number of experiments
NS - not significant

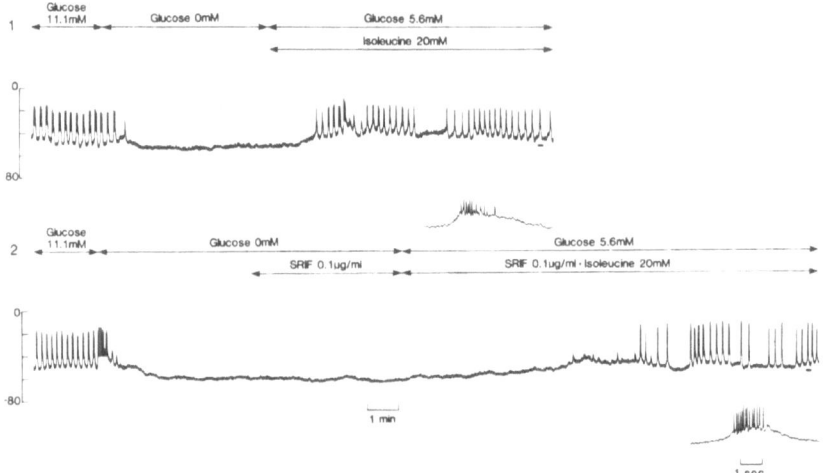

Fig. 3. Influence of preexposure to SRIF on L-isoleucine-induced electrical activity (see Fig. 4).

SOMATOSTATIN: MODE OF ACTION

Somatostatin-receptor interaction may initiate coupling between the receptor and one or more transducing elements residing at the level of the plasma membrane (1). Evidence stemming from electrophysiological and cationic flux studies indicates that SRIF influences the membrane permeability to K^+ and Ca^{++} (1,2,27). SRIF-induced hyperpolarization is most likely due to an increase in P_k to an extent that counteracts the decrease in P_k due to glucose. Consequently, in the absence of adequate depolarization, the influx of Ca^{++} via voltage-sensitive Ca^{++} channels would be

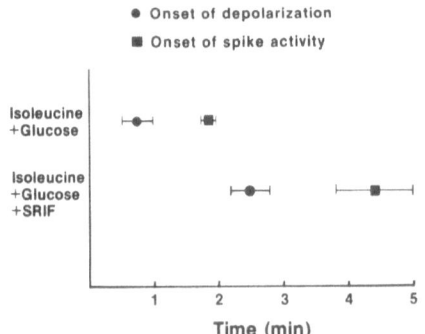

Fig. 4. Effect of SRIF on time delay before onset of depolarization and spike activity induced by L-isoleucine. Each point represents the mean of 3 to 4 observations and the horizontal bars indicate the SEM.

inhibited, as indicated by studies showing that SRIF inhibits spike activity (1,2) and $^{45}CA^{++}$ entry (27). SRIF may decrease Ca^{++} permeability in addition to its effect on P_k. This would account for the decrease in $^{45}Ca^{++}$ entry, but the decrease in intracellular Ca^{++} cannot be responsible for the increase in P_k. According to the available evidence (24,25), an increase in the level of intracellular Ca^{++} activates a Ca^{++}-sensitive P_k leading to hyperpolarization. Evidently SRIF increases P_k independently of the Ca^{++}-sensitive P_k; an alternative mechanism may be that it increases an ATP-sensitive P_k that is insensitive to Ca^{++} as identified by the patch clamp technique (30,31). This may be true of metabolizable substrates glucose and isoleucine, but another mechanism may account for the lack of an effect of SRIF on glyburide-induced electrical activity. It is assumed that SRIF would inhibit glyburide-induced secretory activity since the hormone inhibits tolbutamide-induced insulin secretion in other preparations (6,7,10). It is possible that SRIF inhibits glyburide-induced insulin release by influencing the levels of cyclic AMP or intracellular Ca^{++} (1) without a direct effect on P_k and electrical activity. The inhibitory effect of SRIF on the generation of cyclic AMP may lead to an additional reduction in the level of cytosolic Ca^{++}. The decrease in cyclic AMP and Ca^{++} would disrupt the modulatory influence of these second messengers on other sites in the activation of the secretory complex. Alternatively, it may be that a higher concentration of SRIF than used in our experiments is required to inhibit the electrical activity. Nevertheless, the ability of SRIF to inhibit glucose-, isoleucine-, but not glyburide-induced electrical activity suggests that somatostatin influences the same or different K^+ channels stimulated by glucose and isoleucine, but does not influence that affected by glyburide.

ACKNOWLEDGMENTS

The author is grateful to Kelly Goldsmith for her technical assistance and Lou Pandelis for typing the manuscript. The work was supported by National Institutes of Health Award AM21973 and National Science Foundation Grant PCM-8309252.

REFERENCES

1. Pace CS. Somatostatin: control of stimulus-secretion coupling in pancreatic islet cells. In: Bloom FE, ed. Peptides: integrators of cell and tissue function. New York: Raven Press, 1980.
2. Pace CS, Tarvin JT. Somatostatin: mechanism of action in pancreatic islet B-cells. Diabetes 1981; 37:836-42.
3. Alberti KGMM, Christensen SE, Iversen J, et al. Inhibition of insulin secretion by somatostatin. Lancet 1973; 2:1299-1301.
4. Chideckel EW, Palmer J, Koerker DJ, Ensinck J, Davidson MB, Goodner CJ. Somatostatin blockade of acute and chronic stimuli of the endocrine pancreas and the consequences of this blockage on glucose homeostasis. J Clin Invest 1975; 55:754-62.
5. Efendic S, Luft R. Studies on the mechanism of somatostatin action on insulin release in man. I. Effect of blockade of α-adrenergic receptors. Acta Endocrinol (Copenh) 1975; 78:516-23.
6. Efendic S, Luft R, Claro A. Studies on the mechanism of somatostatin action on insulin release in man. II. Comparison of the effects of somatostatin on insulin release induced by glucose, glucagon and tolbutamide. Acta Endocrinol (Copenh) 1976; 81:743-52.
7. Gerich JE, Lorenzi M, Schneider V, Forsham PH. Effect of somatostatin on plasma glucose and insulin responses to glucagon and tolbutamide in man. J Clin Endocrinol Metab 1974; 39:1057-60.

8. Koerker DJ, Ruch W, Chideckel E, et al. Somatostatin: hypothalamic inhibitor of the endocrine pancreas. Science 1974; 184:482-4.

9. Leblanc H, Anderson JR, Sigel MB, Yen SSC. Inhibitory action of somatostatin on pancreatic α and B-cell function. J Clin Endocrinol Metab 1975; 40:568-72.

10. Iversen J, Hermansen K. Characterization of the inhibitory effect of somatostatin upon insulin and glucagon release in the isolated perfused canine pancreas: evidence for interaction with calcium. Metabolism 1980; 29:151-60.

11. Henquin JC, Meissner HP. Effects of amino acids on membrane potential and ^{86}Rb fluxes in pancreatic B-cells. Am J Physiol 1981; 240:E245-52.

12. Henquin JC, Meissner HP. Opposite effects of tolbutamide and diazoxide on ^{86}Rb fluxes and membrane potential in pancreatic B-cells. Biochem Pharmacol 1982; 31:1407-15.

13. Gylfe E, Hellman B, Sehlin J, Taljedal I-B. Interaction of sulfonylurea with the pancreatic B-cell. Experientia 1984; 40:1126-34.

14. Boschero AC, Malaisse WJ. Stimulus-secretion coupling of glucose-induced insulin release. XXIX. Regulation of ^{86}Rb$^+$ efflux from perifused islets. Am J Physiol 1979; 236:E139-46.

15. Sehlin J, Taljedal I-B. Transport of rubidium and sodium in pancreatic islets. Am J Physiol 1979; 236:E139-46.

16. Boschero AC, Kawazu S, Duncan G, Malaisse WJ. Effect of glucose on K$^+$ handling by pancreatic islets. FEBS Lett 1977; 83:151-4.

17. Henquin JC. D-Glucose inhibits potassium efflux from pancreatic islet cells. Nature 1978; 271:271-3.

18. Malaisse WJ, Boschero AC, Kawazu S, Hutton JC. The stimulus secretion coupling of glucose-induced insulin release. XXVII. Effect of glucose on K$^+$ fluxes in isolated islets. Pflugers Arch 1978; 373: 237-42.

19. Armstrong CM. Interaction of tetraethylammonium ion derivatives with the potassium channels of giant axons. J Gen Physiol 1971; 58:413-37.

20. Hille B. Ionic channels in nerve membranes. Prog Biophys Mol Biol (US) 1970; 21:1-32.

21. Stanfield PR. The effect of the tetraethylammonium ion on the delayed currents of frog skeletal muscle. J Physiol (Lond) 1970; 209:209-29.

22. Henquin JC. Tetraethylammonium potentiation of insulin release and inhibition of rubidium efflux in pancreatic islets. Biochem Biophys Res Commun 1977; 77:551-6.

23. Atwater I, Ribalet B, Rojas E. Mouse pancreatic B-cells: tetraethylammonium blockage of the potassium permeability increase induced by depolarization. J Physiol (Lond) 1979; 288:561-74.

24. Lew VL, Ferreira HG. Variable Ca sensitivity of a K-selective channel in intact red cell membranes. Nature 1976; 263:336-8.

25. Atwater I, Dawson CM, Ribalet B, Rojas E. Potassium permeability activated by intracellular calcium ion concentration in the pancreatic B-cell. J Physiol (Lond) 1979; 288:575-88.

26. Henquin JC, Horemans B, Nenquin M, Verniers J, Lambert AE. Quinine induced modifications of insulin release and glucose metabolism by isolated pancreatic islets. FEBS Lett 1975; 57:280-4.

27. Oliver JR. Inhibition of calcium uptake by somatostatin in isolated rat islets of Langerhans. Endocrinology 1976; 99:910-3.

28. Bent-Hansen L, Capito K, Hedeskov CJ. The effect of calcium on somatostatin inhibition of insulin release and cyclic AMP production in mouse pancreatic islets. Biochem Biophys Acta 1979; 585:240-9.

29. Lin BJ. Effects of somatostatin on insulin biosynthesis, glucose oxidation, and cyclic guanosine monophosphate level. Metabolism 1978; 27(suppl 1):1295-8.

30. Cook DR, Hales CN. Intracellular ATP directly blocks K$^+$ channels in

pancreatic B-cells. Nature 1984; 311:271-3.

31. Rorsman P, Trube G. Glucose dependent K^+ channels in pancreatic B-cells are regulated by intracellular ATP. Pflugers Arch 1985; 405:305-9.

12

MECHANISMS BY WHICH SOMATOSTATIN INHIBITS PITUITARY HORMONE RELEASE*

Agnes Schonbrunn and Bruce D. Koch

Laboratory of Toxicology
Harvard School of Public Health
Boston, Massachusetts

INTRODUCTION

Since somatostatin inhibits secretion in a wide variety of target cells, studies probing its mechanism of action have focused on the involvement of the two intracellular messengers known to regulate secretory processes: cyclic AMP and calcium (see reviews 1-5). It has been hypothesized that somatostatin not only regulates the concentrations of cyclic AMP and cytosolic calcium, but also modifies the effectiveness of a constant amount of each of these intracellular messengers. Although direct evidence showing that somatostatin is able to regulate the effectiveness of either cyclic AMP or calcium is still lacking, recent studies have begun to clarify how somatostatin alters the concentrations of these two intracellular messengers and the extent to which such changes are involved in mediating somatostatin's effects on hormone secretion. This review summarizes studies on the mechanisms by which somatostatin inhibits growth hormone (GH) and prolactin (PRL) secretion from GH pituitary cells. These cells have two major advantages for elucidating the biochemical mediators involved in somatostatin action. First, the effects of somatostatin to inhibit GH and PRL secretion in GH_4C_1 cells parallel its actions in estrogen primed pituitary cells both in primary culture and in vivo (4,6-9). Second, GH_4C_1 cells are clonal in origin and therefore both hormonal and biochemical responses are produced by the same population of target cells and can be quantitatively correlated.

RESULTS

Biological Actions of Somatostatin in GH_4C_1 Cells

Somatostatin inhibits the secretion of PRL and GH by GH_4C_1 cells in a parallel manner and these effects occur at physiological concentrations of peptide ($IC_{50} = 0.7$ nM) (10,11). The biological response is rapid:

---

* The experiments described in this review were supported by a research grant from the NIADDK (AM-32234). BDK was the recipient of an Institutional National Research Service Award (5T32GM07258) and a fellowship from the Albert J. Ryan Foundation, Cincinnati, OH.

Following addition of 100 nM somatostatin, maximal inhibition of hormone secretion is observed within 5 minutes, the earliest time examined (10, unpublished observations). Inhibition remains unabated for at least 3 hours in the continued presence of peptide (10). Somatostatin decreases hormone release under most conditions: it not only inhibits basal secretion, but it also reduces secretion stimulated by secretagogues which utilize a variety of intracellular messengers (10-12). For example, somatostatin noncompetitively inhibits the stimulatory effect of vasoactive intestinal peptide (VIP), which acts by increasing the activity of adenylate cyclase and elevating intracellular cyclic AMP levels (11,13). In addition, somatostatin inhibits stimulation by thyrotropin releasing hormone (TRH) and bombesin which act by increasing phospholipase C activity and thereby elevate intracellular levels of diacylglycerol, inositol polyphosphates and cytosolic free calcium ($[Ca^{2+}]_i$) (12,14-16).

Binding studies with $[^{125}I-Tyr^1]$somatostatin have shown that intact GH_4C_1 cells contain a single class of specific, high-affinity receptors for somatostatin which appear to mediate the biological actions of this peptide (10,17). Unlike most other peptide hormones, receptor-bound somatostatin is not rapidly internalized but remains at the cell surface during the time that secretion is inhibited (18). Therefore, somatostatin must elicit its intracellular effects from the plasma membrane.

Somatostatin Inhibits Hormone Secretion by at Least Two Mechanisms

As with most secretory cells, increasing intracellular cyclic AMP concentrations with any of several pharmacological agents markedly stimulates hormone release by GH_4C_1 cells (11,19,20). Therefore, one potential mechanism for inhibiting secretion is to reduce cyclic AMP levels. In fact, several lines of evidence indicate that somatostatin does inhibit hormone secretion by regulating the intracellular concentration of cyclic AMP. Although somatostatin does not significantly reduce basal intracellular cyclic AMP levels, it consistently inhibits stimulation of cyclic AMP accumulation by VIP (13). Inhibition of VIP-stimulated cyclic AMP accumulation by somatostatin is maximal within 15 seconds, the earliest time tested (13,21). Therefore, this effect appears to be sufficiently rapid to initiate somatostatin's inhibition of VIP-stimulated hormone release. The concentrations of somatostatin which cause half-maximal inhibition of VIP-stimulated cyclic AMP accumulation (IC_{50} = 1.2 nM) and prolactin secretion (IC_{50} = 0.7 nM) are similar (11,13). In addition, somatostatin reduces the effect of maximal concentrations of VIP on both cyclic AMP accumulation and hormone secretion, but it does not significantly alter the dose-response characteristics of VIP for either response (11,13). These results support the conclusion that changes in cyclic AMP levels mediate the inhibitory effect of somatostatin on VIP-stimulated hormone secretion.

In contrast to the close parallel between the effects of somatostatin on VIP-stimulated cyclic AMP accumulation and VIP-stimulated hormone release, there is a clear discrepancy between the ability of somatostatin to inhibit basal hormone secretion and its lack of effect on basal cyclic AMP levels (11,13). If the effect of somatostatin on VIP-stimulated cyclic AMP production indeed has biological significance, this discrepancy must be resolved. Two hypotheses are possible. Somatostatin may cause undetectably small changes in basal cyclic AMP levels which are nonetheless biologically significant and, therefore, it may inhibit both basal and VIP-stimulated secretion by the same mechanism. Alternatively, somatostatin may activate two different mechanisms: inhibition of VIP-stimulated hormone release could be mediated by alterations in cyclic AMP levels, while inhibition of basal hormone release would occur independently of changes in cyclic AMP concentrations. To distinguish between these two hypotheses, we determined whether elevating intracellular cyclic AMP levels pharmacologically blocked somatostatin inhibition of hormone secretion.

Cyclic AMP analogs directly stimulate cyclic AMP-dependent protein kinases and, therefore, elicit cyclic AMP inducible effects at a site distal to the activation of adenylate cyclase (22). We have found that the analog 8-(4-chlorophenylthio)-cyclic AMP [(Cl-ϕ-S)cAMP] causes a dose-dependent stimulation of PRL release in GH_4C_1 cells (23). Somatostatin does not affect the potency of (Cl-ϕ-S)cAMP to increase secretion, but reduces the stimulation produced by maximum concentrations of this secretagogue (23). These results demonstrate that somatostatin can inhibit hormone secretion in the presence of maximally effective intracellular cyclic AMP levels. In this situation, the high (Cl-ϕ-S)cAMP concentrations would overwhelm any undetectably small reduction in cyclic AMP levels which somatostatin might produce in the absence of a stimulator of adenylate cyclase. Therefore, when maximal concentrations of a cyclic AMP analog are present, inhibition of hormone secretion by somatostatin must be independent of changes in cyclic AMP levels: i.e., somatostatin must have a cyclic AMP-independent mechanism of action. This conclusion is supported by similar experiments in which cyclic AMP levels were pharmacologically increased by another cyclic AMP analog, 8-Br-cAMP, and by forskolin, a very effective activator of adenylate cyclase (4,11).

Having established that somatostatin inhibits hormone secretion by a cyclic AMP-independent mechanism, we wanted to determine whether its action to reduce VIP-stimulated cyclic AMP accumulation was biologically significant. The results in Figure 1 show that somatostatin was more effective at inhibiting the stimulatory effect of maximal concentrations of VIP than of (Cl-ϕ-S)cAMP, consistent with somatostatin decreasing cyclic AMP levels only in the presence of VIP. Furthermore, when maximum concentrations of VIP and (Cl-ϕ-S)cAMP were added together, somatostatin decreased PRL secretion less than in the presence of VIP. Thus, (Cl-ϕ-S)cAMP reduced, but did not prevent, somatostatin inhibition of VIP-stimulated hormone release. These results clearly indicate that inhibition of VIP-stimulated cyclic AMP accumulation is at least partially responsible for somatostatin's reduction of VIP-stimulated hormone secretion. This conclusion is substantiated by similar experiments using forskolin, instead of (Cl-ϕ-S)cAMP, to elevate intracellular cyclic AMP levels (4,11).

In summary, our results show that somatostatin acts by at least two different mechanisms: inhibition of VIP-stimulated hormone secretion is largely due to inhibition of VIP-stimulated cyclic AMP accumulation, whereas inhibition of (Cl-ϕ-S)cAMP-stimulated hormone secretion, and probably also basal hormone secretion, are independent of changes in intracellular cyclic AMP levels.

Somatostatin Reduces Intracellular Cyclic AMP by Inhibiting Adenylate Cyclase

Somatostatin could decrease cyclic AMP accumulation either by stimulating cyclic AMP degradation or by inhibiting cyclic AMP synthesis. To identify the primary site of somatostatin action in intact GH_4C_1 cells, we determined the degree to which somatostatin inhibited VIP-stimulated cyclic AMP accumulation in the presence of varying concentrations of the phosphodiesterase inhibitor 3-isobutyl-1-methylxanthine (IBMX) (13). Although increasing IBMX concentrations markedly elevated cyclic AMP levels, both in the absence and presence of VIP, the degree to which somatostatin inhibited VIP stimulation was not altered (13). If somatostatin acts to stimulate phosphodiesterases, pharmacological inhibition of these enzymes should block reduction of cyclic AMP levels. Since somatostatin's effect was not reduced by IBMX, the peptide must decrease cAMP concentrations primarily by inhibiting adenylate cyclase.

To investigate the mechanism by which somatostatin regulates adenylate cyclase, we examined the interaction between the somatostatin receptor and components of the adenylate cyclase system (21,24). In parallel with the lack of effect of somatostatin on basal cyclic AMP levels in cells, somatostatin did not significantly alter unstimulated adenylate cyclase activity in GH_4C_1 cell membranes (24). However, in both membranes and cells somatostatin decreased the maximal stimulatory effect of VIP, without changing its potency. Half-maximal inhibition of adenylate cyclase was produced by 2.3 nM somatostatin, which is close to the IC_{50} for somatostatin inhibition of cyclic AMP accumulation in intact cells (1.2 nM) (13,24). Furthermore, several somatostatin analogs were shown to have similar relative potencies to inhibit cyclic AMP production in cells and adenylate cyclase activity in membrane preparations (13,24). Thus, there is a close parallel between the effects of somatostatin on cyclic AMP accumulation in intact cells and on adenylate cyclase activity in membranes.

Like other receptors which regulate adenylate cyclase activity (25), the somatostatin receptor is coupled to this enzyme by a guanine nucleotide binding protein. Thus, both GTP and the nonhydrolyzable GTP analog Gpp(NH)p, decreased the saturable binding of $[^{125}I\text{-}Tyr^1]$somatostatin to GH_4C_1 cell membranes, whereas the nonhydrolyzable ATP analog App(NH)p had no effect (24). GTP did not alter the number of somatostatin receptors in GH_4C_1 cell membranes; rather, it reduced the affinity of these sites for somatostatin (24). Furthermore, the decrease in binding affinity induced by guanine nucleotides could be explained by an increase in the rate constant for somatostatin dissociation (24). In fact, results from kinetic experiments indicated that somatostatin receptors exist in two interconvertible forms with different affinities for agonists. Guanine nucleotides regulate conversion of the receptor between a slowly dissociating, high affinity form, and a rapidly dissociating, low affinity form

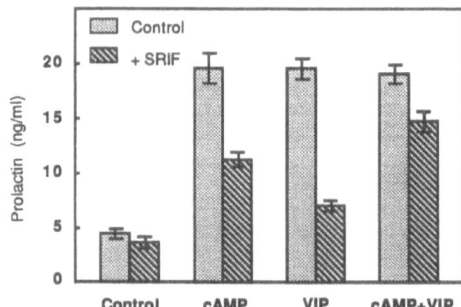

Fig. 1. Effect of (Cl-ϕ-S)cAMP on somatostatin inhibition of VIP-stimulated PRL secretion. GH_4C_1 cells were incubated with or without 100 nM somatostatin (SRIF) either in the absence of any secretagogue (control) or in the presence of 1 mM (Cl-ϕ-S)cAMP, 100 nM VIP, or both agents. The amount of PRL released into the medium in 30 min was measured by RIA.

(24). This behavior mimics that of beta-adrenergic receptors, which stimulate cyclase (26), and indicates that a guanine nucleotide binding protein mediates inhibition of adenylate cyclase by the somatostatin receptor in a manner analogous to the action of stimulatory receptors (24).

To determine whether the guanine nucleotide binding protein which couples the somatostatin receptor to adenylate cyclase is N_i, a protein which mediates inhibition of this enzyme by other receptors, we utilized the Bordetella pertussis toxin, islet-activating protein (27-29). Pertussis toxin catalyzes the transfer of ADP-ribose from NAD to a 41,000-Da membrane-associated guanine nucleotide binding protein which is the alpha subunit of N_i. This covalent modification prevents inhibition of adenylate cyclase by a variety of hormones and neurotransmitters (27-29). Pretreatment of GH_4C_1 cells with this toxin completely blocked somatostatin inhibition of VIP-stimulated cyclic AMP accumulation (21). Furthermore, somatostatin inhibition of VIP-stimulated adenylate cyclase activity was reduced in membranes prepared from pertussis toxin pretreated cells (21). The only substrate for pertussis toxin catalyzed ADP-ribosylation in GH cell membranes is a 41,000-Da protein (30,31; R. Huff, B. Koch, E. Neer and A. Schonbrunn, unpublished observations). Therefore, our results suggest that inhibition of VIP-stimulated adenylate cyclase by the occupied somatostatin receptor is mediated by the inhibitory guanine nucleotide binding protein, N_i.

Both Mechanisms of Somatostatin Action are Blocked by Pertussis Toxin

Since pertussis toxin treatment prevented somatostatin inhibition of VIP-stimulated adenylate cyclase and cyclic AMP accumulation, we expected that it should also block those biological actions of somatostatin which result from this inhibition. The data in Figure 2 demonstrate that pertussis toxin pretreatment did prevent somatostatin inhibition of VIP-stimulated PRL release (21). Surprisingly, somatostatin inhibition of basal hormone secretion, although small in the amino-acid free buffer used in this experiment, was also blocked in pertussis toxin-treated cells (Fig. 2). Similarly, pertussis toxin pretreatment prevented the more substantial inhibition of basal hormone secretion produced by somatostatin in serum free growth medium (21).

To further characterize the effect of pertussis toxin treatment on the cyclic AMP-independent actions of somatostatin, we used four secretagogues which do not regulate adenylate cyclase activity (Fig. 2). 8-Br-cAMP, like (Cl-ϕ-S)cAMP, directly activates cyclic AMP-dependent protein kinases and thereby circumvents the adenylate cyclase system. High extracellular K^+ is believed to stimulate hormone release by depolarizing the plasma membrane, opening voltage-sensitive Ca^{2+} channels, and increasing intracellular free Ca^{2+} concentrations ($[Ca^{2+}]_i$). Elevated extracellular K^+ does not affect intracellular cyclic AMP levels in GH_4C_1 cells at any time from 30 s to 30 min either in the presence or in the absence of somatostatin (21). TRH and bombesin also do not reproducibly alter cyclic AMP levels in GH_4C_1 cells (13), and have been proposed to stimulate secretion by increasing the hydrolysis of polyphosphatidyl inositols and subsequently elevating $[Ca^{2+}]_i$ and diacylglycerol (14-16). Somatostatin does not alter cyclic AMP levels in the presence of either of these peptides (13). The results in Figure 2 show that pertussis toxin treatment did not affect the degree to which 8-Br-cAMP, K^+, TRH or bombesin increased prolactin release. However, the toxin blocked somatostatin inhibition of hormone secretion under all conditions (21,31). The ability of pertussis toxin to prevent somatostatin inhibition of hormone secretion stimulated by a variety of pharmacological and physiological secretagogues which do not affect adenylate cyclase, suggests that the cyclic AMP-independent mechanism by which somatostatin inhibits hormone secretion requires N_1 or another pertussis toxin-sensitive guanine nucleotide binding protein.

It is not known how many pertussis toxin sensitive GTP-binding proteins interact with the somatostatin receptor. Although pertussis toxin ADP-ribosylates only a single 41,000 dalton protein in GH_4C_1 cell membranes (R. Huff, B. Koch, E. Neer and A. Schonbrunn, unpublished observations), it is certainly possible that the toxin has multiple targets in intact cells. In fact, even though the alpha subunit of N_1 is either the sole or the major protein modified by pertussis toxin in most membrane preparations, three other GTP-binding proteins can be ADP-ribosylated by pertussis toxin in some systems (32-34). Furthermore, two different pertussis toxin substrates, N_1 and N_o, have been shown to couple to the same receptor in reconstitution experiments (35). Unfortunately, there is no practical method for detecting those pertussis toxin substrates which are ADP-ribosylated only in whole cells. The assay used to determine whether a particular protein is ADP-ribosylated in cells involves preparing membranes from control and toxin-treated cultures and then comparing the extent to which pertussis toxin can transfer $[^{32}P]$ADP-ribose from $[^{32}P]$NAD to different molecular weight proteins in the two preparations (27-29). Therefore, the only in vivo effects of the toxin which can be detected are those which prevent pertussis toxin catalyzed ADP-ribosylation in membranes.

To explore the possibility that the somatostatin receptor was coupled to more than one type of GTP-binding protein, we took advantage of the observation that different guanine nucleotide binding proteins are ADP-ribosylated with different efficiencies by pertussis toxin (32). Thus, we

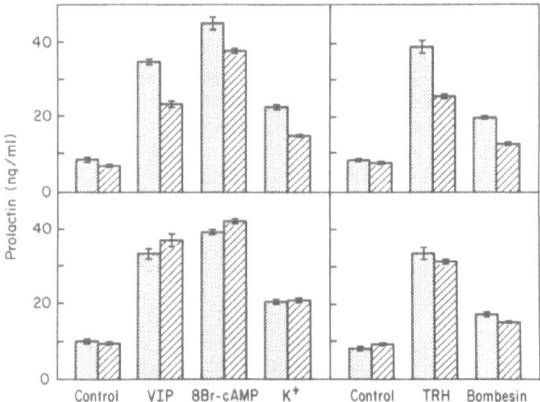

Fig. 2. Effect of pertussis toxin on somatostatin inhibition of PRL release. Cells were pretreated overnight without (upper panels) or with (lower panels) 50 ng/ml pertussis toxin. PRL release was then determined during a 30-min incubation either in the absence (☐) or presence (▨) of 100 nM somatostatin and the secretagogues shown (21). The concentrations of secretagogues used were as follows: VIP, 100 nM; 8-Br-cAMP, 5 mM; K^+, 11 mM; TRH, 1 μM; bombesin, 100 nM.

determined the concentration dependence for pertussis toxin blockage of somatostatin inhibition of VIP-stimulated as well as K^+-stimulated prolactin secretion (21). Both effects of somatostatin were completely blocked by pertussis toxin with the same potency (ED_{50} = 0.3 ng/ml) (21). Although not definitive, these results suggest that the toxin acts at a single, common site to prevent these two actions of somatostatin and, therefore, that N_i may be involved in both the cyclic AMP-dependent and the cyclic AMP-independent mechanism by which somatostatin inhibits secretion.

Equilibrium binding studies with $[^{125}I\text{-}Tyr^1]$somatostatin and intact GH_4C_1 cells have shown that these cells contain a single class of high-affinity binding sites for somatostatin (10). Furthermore, the potencies of somatostatin and 19 somatostatin analogs to inhibit VIP-stimulated cyclic AMP production and basal PRL secretion correlated closely with their receptor binding affinities (17). These results indicate that the characterized binding sites represent the biologically relevant receptors that mediate the actions of somatostatin by both the cyclic AMP dependent and cyclic AMP independent mechanisms. Therefore, the simplest hypothesis which explains the currently available data is that somatostatin initiates both its mechanisms by binding to a single class of receptors which interact with a single type of pertussis toxin sensitive GTP-binding protein, probably N_i.

Somatostatin Causes Membrane Hyperpolarization and Decreases $[Ca^{2+}]$ by a cAMP Independent Mechanism

The biochemical events involved in somatostatin's inhibition of hormone secretion by the cyclic AMP-independent mechanism are unknown. It is unlikely that changes in phosphatidylinositol turnover are involved since somatostatin does not affect basal or TRH-stimulated $^{32}PO_4$ incorporation into phospholipids (16) or diacylglycerol production (31). However, several independent lines of evidence have indicated that regulation of $[Ca^{2+}]_i$ might be involved in at least some of somatostatin's biological actions (1-5). Recently, somatostatin has been shown to decrease $[Ca^{2+}]_i$ and hyperpolarize GH cells (21,36). These effects are shown in Figure 3. Changes in the membrane potential were monitored with the fluorescent dye bisoxonol (37-39). Because bisoxonol is a lipophilic anion which freely permeates the cells, its distribution across the plasma membrane is dependent upon the membrane potential (37-39). Upon binding of bisoxonol to hydrophobic molecules, an increase in the quantum efficiency of the dye occurs, leading to a larger fluorescence signal (37). Thus, an increase in bisoxonol fluorescence indicates that the membrane potential has depolarized, allowing more of this negatively charged dye to enter the cells. The concentration of intracellular free calcium in GH_4C_1 cells was measured by following the fluorescence of the calcium sensitive dye, Quin-2 (21). The experiment shown in Figure 3 demonstrates that somatostatin causes both a hyperpolarization and a decrease in $[Ca^{2+}]_i$ within 30 seconds.

Since somatostatin does not significantly decrease intracellular cyclic AMP levels in the absence of a stimulator of adenylate cyclase (13,21), its ionic effects are unlikely to result from changes in cyclic AMP concentrations. Nonetheless, it was possible that undetectably small changes in basal cyclic AMP levels mediated somatostatin's effects on the membrane potential and/or on the $[Ca^{2+}]_i$. Therefore, we determined whether supramaximal cyclic AMP concentrations blocked somatostatin's ability to elicit these ionic changes (Fig. 4, 23). Addition of 0.5 mM (Cl-ϕ-S)cAMP to cells raised the $[Ca^{2+}]_i$, but further increasing the (Cl-ϕ-S)cAMP concentration to 1 mM had no additional effect (Fig. 4). This result indicates that either 1 mM (Cl-ϕ-S)cAMP constituted a maximally effective concentration or the response to (Cl-ϕ-S)cAMP had desensitized. Somatostatin added after the cyclic AMP analog still decreased $[Ca^{2+}]_i$ (Fig. 4). Similarly, somatostatin was able to cause membrane hyperpolarization in the presence of a maximal concentration of (Cl-ϕ-S) cAMP (23). Since somatostatin elicited both ionic effects in the presence of maximal, as well as basal, cyclic AMP_2 levels, it must produce the hyperpolarization and the reduction in $[Ca^{2+}]_i$ by cyclic AMP-independent mechanisms.

Pertussis Toxin Blocks the Somatostatin Induced Hyperpolarization and Reduction in $[Ca^{2+}]_i$

Previous results showed that pretreatment of GH_4C_1 cells with pertussis toxin prevented the cyclic AMP-independent mechanism by which somatostatin inhibits hormone secretion (Fig. 2, 21). Therefore, if the ionic effects of somatostatin mediate its cyclic AMP-independent biological actions, they should also be inhibited by pertussis toxin. The results in Figure 5 show that pertussis toxin blocked the reduction of both basal and K^+-elevated $[Ca^{2+}]_i$ by somatostatin (21). In addition, the membrane hyperpolarization produced by somatostatin was also prevented by toxin pretreatment (40). These results indicate that N_i, or another related GTP-binding protein, couple the somatostatin receptor to a reduction in the $[Ca^{2+}]_i$ and membrane hyperpolarization and that this coupling mechanism bypasses the adenylate cyclase system. Furthermore, because the effects of somatostatin on the $[Ca^{2+}]_i$ and the membrane potential are independent of changes in cyclic AMP concentrations, they may provide the biophysical basis for the cyclic AMP-independent mechanism by which somatostatin inhibits hormone secretion.

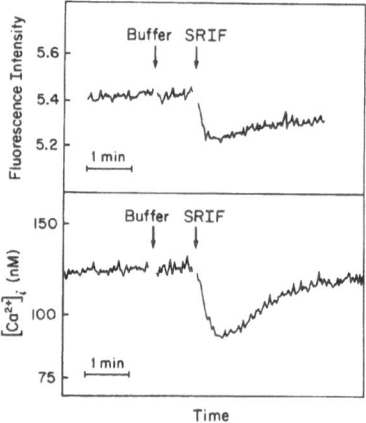

Fig. 3. Effect of somatostatin upon the membrane potential and $[Ca^{2+}]_i$. Top panel: Changes in the membrane potential were monitored by measuring the fluorescence of bisoxonol in the presence of GH_4C_1 cells (37). Bottom panel: The $[Ca^{2+}]_i$ was determined in cells by monitoring the fluorescence of intracellular Quin-2. $[Ca^{2+}]_i$ were calculated from the intensity of the fluorescent signal as previously described (21). In both panels, arrows show the addition of buffer (2 mM acetic acid, 0.1% BSA) or 100 nM somatostatin.

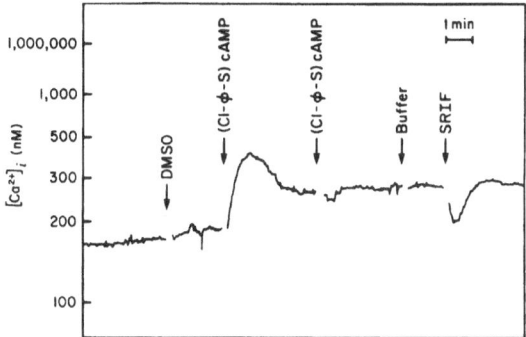

Fig. 4. Effect of (Cl-ϕ-S)cAMP on the decrease in $[Ca^{2+}]_i$ produced by somatostatin. The $[Ca^{2+}]_i$ was determined by monitoring the fluorescence of intracellular Quin-2 as previously described (21). Arrows show two sequential additions of 0.5 mM (Cl-ϕ-S)cAMP, buffer, and 100 nM somatostatin.

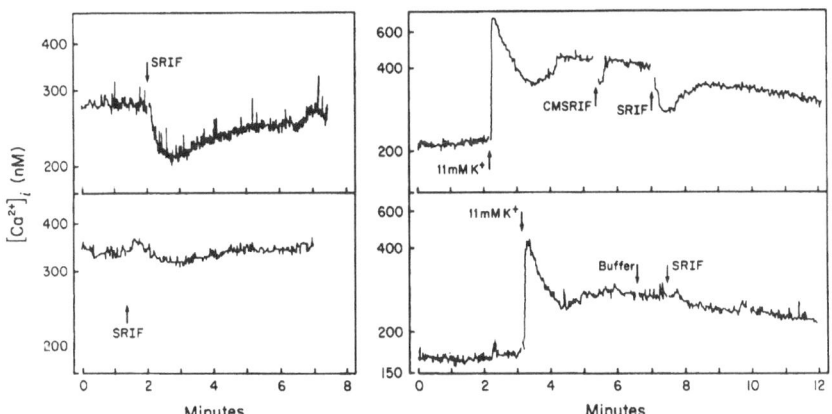

Fig. 5. Effect of pertussis toxin on somatostatin regulation of $[Ca^{2+}]_i$. Cells were incubated overnight with either medium alone (top panels) or with maximum concentrations of pertussis toxin (lower panels). Changes in $[Ca^{2+}]_i$ were determined by monitoring the fluorescence of intracellular Quin-2 as previously described (21). Arrows mark the addition of 11 mM K^+, 100 nM somatostatin (SRIF), 100 nM dicarboxymethyl somatostatin (CMSRIF, a relatively inactive analog), or buffer. The left two panels show the effects of somatostatin on basal $[Ca^{2+}]_i$ and the right two panels show the effects of somatostatin on $[Ca^{2+}]_i$ elevated by 11 mM $[K^+]_e$ (21).

Somatostatin's Cyclic AMP Independent Actions Require a Transmembrane
Potassium Ion Gradient

Since GH_4C_1 cells are electrically active (41), their membrane
potential is controlled primarily by the concentration gradients and
relative permeabilities of K^+, Na^+, Ca^{2+}, and Cl^-. Therefore, to determine whether the transmembrane movement of these ions is necessary for
somatostatin to elicit either the hyperpolarization or the reduction in
$[Ca^{2+}]_i$, we examined the integrity of these somatostatin responses when
the concentration gradients of these ions were altered (23). Substitution
of choline for all extracellular Na^+ had no effect on either the hyperpolarization or the decrease in $[Ca^{2+}]_i$ induced by somatostatin. Although
decreasing the extracellular Cl^- concentration did inhibit the hyperpolarization and the decrease in $[Ca^{2+}]_i$ to some extent, it did not block
these responses in a manner consistent with a requirement for a transg-
membrane Cl^- gradient (23). In contrast, decreasing extracellular Ca^{2+}
from 1 mM to 250 nM abolished somatostatin's reduction of the $[Ca^{2+}]_i$, but
did not block the hyperpolarization response. These results indicate that
the somatostatin induced hyperpolarization is not primarily due to changes
in the conductances of Na^+, Cl^-, or Ca^{2+}. However, the somatostatin
induced decrease in $[Ca^{2+}]_i$ requires Ca^{2+} influx, although it is also
independent of the Na^+ and Cl^- gradients.

Somatostatin's actions were most markedly affected by changes in the
K^+ gradient. Elevating extracellular K^+ concentrations from 4.6 to 50 mM
completely blocked both the somatostatin-induced hyperpolarization and the
reduction in $[Ca^{2+}]_i$. Furthermore, the magnitude of the hyperpolarization
response decreased exponentially with increasing extracellular $[K^+]$,
consistent with it being directly dependent upon the K^+ gradient.
Together, these results support the conclusion that the primary cyclic
AMP-independent effect of somatostatin is to increase K^+ conductance, and
that the effect on $[Ca^{2+}]_i$ is secondary to this change (23). Therefore,
our studies indicate that the somatostatin-induced hyperpolarization
probably causes the decrease in $[Ca^{2+}]_i$ by reducing Ca^{2+} influx through
the voltage-dependent Ca^{2+} channels which exist in GH cells (41,42).

Using voltage-clamp techniques, Barker and Dufy found that somatostatin activates a transient outward current in GH cells (43). These
results support the conclusion that somatostatin increases a K^+ conductance. Furthermore, somatostatin reduced spontaneous Ca^{2+} action potentials (43). It seems likely that the decrease in the rate of Ca^{2+} action
potentials reduces Ca^{2+} influx sufficiently to account for the decrease in
$[Ca^{2+}]_i$ produced by somatostatin.

Since a K^+ gradient was required for the cyclic AMP-independent
effects of somatostatin on the membrane potential and the $[Ca^{2+}]_i$, we
explored the importance of this ion in the peptide's cyclic AMP-
independent inhibition of hormone secretion (23). High extracellular K^+
concentrations ($\geq$ 50 mM) completely reversed somatostatin inhibition of
secretion (23), indicating that the cAMP-independent mechanism of somatostatin action is mediated by an increase in K^+ conductance.

SUMMARY

Somatostatin inhibits hormone secretion from GH cells by two mechanisms which appear to be triggered by a single class of receptors (Fig.
6). One mechanism involves inhibition of stimulated adenylate cyclase
activity. Inhibition of this enzyme by somatostatin reduces the cyclic
AMP generated by VIP and other secretagogues which activate adenylate
cyclase and consequently decreases stimulation of secretion. Somatostatin

130

also inhibits hormone secretion by a cyclic AMP-independent mechanism. In addition, somatostatin causes membrane hyperpolarization and reduces $[Ca^{2+}]_i$ independently of any changes in cyclic AMP levels. Our results indicate that an increase in K^+ conductance is the biophysical event responsible for somatostatin's cyclic AMP-independent effects on the membrane potential, on the $[Ca^{2+}]_i$, and on hormone secretion. Interestingly, the somatostatin receptor appears to be coupled both to inhibition of adenylate cyclase and to an increase in K^+ conductance by a pertussis toxin sensitive GTP-binding protein, probably N_i.

Accumulating evidence indicates that the mechanism of somatostatin action in somatotrophs is similar to that in GH_4C_1 cells. Although somatostatin consistently inhibits basal GH secretion, its effects on basal cyclic AMP levels in normal pituitary cells are variable and often not significant (44-48). In contrast, somatostatin inhibits prostaglandin- and growth hormone releasing factor (GRF)-stimulated cyclic AMP accumulation and GH release in parallel (49-51). Furthermore, somatostatin partially blocks prostaglandin and GRF stimulation of adenylate cyclase activity in rat anterior pituitary membranes (51,52). Finally, pretreatment of primary cultures of rat pituitary cells with pertussis toxin antagonizes somatostatin inhibition of both basal and GRF-stimulated GH release (53). These results indicate that the somatostatin receptor is

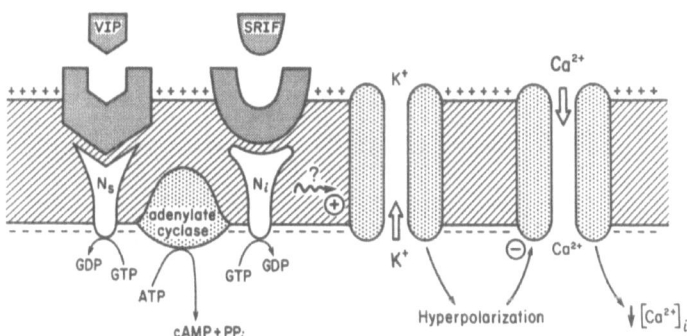

Fig. 6. Signal transduction mechanisms activated by somatostatin. This model shows the fewest components necessary to explain the two independent mechanisms by which somatostatin inhibits hormone release in GH_4C_1 cells. The receptors for VIP and somatostatin (SRIF) interact with two different GTP-binding proteins: N_s and N_i. These are the guanine nucleotide regulatory subunits which couple adenylate cyclase to stimulatory and inhibitory receptors, respectively. Activation of the somatostatin receptor causes inhibition of VIP-stimulated adenylate cyclase as well as enhancement of a K^+-conductance. Both of these actions are mediated by N_i, or another pertussis toxin sensitive GTP-binding protein. The decrease in intracellular cyclic AMP levels resulting from inhibition of adenylate cyclase produces the cyclic AMP-dependent actions of somatostatin. The increase in K^+ conductance results in hyperpolarization of the cell and therefore decreases Ca^{2+} influx through voltage sensitive channels. The resulting decrease in $[Ca^{2+}]_i$ is responsible for the cyclic AMP-independent actions of somatostatin.

coupled to the guanine nucleotide binding protein N_i in normal pituitary cells and that inhibition of adenylate cyclase may be responsible for somatostatin inhibition of GRF and prostaglandin-stimulated GH secretion. However, because somatostatin blocks GRF-stimulated GH release completely, but only partially inhibits GRF-stimulated cyclic AMP accumulation, a second mechanism has been postulated for somatostatin (51).

Very recently Yamashita et al. reported that, under current clamp conditions, somatostatin hyperpolarizes the membrane potential of human GH secreting adenoma cells (54). This effect coincides with both an increase in K^+ conductance and an inhibition of spontaneous action potential activity. The authors concluded that somatostatin increases a K^+ conductance, thereby hyperpolarizing the cells, and thus decreasing the frequency of Ca^{2+} action potentials by making the membrane potential more negative than threshold. A reduction in the frequency of Ca^{2+} action potentials could cause a reduction in $[Ca^{2+}]_i$. However, the effect of somatostatin on $[Ca^{2+}]_i$ has not yet been determined in somatotrophs.

In summary, somatostatin appears to regulate two membrane activities in both GH cells and somatotrophs: adenylate cyclase and a K^+ channel. We have shown that these two effects occur independently in GH cells and have provided evidence that they both play a role in somatostatin's effects on hormone secretion. However, in somatotrophs the relationship between somatostatin inhibition of adenylate cyclase and its stimulation of a K^+ conductance has yet to be critically examined. Furthermore, the nature of the K^+ channel regulated by somatostatin and the mechanisms by which it is coupled to the somatostatin receptor remains to be elucidated in any target cell. Finally, since several classes of somatostatin receptors may exist, it will be important to determine whether they activate the same or different membrane events. Thus, although the molecular mechanism of somatostatin action has certainly become better understood in the last few years a great deal remains to be learned.

ACKNOWLEDGMENTS

We thank W. Peter Burhoe for expert technical assistance, Dr. Marjorie Norman for critical comments on this manuscript, and Rebecca Siebens for secretarial help.

REFERENCES

1. Reichlin S. Somatostatin. N Engl J Med 1983; 309:1495 and 1556.
2. Gottesman IS, Mandarino LJ, Gerich JE. Somatostatin: its role in health and disease. In: Cohen MP, Foa PP, eds. Special topics in endocrinology and metabolism, vol 4. New York: Alan R. Liss Inc., 1982:177.
3. Pace CS. Somatostatin: control of stimulus-secretion coupling in pancreatic islet cells. In: Bloom FE, ed. Peptides: integrators of cell and tissue function. New York: Raven Press, 1980:163.
4. Schonbrunn A, Dorflinger LJ, Koch BD. Mechanisms of somatostatin action in pituitary cells. In: Patel Y, Tannenbaum G, eds. Somatostatin. New York: Plenum Press, 1985:305.
5. Patel YC, Srikant CB. Somatostatin mediation of adenohypophysial secretion. Annu Rev Physiol 1986; 48:551.
6. Vale W, Rivier C, Brazeau P, Guillemin R. Effects of somatostatin on the secretion of thyrotropin and prolactin. Endocrinology 1974; 95:968.
7. Drouin J, De Lean A, Rainville D, Lachance R, Labrie F. Characteristics of the interaction between thyrotropin-releasing hormone and

somatostatin for thyrotropin and prolactin release. Endocrinology 1976; 98:514.

8. Enjalbert A, Epelbaum J, Arancibia S, Tapia-Arancibia L, Blute-Pajot M-T, Kordon C. Reciprocal interactions of somatostatin with thyrotropin-releasing hormone and vasoactive intestinal peptide on prolactin and growth hormone secretion in vitro. Endocrinology 1982; 111:42.

9. Cooper GR, Shin SH. Somatostatin inhibits prolactin secretion in the estradiol primed male rat. Can J Physiol 1981; 59:1082.

10. Schonbrunn A, Tashjian AH Jr. Characterization of functional receptors for somatostatin in rat pituitary cells in culture. J Biol Chem 1978; 253:6473.

11. Dorflinger LJ, Schonbrunn A. Somatostatin inhibits basal and vasoactive intestinal peptide stimulated hormone release by different mechanisms in GH pituitary cells. Endocrinology 1983; 113:1551.

12. Westendorf JM, Schonbrunn A. Bombesin stimulates prolactin and growth hormone release by pituitary cells in culture. Endocrinology 1982; 110:352.

13. Dorflinger LJ, Schonbrunn A. Somatostatin inhibits vasoactive intestinal peptide-stimulated cyclic adenosine monophosphate accumulation in GH pituitary cells. Endocrinology 1983; 113:1541.

14. Gershengorn MC. Mechanism of thyrotropin releasing hormone stimulation of pituitary hormone secretion. Annu Rev Physiol 1986; 48:515.

15. Williams JA. Regulatory mechanisms in pancreas and salivary acini. Annu Rev Physiol 1984; 46:361.

16. Sutton CA, Martin TFJ. Thyrotropin releasing hormone (TRH) selectively and rapidly stimulates phosphatidylinositol turnover in GH pituitary cells: a possible second step of TRH action. Endocrinology 1982; 110:1273.

17. Schonbrunn A, Rorstad OP, Westendorf JM, Martin JB. Somatostatin analogs: correlation between receptor binding affinity and biological potency in GH pituitary cells. Endocrinology 1983; 113:1559.

18. Presky DH, Schonbrunn A. Receptor-bound somatostatin and epidermal growth factor are processed differently in GH_4C_1 rat pituitary cells. J Cell Biol 1986; 102:878.

19. Dannies PS, Gautvik KM, Tashjian AH Jr. A possible role of cyclic AMP in mediating the effects of thyrotropin-releasing hormone on prolactin release and on prolactin and growth hormone synthesis in pituitary cells in culture. Endocrinology 1976; 98:1147.

20. Dannies PS, Tashjian AH Jr. Action of cholera toxin on hormone synthesis and release in GH cells: evidence that adenosine 3'5'-monophosphate does not mediate the decrease in growth hormone synthesis caused by thyrotropin-releasing hormone. Endocrinology 1980; 106:1532.

21. Koch BD, Dorflinger LJ, Schonbrunn A. Pertussis toxin blocks both cyclic AMP-mediated and cyclic AMP-independent actions of somatostatin: evidence for coupling of N_i to decreases in intracellular free calcium. J Biol Chem 1985; 260(24):13138-45.

22. Miller JP. Cyclic nucleotide analogues. In: Cramer H, Schultz J, eds. Cyclic 3'5' nucleotides: mechanism of action. New York: John Wiley and Sons, 1977:77.

23. Koch BD, Schonbrunn A. A transmembrane K^+ gradient is required for somatostatin to decrease intracellular free $[Ca^{2+}]$ and inhibit hormone release via a cAMP-independent mechanism. Proceedings of the 16th Meeting of the Society for Neuroscience, 1986:734.

24. Koch BD, Schonbrunn A. The somatostatin receptor is directly coupled to adenylate cyclase in GH_4C_1 pituitary cell membranes. Endocrinology 1984; 114:1784.

25. Gilman AG. G proteins and dual control of adenylate cyclase. Cell 1984; 36:577.

26. De Lean A, Stadel JM, Lefkowitz RJ. A ternary complex model explains

the agonist-specific binding properties of the adenylate cyclase-coupled B-adrenergic receptor. J Biol Chem 1980; 255:7108.

27. Ui M, Katada T, Murayama T, et al. Islet-activating protein, pertussis toxin: a specific uncoupler of receptor-mediated inhibition of adenylate cyclase. In: Greengard P, ed. Advances in cyclic nucleotide and protein phosphorylation research, vol 17. New York: Raven Press, 1984:145.

28. Hewlett EL, Cronin MJ, Moss J, Anderson H, Myers GH, Pearson RD. Pertussis toxin: lessons from biological and biochemical effects in different cells. In: Greengard P, ed. Advances in cyclic nucleotide and protein phosphorylation research, vol 17. New York: Raven Press, 1984:173.

29. Sekura RD. Pertussis toxin: a tool for studying the regulation of adenylate cyclase. Methods Enzymol 1985; 109:588.

30. Wojcikiewicz RJH, Dobson PRM, Irons LQ, Robinson A, Brown BL. The relationship between pertussis-toxin induced ADP-ribosylation of a plasma-membrane protein and reversal of muscarinic inhibition of prolactin secretion in GH3 cells. Biochem J 1984; 224:339.

31. Yajima, Akita Y, Saito T. Pertussis toxin blocks the inhibitory effects of somatostatin on cAMP-dependent vasoactive intestinal peptide and cAMP-independent thyrotropin releasing hormone-stimulated prolactin secretion in GH3 cells. J Biol Chem 1986; 261:2684.

32. Neer EJ, Lok JM, Wolf LG. Purification and properties of the inhibitory guanine nucleotide regulatory unit of brain adenylate cyclase. J Biol Chem 1984; 259:14,222.

33. Van Dop C, Yamanaka G, Steinberg F, et al. ADP-ribosylation of transducin by pertussis toxin blocks the light-stimulated hydrolysis of GTP and cGMP in retinal photoreceptors. J Biol Chem 1984; 259:23.

34. Gierschik P, Falloon J, Milligan G, Pines M, Gallin JI, Spiegel A. Immunochemical evidence for a novel pertussis toxin substrate in human neutrophils. J Biol Chem 1986; 261:8058.

35. Florio VA, Sternweis PC. Reconstitution of resolved muscarinic cholinergic receptors with purified GTP-binding proteins. J Biol Chem 1985; 260:3477.

36. Schlegel W, Wuarin F, Wollheim CB, Zahnd GR. Somatostatin lowers the cytosolic free Ca^{2+} concentration in clonal rat pituitary cells (GH3 cells). Cell Calcium 1984; 5:223.

37. Rink TJ, Montecucco C, Hesketh TR, Tsien RY. Lymphocyte membrane potential assessed with fluorescent probes. Biochim Biophys Acta 1980; 595:15.

38. Rink TJ. Measurement of membrane potential with chemical probes. Lipid Membr Biochem 1982; B423:1.

39. Waggoner AS. Dye indicators of membrane potential. Annu Rev Biophys Bioeng 1979; 8:47.

40. Schlegel W, Wuarin F, Zbaren C, Wollheim CB, Zahnd GR. Pertussis toxin selectively abolishes hormone induced lowering of cytosolic calcium in GH_3 cells. FEBS Lett 1985; 189:27.

41. Taraskevich PS, Douglas WW. Electrical behaviour in a line of anterior pituitary cells (GH cells) and the influence of the hypothalamic peptide, thyrotrophin releasing factor. Neuroscience 1980; 5:421.

42. Dubinsky JM, Oxford GS. Ionic currents in two strains of rat anterior pituitary tumor cells. J Gen Physiol 1984; 83:309.

43. Barker JL, Dufy B. Peptide and amino acid electropharmacology of cultured mammalian central neurons and clonal pituitary cells. Regul Pept 1985; 4(suppl):14.

44. Borgeat P, Labrie F, Drouin J, et al. Inhibition of adenosine 3',5'-monophosphate accumulation in anterior pituitary gland in vitro by growth-hormone-release-inhibiting hormone. Biochem Biophys Res Commun 1974; 56:1052.

45. Kaneko T, Oka H, Munemura M, Suzuki S, Yasuda H, Oda T. Stimulation

of guanosine 3',5'-cyclic monophosphate accumulation in rat anterior pituitary gland in vitro by synthetic somatostatin. Biochem Biophys Res Commun 1974; 61:53.

46. Schofield JG, Mira-Moser F, Schorderet M, Orci L. Somatostatin inhibition of rat growth hormone release in vitro in the presence of BaCl$_2$ or 3-isobutyl-1-methylxanthine. FEBS Lett 1974; 46:171.

47. Lippmann W, Sestanj J, Nelson VR, Immer HU. Antagonism of prosta-glandin-induced cyclic AMP accumulation in the rat anterior pituitary in vitro by somatostatin analogs. Experientia 1976; 32:1034.

48. Sheppard MS, Spence JW, Kraicer J. Release of growth hormone from purified somatotrophs: role of adenosine 3',5'-monophosphate and guanosine 3',5'-monophosphate. Endocrinology 1979; 105:261.

49. Bilezikjian LM, Vale WW. Stimulation of adenosine 3',5'-monophos-phate production by growth hormone-releasing factor and its inhibi-tion by somatostatin in anterior pituitary cells in vitro. Endo-crinology 1983; 113:1726.

50. Michel D, Lefebvre G, Labrie F. Interactions between growth hormone-releasing factor, prostaglandin E$_2$ and somatostatin on cyclic AMP accumulation in rat adenohypophyseal cells in culture. Mol Cell Endocrinol 1983; 33:255.

51. Harwood JP, Grewe C, Aguilera G. Actions of growth hormone releasing factor on somatostatin adenylate cyclase and GH release in rat anterior pituitary. Mol Cell Endocrinol 1984; 37:277.

52. Rouleau D, Barden N. Inhibition of anterior pituitary prostaglandin-stimulated adenylyl cyclase activity by somatostatin. Can J Biochem 1981; 59:307.

53. Cronin MJ, Rogol AD, Myers GA, Hewlett EL. Pertussis toxin blocks the somatostatin-induced inhibition of growth hormone release and adenosine 3',5'-monophosphate accumulation. Endocrinology 1983; 113:209.

54. Yamashita N, Shibuya N, Ogata E. Hyperpolarization of the membrane potential caused by somatostatin in dissociated human pituitary adenoma cells that secrete growth hormone. Proc Natl Acad Sci USA 1986; 83:6198.

13

MOLECULAR MECHANISMS OF SOMATOSTATIN INHIBITION OF

HORMONE RELEASE FROM AtT-20 CELLS

Lawrence C. Mahan* and Terry Reisine

*Laboratory of Cell Biology
National Institute of Mental Health
Bethesda, MD, and

Department of Pharmacology
University of Pennsylvania
Philadelphia, PA

INTRODUCTION

Somatostatin (SRIF), a tetradecapeptide initially isolated from the hypothalamus and characterized for its ability to inhibit the secretion of growth hormone, regulates the secretion of a variety of hormones from tissues including the pituitary, pancreas and intestine (1-4). The widespread distribution of SRIF and its receptor in nervous tissue is well described, implicating a role in neurotransmission as well (5,6). A number of cell lines exist which have been utilized to facilitate our understanding of the biochemical mechanisms involved in the inhibitory actions of SRIF. Of particular advantage is the tumor cell, AtT-20/D16-16, which consists of a homogeneous population of corticotrophs (7). The secretion of adrenocorticotropin (ACTH) from AtT-20 cells is under "multi-hormonal" control (8,9). Secretagogues include corticotropin releasing factor (CRF), vasoactive intestinal peptide (VIP) and beta-adrenergic agonists, all of which act through the activation of adenylate cyclase and the generation of cAMP (10). Secretion of ACTH is also stimulated by the membrane-depolarizing cation K^+, which increases Ca^{++} influx and intracellular Ca^{++} mobilization (11-13). More recently, it has been shown that lithium and phorbol esters promote the secretion of ACTH in these cells, perhaps through a stimulation of phosphoinositide metabolism or the activation of protein kinase C (14). Thus it is evident that more than one intracellular pathway exists for the secretion of ACTH in AtT-20 cells.

By analogy, SRIF appears to inhibit the secretion of ACTH in AtT-20 cells through "multi-transductional" pathways. That is, SRIF inhibits ACTH release in response to secretagogues acting through distinct intracellular processes (15,16). It is evident, however, that the inhibitory capabilities of SRIF are dependent on receptor interactions with the inhibitory guanine nucleotide-binding protein(s), termed N_i, and possibly the more recently described N_o (17). The following studies were carried out in order to define more clearly these distinct coupling pathways of the SRIF receptor and to gain insight into the mechanism of action of SRIF in the regulation of hormone secretion in AtT-20 cells.

SOMATOSTATIN RECEPTORS AND ADENYLATE CYCLASE

Perhaps the best understood of SRIF's actions is its ability to inhibit the release of ACTH stimulated by secretagogues that activate adenylate cyclase. The effects of these agents are mediated by specific receptors (CRF, VIP, and B-agonists) on AtT-20 cells or by hormone-independent activation of adenylate cyclase (forskolin and cholera toxin). This pathway requires interaction with the stimulatory guanine-nucleotide binding protein(s), N_s, a heterotrimer of α_s, (45,000 daltons), β (35,000 daltons) and γ (10,000 daltons) subunits (18). The α subunit in AtT-20 cells has been identified by NAD-dependent ADP-ribosylation by cholera toxin (unpublished observations). In addition, these cells contain the 41,000 dalton subunit, α_i, identified by the NAD-dependent ADP-ribosylation by the toxin of Bordetella pertussis (19,20). This inhibitory guanine nucleotide-binding protein shares the β and γ subunits of N_s to form the regulatory complex of adenylate cyclase.

Stimulation of adenylate cyclase and increases in intracellular cAMP lead to the activation of cAMP-dependent protein kinase AtT-20 cells. Several proteins have been identified in these cells as phosphorylation substrates of cAMP-dependent protein kinase that may be the link between the intracellular actions of cAMP and the secretion of ACTH (21). Direct evidence that the secretion of ACTH is dependent upon the activation of cAMP-dependent protein kinase was demonstrated in AtT-20 cells by the use of liposome-mediated injection of the inhibitor protein (PKI) of this kinase (22). PKI-containing liposomes, covalently coated with protein A, bound to cells previously labeled with antibodies against the cell adhesion glycoprotein N-CAM. Binding of liposomes induced fusion with AtT-20 cells resulting in the insertion of PKI into the cells. This manipulation resulted in the complete inhibition of ACTH secretion stimulated by CRF or beta-adrenergic agonists, the diterpene forskolin, and 8-bromo-cAMP. In addition, phosphorylation of protein substrates for cAMP-dependent protein kinase was markedly inhibited (23,24).

Somatostatin receptors on AtT-20 cells, as well as a number of other cell types such as S49 T-lymphoma cells and GH_4C_1 clonal pituitary tumor cells, have been shown to be functionally coupled to the inhibition of adenylate cyclase (15,25,26). In AtT-20 cells, SRIF as well as somatostatin-28 and other SRIF analogues were all equally efficacious in inhibiting the intracellular accumulation of cAMP in response to CRF, isoproterenol and forskolin. The potencies and rank order of these agonist analogues in blocking this response were similar to those observed for their inhibition of both secretion of ACTH and binding of either radiolabeled [^{125}I]CGP-23996, a degradation-resistant analogue of SRIF, or [^{125}I-Tyr^{11}]SRIF to receptors in membrane preparations (27). SRIF reduced hormone-stimulated accumulation of cAMP to nearly basal levels (in the presence of a phosphodiesterase inhibitor) with little or no effect on the basal accumulation.

In addition to the ability of SRIF to inhibit the activation of adenylate cyclase, SRIF is able to inhibit ACTH secretion beyond the activation of adenylate cyclase. 100 μM 8-bromo-cAMP has been shown to be equally efficacious as hormones such as CRF in promoting secretion of ACTH from intact AtT-20 cells (10). This membrane-permeant cAMP analogue has been shown to activate cAMP-dependent protein kinases in a variety of cells including AtT-20 cells (12,28). Addition of SRIF resulted in a potent inhibition of 8-bromo-cAMP-mediated secretion of ACTH (16). The mechanism by which SRIF blocks 8-bromo-cAMP induced release of ACTH is not known. Conceivably SRIF blocks protein kinase-mediated protein phosphorylation to prevent the stimulation of ACTH release. This would be consistent with recent data on the effect of SRIF on protein phosphorylation in GH pituitary tumor cells (29).

Role of Guanine Nucleotide-binding Protein(s)

Treatment of intact AtT-20 cells with pertussis toxin (50 ng/ml) completely abolished the inhibitory actions of SRIF in the adenylate cyclase-mediated secretion of ACTH (20). Similar results have been reported for the effects of pertussis toxin on SRIF-mediated inhibition of VIP stimulated cAMP accumulation and prolactin release from GH_4C_1 cells (30). These results are consistent with the hypothesis that pertussis toxin treatment specifically blocks the interaction of somatostatin receptors on AtT-20 cells with the inhibitory guanine nucleotide-binding complex, N_i, through the ADP ribosylation and subsequent inactivation of the 41,000 dalton α_i subunit.

Prior treatment of cells with pertussis toxin reduced both the potency (~50 fold) and efficacy (40-50%) of SRIF's inhibition of ACTH secretion in response to 8-bromo-cAMP (16). Although this effect is not as marked as the complete attenuation of SRIF's inhibition of hormone or forskolin-mediated secretion, it does implicate a role for a GTP-binding, pertussis toxin-sensitive substrate (perhaps N_i or N_o) in the direct inhibition of cAMP-dependent protein kinase or events distal to its activation such as protein phosphorylation in AtT-20 cells.

SOMATOSTATIN RECEPTORS AND Ca^{++} MOBILIZATION

Ca^{++} has an essential role in stimulus-secretion coupling in AtT-20 cells as evidenced by the cessation of ACTH release in the absence of extracellular Ca^{++} (11). Ca^{++} mobilization, either through Ca^{++} channels in the plasma membrane or from intracellular storage sites, may be a common mechanism in the secretion pathway for agents that stimulate release of ACTH in AtT-20 cells. It follows that interference in Ca^{++} mobilization would be a likely mechanism in the "multi-transductional" inhibition of ACTH secretion by SRIF.

Basal Cytosolic Ca^{++} Levels

In the absence of stimulated Ca^{++} influx, 0.1 µM SRIF rapidly decreased basal cytosolic Ca^{++} in AtT-20 cells measured with the fluorescent Ca^{++}-chelating probe, Quin 2. In whole-cell patch clamp experiments, 0.01-1.0 µM SRIF produced a 30-40% decrease in the magnitude of voltage-dependent Ca^{++} current with no change in the threshold for activation of the Ca^{++} current or the voltage of maximal current amplitude (31). This inhibition was rapid (~2 min) but transient (~5 min to recovery). The response to addition of the voltage-dependent Ca^{++} channel blocking agent, nifedipine, at a time of maximal inhibition of current by SRIF was non-additive suggesting a common mechanism of action. Thus SRIF is able to partially block spontaneous Ca^{++} currents in these cells which may account for the lowering of basal ACTH release observed using high concentrations of SRIF. Virtually identical findings have been observed for the inhibition of SRIF of basal intracellular Ca^{++} levels and prolactin release in GH_4C_1 cells (30).

Ca^{++} and cAMP-Dependent Pathways

Hormone secretagogues that activate adenylate cyclase and increase intracellular cAMP increase cytosolic Ca^{++} in AtT-20 cells (13,32). The complete sequence of molecular events between an increase in cAMP levels and Ca^{++} mobilization, however, are unknown. Activation of cAMP-dependent protein kinase in AtT-20 cells is required: (1) 8-bromo-cAMP mimicked the increase in cytosolic Ca^{++} produced by CRF, VIP, beta-adrenergic agonists or forskolin (32); (2) fusion of PKI-containing liposomes with intact cells markedly attenuated the rise in cytosolic Ca^{++} produced by secretagogues that activate cAMP-dependent protein kinase but not by those that stimulated Ca^{++} mobilization by other mechanisms (33). The source of the increased cytosolic Ca^{++} appears in part to be extracellular and requires functional voltage-dependent Ca^{++} channels (31). Chelation of extracellular Ca^{++} with EGTA or inclusion of Ca^{++} channel blockers [nifedipine (10 μM), verapamil (10 μM) or nisoldipine (0.1 μM)] inhibited the rise in cytosolic Ca^{++} produced by all secretagogues that activate cAMP-dependent protein kinase.

Recent studies have shown that cAMP-dependent protein kinase regulates the phosphorylation of a component of the Ca^{++} channel in heart cells (34). In addition, using patch clamp techniques, 8-bromo-cAMP has been shown to directly activate Ca^{++} conductance channels in AtT-20 cells (32). Thus the activation of cAMP-dependent protein kinase could catalyze the phosphorylation of a voltage-sensitive Ca^{++} channel in AtT20 cells to raise intracellular Ca^{++} and promote secretion of ACTH. An alternative hypothesis has been suggested by whole-cell patch clamp experiments in which isoproterenol slowed the frequency of openings of K^+ conductance (hyperpolarizing) channels in AtT-20 cells (35). Addition of cAMP to excised patches also suppressed the activity of this channel. These results imply that cAMP-dependent protein kinase could phorphorylate the K^+ channel directly, reducing its frequency of opening, and enhance the generation of action potentials. Such increases in action potentials in AtT-20 cells have been directly related to the ability of beta-adrenergic agonists to stimulate ACTH release. Since AtT-20 cells contain voltage-dependent Ca^{++} channels, increased frequency of depolarization could promote Ca^{++} influx and stimulate secretion of ACTH (36).

The rise in cytosolic Ca^{++} measured with Quin 2 in response to CRF, VIP, isoproterenol and forskolin was completely abolished by 0.1-10 μM SRIF (32,37). Surprisingly, in these experiments SRIF had little or no effect on the rise in cytosolic Ca^{++} produced by 8-bromo-cAMP. In experiments utilizing whole-cell patch clamp technique, however, SRIF inhibited 8-bromo-cAMP stimulated Ca^{++} currents (31). Similar results were obtained in cells to which 100 μM cAMP and 1 mM IBMX, a potent inhibitor of cAMP phosphodiesterase, were injected into AtT-20 cells to maximally activate cAMP-dependent protein kinase.

How can these results be reconciled with the potent ability of SRIF to inhibit 8-bromo-cAMP stimulated release of ACTH? One explanation might be that Ca^{++} mobilized (as measured in Quin 2 studies) stimulated by cAMP-dependent protein kinase could involve additional sources of released Ca^{++} besides that resulting from enhanced voltage-dependent Ca^{++} channel conductance. The relationship between the prolonged (hrs) ability of SRIF to inhibit ACTH release and the transient (min) inhibition of Ca^{++} channel activity has yet to be clarified. Perhaps SRIF-induced inhibition of Ca^{++} currents represents one of a number of actions of SRIF to block Ca^{++}-dependent events in the secretory process. Repetitive transient rises in cytosolic Ca^{++} are thought to promote sustained, $alpha_1$-adrenergic stimulation of glucose release in hepatocytes (38). Interaction of SRIF with a repetitive Ca^{++} mobilization that could inhibit sustained ACTH release has yet to be investigated in AtT-20 cells. Thus the exact mechanism by which SRIF inhibits ACTH release stimulated by 8-bromo-cAMP remains unclear.

Ca^{++} and cAMP-Independent Pathways

While it is clear that inhibition of cyclic nucleotide production is a predominant mechanism by which SRIF inhibits the release of ACTH in AtT-20 cells, it is also apparent that SRIF acts through cAMP-independent pathways. The ability of SRIF to inhibit basal Ca^{++} channel activity in AtT-20 cells was unrelated to changes in intracellular cAMP (11,16). Furthermore, while high concentrations (50-100 mM) of extracellular K^+ depolarize AtT-20 cells and cause secretion of ACTH, SRIF potently inhibited this effect (31,37). Neither the ability of K^+ to induce secretion nor the ability of SRIF to inhibit depends on changes in intracellular cAMP. K^+-induced depolarization was associated with a very rapid and pronounced elevation of cytosolic Ca^{++} that was temporally related to ACTH release in superfusion studies (13). Prior to simultaneous addition of 0.1 μM SRIF did not attenuate this increase in cytosolic Ca^{++} more than that accounted for by the magnitude of decrease in basal cytosolic Ca^{++} alone, but completely abolished the early (<10 min) release of ACTH (37).

SRIF has been shown to increase K^+ conductance in GH pituitary tumor cells. This resulted in a hyperpolarization of the membrane potential, an effect that could counteract depolarization-induced hormone secretion (39). As stated, secretagogues such as isoproterenol increase the frequency of action potentials in AtT-20 cells. This is due to a shortening of the after-hyperpolarization induced by K^+ efflux. SRIF could block stimulus-secretion coupling by simply activating K^+ conductance channels. This would prolong after-hyperpolarization, decrease the frequency of action potentials, and suppress Ca^{++} influx in AtT-20 cells. Such a mechanism could be responsible for SRIF's inhibition of both K^+- and 8-bromo-cAMP-stimulated ACTH release and could explain the apparently contradictory results found with measurements of Ca^{++} conductance and Ca^{++} mobilization. Evidence for an effect of SRIF on K^+ conductance in AtT-20 cells, however, is not presently available.

Role of Guanine Nucleotide-Binding Proteins

Guanine nucleotide-binding protein(s) appear to play a role in both cAMP-dependent and cAMP-independent pathways of ACTH secretion in AtT-20 cells. Incubation of AtT-20 cells with pertussis toxin (50-100 ng/ml) blocked the inhibition by 0.1 μM SRIF of increased cytosolic Ca^{++} (measured with Quin 2) in response to forskolin. As discussed, this effect is probably a consequence of the inactivation of N_i. Pertussis toxin also abolished the inhibitory effect of SRIF on basal intracellular Ca^{++} levels and voltage-dependent Ca^{++} currents (37,40). Intracellular addition of the hydrolysis-resistant guanine nucleotide analogue, GTPγs, alone or in combination with SRIF produced irreversible inhibition of Ca^{++} current. As stated, SRIF has little or no effect on the rise in cytosolic Ca^{++} produced by 8-bromo-cAMP, and as expected pertussis toxin treatment had no effect (37). Pertussis toxin treatment reduced the potency ($\cong$100 fold) of SRIF to inhibit K^+-induced ACTH release; however, it did not alter the level of time course of the rise in cytosolic Ca^{++} (16,37).

These data suggest that pertussis toxin-sensitive, guanine nucleotide binding protein(s) mediate the inhibitory action of SRIF in cAMP-independent pathways of secretion, possibly through some initial (transient?) event in Ca^{++} mobilization in AtT-20 cells. GTP-binding proteins appear to be involved in inhibition of cAMP-independent pathways of prolactin secretion by SRIF or dopamine in GH_4C_1 cells (30) and pituitary tumor lactotrophs (41), respectively. Recent studies have demonstrated a role for GTP-binding proteins in GABA- and norepinephrine-induced inhibition of voltage-dependent Ca^{++} channels in dorsal root ganglion neurons as well as in the stimulation of Ca^{++} release from endoplasmic reticulum in N1E-115 neuronal cells (42,43). Furthermore, GTP-binding proteins are believed to couple muscarinic receptors to a K^+ channel in heart cells (44). Whether these regulations occur through an interaction with N_i or N_o cannot yet be distinguished in these experiments or in AtT-20 cells. Similarly, whether pertussis toxin inactivates N_i (or N_o) interaction with Ca^{++} or other ionic channels or only with receptors for SRIF has yet to be determined.

SOMATOSTATIN AND ADDITIONAL cAMP-INDEPENDENT PATHWAYS OF ACTH RELEASE

Lithium and phorbol esters also stimulate the secretion of ACTH in AtT-20 cells (14,45). Roles for both agents have been implicated in hormone-stimulated phosphatidylinositol metabolism. This pathway is thought to trigger Ca^{++} mobilization and the activation of protein kinase C (46). Lithium is a potent inhibitor of the phosphatase that cleaves inositol 1-phosphate to inositol. This inhibition leads to increases in inositol mono-, bis- and trisphosphates. Inositol triphosphate (IP_3) is believed to act through specific intracellular receptors to cause an increase in free cytosolic Ca^{++} by release of Ca^{++} from intracellular stores. In addition to the increase in cytosolic Ca^{++}, concomitant release of diacylglycerol is thought to synergistically activate protein kinase C and lead to enhanced protein phosphorylation.

10 mM lithium stimulated secretion of ACTH in AtT-20 cells comparable to that obtained with CRF (14). Lithium also stimulated the production (~3-fold) of inositol phosphates, in particular IP_1 and IP_2. Inclusion of 0.3 μM SRIF during lithium stimulation caused a 30% and 60-75% decrease in ACTH release and IP_1 respectively. Pretreatment with lithium strongly desensitized the release of ACTH that can be elicited by phorbol myristate acetate (PMA). This suggests that lithium may act through the activation of protein kinase C. Lithium, however, failed to promote the translocation of protein kinase C activity from cytosol to membrane-bound compartments, an event regarded as indicative of the activation of this enzyme (47). Thus it is interesting to speculate that the predominant mechanism of lithium's ability to stimulate secretion of ACTH may be the release of Ca^{++} from intracellular stores through the activation of phosphatidylinositol metabolism. Experiments to determine the effects of lithium on mobilization of Ca^{++} and of the role of SRIF and guanine nucleotide-binding proteins are currently under investigation.

SOMATOSTATIN RECEPTORS IN AtT-20 CELLS

Does SRIF act through a single receptor to affect the multi-transductional inhibition of ACTH secretion in AtT-20 cells? Existence of subtypes of SRIF receptors have been proposed in brain based upon radiolabeled agonist binding alone (48). However, by this criterion, only a single type of receptor was observed in pituitary membranes. SRIF receptors have been identified in membrane preparations from AtT-20 cells using [^{125}I-Tyr^{11}]SRIF or, more recently, with the agonist analogue [^{125}I]CGP-23996 which is resistant to degradation (27,49). These radiolabeled agonists bind to a single class of high affinity (~1-3 nM) sites with a density of approximately 0.8-1.2 pmole/mg protein. Agonist binding to several types of receptors, such as those for opiates, dopamine and muscarinic agonists that have been linked to the inhibition of adenylate cyclase, is regulated by Na^+ ions and GTP. SRIF receptors in membranes from AtT-20 cells showed similar regulation (49). Addition of Na^+ or GTP promoted rapid dissociation of [^{125}I]CGP-23996 bound to AtT-20 membranes. Complete dissociation of agonist in the presence of both Na^+ and GTP was even more rapid (t1/2 < 2 min). This effect was specific for Na^+ ions and has an IC_{50} for Na^+ of ~25 mM. This regulation is thought to represent the uncoupling of receptors from N_i and subsequent formation of a receptor with low affinity for agonist. These data suggest that if SRIF receptors are coupled to distinctly different GTP-binding proteins (e.g., N_i and

N_o), these proteins share similar regulation by Na and GTP. A caveat to this speculation is that agonists must bind with equal affinity to receptors coupled to either GTP-binding protein in membrane preparations.

Treatment of intact cells with pertussis toxin caused a decrease in both binding of [^{125}I]CGP-23996 and affinity of SRIF for receptors in membrane preparations (37). Decreased agonist binding in membranes of GH_4C_1 cells after treatment with pertussis toxin has also been reported (30). Since the affinity of SRIF-agonist probes for receptors can be markedly affected by apparent coupling of receptors to GTP-regulatory proteins, alterations in affinity, and not receptor density, probably account for the effects of toxin. This alone could explain the common sensitivity of the diverse inhibitory pathways of SRIF to treatment with pertussis toxin.

Prolonged exposure (hrs) of AtT-20 cells to SRIF results in functional desensitization of SRIF's ability to inhibit cAMP accumulation and ACTH release (50,51). Desensitization of receptors to SRIF resulted in a supersensitivity to secretagogues that stimulate adenylate cyclase. This suggests that a tonic inhibitory influence may exist in AtT-20 cells, at least between the stimulatory and inhibitory subunits of the guanine nucleotide-binding regulatory complex associated with adenylate cyclase. A decrease in agonist binding, attributed to changes in receptor density (i.e., downregulation) and not affinity, has been reported in desensitized cells (52). It is not clear, however, in these experiments that a clear discrimination between a marked loss in receptor affinity (i.e., uncoupling) for SRIF and true loss of receptors from the plasma membrane was made. Likewise, the dependence of receptor recovery on protein synthesis was not examined. Thus the exact fate of receptors for SRIF after prolonged exposure to agonist and the effect on cAMP-independent pathways of transduction remain to be elucidated.

CONCLUSION

Somatostatin plays an important role as a neurotransmitter in the brain and as a hormone in the anterior pituitary and other tissues. In the CNS, SRIF modulates the release of other neurotransmitters such as dopamine, serotonin and norepinephrine and has been shown to depolarize brain neurons in primary culture (53,54). Furthermore, SRIF was shown to increase cAMP generation in brain astrocytes (55). In contrast, this peptide blocks the secretion of several hormones of the anterior pituitary, ACTH release in AtT-20 cells, and prolactin release in GH pituitary cells. The molecular mechanisms that differentiate such apparently opposite actions of SRIF in brain and pituitary are still unclear. Ligand binding studies with radiolabeled agonists to date have not been able to clearly resolve differences in receptors for SRIF in brain or pituitary that correlate with distinct functional coupling pathways.

Our results in AtT-20 cells suggest that guanine nucleotide-binding regulatory proteins link receptors for SRIF to multiple effector systems. If similar multi-transductional pathways exist in the brain, it is conceivable that a number of distinct regulatory proteins could couple SRIF receptors to a diverse array of physiological responses. Although our studies, as well as those of others, have provided some basic clues to the molecular mechanisms of the action of SRIF, a number of fascinating questions remain to be answered.

REFERENCES

1. Brazeau P, Rivier J, Vale W. Endocrinology 1974; 94:184.
2. Vale W, Rivier J, Brazeau P, Guillemin R. Endocrinology 1974; 95:968.
3. Curry D, Bennett L. Proc Natl Acad Sci, USA 1976; 73:248.
4. Konturck S, Tasler J, Jaworek J, et al. Proc Natl Acad Sci USA 1981; 78:1967.
5. Reichlin S. In: Krieger DT, Brownstein MJ, Martin JB, eds. Brain peptides. New York: John Wiley & Sons, 1983:711-25.
6. Reubi JC, Maurer R. Neuroscience 1985; 15:1183.
7. Richardson UI. Endocrinology 1978; 102:910.
8. Hook VYH, Heisler S, Sabol SL, Axelrod J. Biochem Biophys Res Comm 1982; 106:1364.
9. Reisine TD, Heisler S, Hook VYH, Axelrod J. Biochem Biophys Res Comm 1982; 108:1251.
10. Axelrod J, Reisine TD. Science 1984; 224:452.
11. Richardson UI. Endocrinology 1983; 113:62.
12. Litvin Y, Pasmantier R, Fleischer N, Erlichman J. J Biol Chem 1984; 259:10296.
13. Guild S, Itoh Y, Kebabian J, Luini A, Reisine TD. Endocrinology 1986 (in press).
14. Zatz M, Reisine TD. Proc Natl Acad Sci USA 1985; 82:1286.
15. Heisler S, Reisine TD, Hook VYH, Axelrod J. Proc Natl Acad Sci USA 1982; 79:6502.
16. Reisine TD. Endocrinology 1985; 116:2259.
17. Sternweis PC, Robishaw JD. J Biol Chem 1984; 259:13806.
18. Gilman AG. Cell 1984; 36:577.
19. Bokoch GM, Katada T, Northup JK, Ui M, Gilman AG. J Biol Chem 1984; 259:3560.
20. Reisine TD, Zhang Y, Sekura R. J Pharmacol Exp Ther 1985; 232:275.
21. Rougon G, Barbet J, Affolter H-U, Reisine TD. Soc Neurosci Abst 1985; 11:1093.
22. Reisine TD, Rougon G, Barbet J. J Cell Biol 1986 (in press).
23. Reisine TD, Rougon G, Barbet J, Affolter H-U. Proc Natl Acad Sci USA 1985; 82:8261.
24. Affolter H-U, Rougon G, Reisine TD. DNA 1986; 5:86.
25. Jakobs KH, Aktories K, Schultz G. Eur J Biochem 1984; 140:177.
26. Dorflinger LJ, Schonbrunn A. Endocrinology 1983; 113:1551.
27. Srikant CB, Heisler S. Endocrinology 1985; 117:271.
28. Miyazaki K, Reisine TD, Kebabian J. Endocrinology 1984; 115:1933.
29. Sobel A, Tashijian A. J Biol Chem 1984; 258:10312.
30. Koch BD, Dorflinger LJ, Schonbrunn A. J Biol Chem 1985; 260:13138.
31. Luini A, Lewis D, Guild S, Schofield G, Weight F. J Neuroscience 1986 (in press).
32. Luini A, Lewis D, Guild S, Corda D, Axelrod J. Proc Natl Acad Sci USA 1985; 82:8034.
33. Reisine TD, Guild S. Soc Neurosci Abst 1986 (in press).
34. Curtis B, Catterall W. Proc Natl Acad Sci, USA 1985; 82:2528.
35. Nowycky M, Reisine TD. Soc Neurosci Abst 1986 (in press).
36. Suprenant A. J Cell Biol 1982; 95:559.
37. Reisine TD, Guild S. J Pharmacol Exp Ther 1985; 235:551.
38. Woods NM, Cuthbertson KSR, Cobbold PH. Nature 1986; 319:600.
39. Barker JL, Dufy B. Regul Pept [suppl] 1985; 4:14.
40. Lewis D, Weight F, Luini A. International Conference on Somatostatin, Washington, DC, 1986; Abstract I-17:45.
41. Delbeke D, Scammell JG, Martinez-Campos A, Dannies PS. Endocrinology 1986; 118:1271.
42. Holz GG IV, Rane SG, Dunlap K. Nature 1986; 319:670.
43. Gill DL, Ueda T, Sheau-Huei C, Noel MW. Nature 1986; 329:461.
44. Pfaffinger PJ, Martin JM, Hunter DD, Nathanson NM, Hille B. Nature 1985; 317:536.

45. Phillips M, Jaken S. J Biol Chem 1983; 258:2875.
46. Nishizuka Y. Trends Biochem Sci 1983; 8:13.
47. Zatz M, Mahan LC, Reisine TD. J Neurochem (submitted 1986).
48. Tran VT, Beal MF, Martin JB. Science 1985; 228:492.
49. Mahan LC, Reisine TD, Axelrod J. Soc Neurosci Abst 1986 (in press).
50. Reisine TD, Axelrod J. Endocrinology 1983; 113:811.
51. Reisine TD. J Pharmacol Exp Ther 1984; 229:14.
52. Heisler S, Srikant CB. Endocrinology 1985; 117:217.
53. Chesselet M-F, Reisine TD. J Neuroscience 1983; 3:232.
54. Delf J, Dichter M. J Neuroscience 1983; 3:1176.
55. Rougon G, Noble M, Mudge A. Nature 1983; 305:715.

III. ROLE OF SOMATOSTATIN IN NERVOUS SYSTEM FUNCTION AND
CONTROVERSIES IN SOMATOSTATIN RESEARCH

14

REGULATION OF HYPOTHALAMIC SOMATOSTATIN SECRETION

Richard Robbins

Section of Neuroendocrinology
Departments of Medicine and OB/GYN
Yale University School of Medicine

The secretion of somatostatin (SS) from nerve terminals of hypothalamic neurons can be measured in several different experimental models. Direct measurement of peptide release by radioimmunoassay is generally held to be the most reliable method. Indirect estimates of the release of SS have been estimated from changes in serum levels of growth hormone (GH) either basally or in response to a secretogogue. Changes in SS receptor populations on pituitary membranes have also been suggested as a means of estimating endogenous SS secretion. Finally, changes in hypothalamic SS levels in the anterior hypothalamus or in the median eminence have been used as markers of the secretory activity of these neurons. In this review I will attempt to summarize studies examining the factors which regulate hypothalamic SS secretion utilizing direct measurements of SS levels. Studies on SS secretion from neurons outside the hypothalamus will not be primarily considered.

SYSTEMS USED TO EXAMINE THE SECRETION OF SOMATOSTATIN

The most common system used to measure SS secretion has been the explanted median eminence or basal hypothalamus. The main drawback of the explant model is that cells in the interior of the tissue may be undergoing degeneration due to poor oxygenation or intracellular changes in ions including pH. In addition, many of the nerve terminals which are releasing SS have been severed from their cell bodies and they are slowly dying. It is generally accepted, however, that thin slices of the median eminence are viable and reliable for several hours after preparation if kept at the appropriate temperature and oxygenation in physiologic buffers.

Dissociated cell cultures of hypothalamic cells have also proven to be valuable in that rapid stable SS secretion can be achieved in a totally defined environment. A different set of reservations apply to cell cultures. Since these cells are fetal or neonatal, in general, they may not have developed normal receptors or intracellular trafficking patterns necessary for a mature neuron to respond to the appropriate signal. Furthermore, the normal intercellular connections, which presumably have major influences over the activity of a cell, are lost or should be presumed lost unless otherwise demonstrated. This last caveat is only included in that reaggregation of dispersed cells probably does not occur entirely randomly. The existence of specific nerve cell adhesion molecules and comparable molecules on glial cells makes it likely that some level of selective reaggregation occurs in all dispersed cell preparations.

Cell cultures, however, have certain advantages over explants. They are intact viable cells. Their environment can be totally or near-totally defined and regulated, and the problems with diffusion of secretogogues in and diffusion of SS out is largely eliminated.

The most attractive models for studying SS secretion, however, with respect to normal physiology are those in which the hypothalamic cells are fully developed, have normal cellular interconnections, and can be sampled rapidly. The two techniques which approach this ideal are the push-pull cannula and hypophyseal portal vessel cannulation. The major drawbacks of these systems include the need for anesthetics which have neuromodulatory effects, and mechanical or surgical distortion of the normal anatomical interrelationships.

The preparation with the least physiological relevance is the synaptosome. This method examines secretion from pinched-off nerve terminals. It has the advantage of being the most "biochemical" in that many exact replicate tubes can be prepared and no attempts to demonstrate viability are necessary. These preparations have been most useful in examining the roles of ionic channel modulation by chemical probes.

In summary, a number of very different methods to directly measure SS secretion or release have been developed. Each has its unique advantages and drawbacks. When taken together, however, these techniques have provided us with an understanding of the mechanisms which govern the activity of hypothalamic SS neurons.

THE EFFECTS OF NEUROTRANSMITTERS (Table 1)

Dopamine (DA) has been found to stimulate SS release by many different investigators. The one exception comes from the work of Bennett et al. (1) who noted that dopamine decreased the release of immunoreactive somatostatin (IRS) from hypothalamic synaptosomes. Wakabayashi and co-workers (2), however, found that DA stimulated SS secretion from a similar preparation. In work employing hypothalamic explants, DA has uniformly been reported to stimulate the release of IRS. Most recently Lewis and collaborators (3) have found that this action is predominantly mediated by D2 receptors. In their report D2 antagonists such as metoclopramide and domperidone effectively blocked the action of DA whereas D1 antagonists did not. Similarly, D2 agonists (e.g., LY 171555), but not D1 agonists (e.g., SKF 38393A) stimulated IRS secretion. Interestingly octacosapeptide somatostatin (SS-28) production was much higher than that of tetradecapeptide somatostatin (SS-14) in response to DA.

Chihara et al. (4) have reported that DA directly stimulates SS release into rat hypophyseal portal blood. Developing hypothalamic cells in culture also respond to DA indicating that this response may also be important in hypothalamic formation (5). The ability of PGE_2 to block the stimulatory action of DA on SS neurons was first reported by Ojeda et al. (6).

Although norepinephrine (NE) has also been reported to be stimulatory to hypothalamic SS neurons, its effects are less dramatic and are not present in several systems. Bennett et al. (1) reported that NE decreases IRS release. No change in IRS release from hypothalamic explants were re-

Table 1. Hypothalamic somatostatin release:
neurotransmitters (references)

Substance	Increase	Decrease	No effect
Potassium	2,5,23,24,37	-	-
Veratridine	1,7,26	-	-
Dopamine	2,3,4,5,6 7,10	1	8
Norepinephrine	4,9,10	1	7,8
Serotonin	-	1,7	4,7
Acetylcholine	4	12	7,8
GABA	-	14,15	8,13
Melatonin	11		
Taurine	30		

ported by Maeda and Frohman (7) or by Terry et al. (8). Epelbaum et al. (9), on the other hand, found that NE could stimulate IRS release from explants via an alpha adrenergic mechanism. This effect was only present in explants which contained SS cell bodies, and did not occur in those which only contained nerve terminals. Negro-Vilar et al. (10) also found that the NE effect could be blocked by an alpha adrenergic antagonist. Chihara et al. (4) noted that NE increased IRS release into the hypophyseal portal circulation, although less potently than DA.

The effects of serotonin on SS secretion have been studied in several systems. This indolamine did not cause any significant change in portal blood levels of IRS (4), nor did it change IRS release from hypothalamic explants (7). Both Bennett et al. (1) and Richardson et al. (11) found that serotonin decreased IRS secretion from two different hypothalamic in vitro preparations.

Acetylcholine (ACh) was found to increase rat hypophyseal portal IRS levels (4). Direct exposure of isolated hypothalamic neurons to cholinergic stimuli, however, did not result in any change in IRS release (7,8) or resulted in decreased release (12).

The inhibitory amino acid GABA was found to have no effect on IRS release from hypothalamic explants by Terry et al. (8) or by Epelbaum et al. (13). GABA has been reported to inhibit IRS release (14) and to decrease SS levels in the hypothalamus (15).

EFFECTS OF PITUITARY HORMONES

These studies are directed at the question of "short-loop" feedback mechanisms by which the pituitary may modulate the activity of hypothalamic SS neurons. The recognition of high levels of pituitary hormones in portal blood provides a basis for this hypothesis.

151

CH is the pituitary hormone most extensively studied for possible SS regulatory capability. Both Kanatsuka et al. (16) and Patel (17) found that GH could increase hypothalamic IRS content. These studies confirmed the earlier studies of Hoffman and Baker (18) which discovered that histochemically localized IRS was partially restored to the median eminence of hypophysectomized rats after treatment with GH. The possibility that GH effects were mediated indirectly (e.g., by somatomedins) could not be excluded in these studies. When directly applied to isolated hypothalamic neurons, GH stimulated IRS secretion in both adult (19,20,21) and neonatal (5) tissues. In monolayer hypothalamic cell cultures, GH at concentrations as low as 3 micromolar were able to increase cellular IRS levels (5). The GH effect was not present prior to 12 hours of exposure to GH suggesting a complex indirect action. When compared to equimolar concentrations of other pituitary hormones, GH was the only factor capable of increasing intracellular stores and secretion. TSH stimulated IRS release but depleted cellular IRS levels; PRL had no effect and an ACTH analog reduced synthesis and secretion. Previous studies on the influence of TSH on IRS release from adult hypothalamic fragments found either no effect (21) or a nonsignificant increase in IRS release (22).

EFFECTS OF OTHER FACTORS

In addition to increased IRS release induced by depolarizing levels of potassium (2,5,23,24), activation of sodium channels with the drug veratridine also increases IRS secretion (1,7,14,25,26). Extracellular glucose concentrations also seem to regulate the rate of IRS release. Sudden decreases in glucose stimulates IRS release from hypothalamic explants (27,28). In a complimentary study, Chihara et al. (4) noted that elevation of serum glucose resulted in an increase in hypophyseal portal blood IRS levels.

A number of other agents have been found to increase hypothalamic SS secretion. These include cysteamine (29,30), triiodothyronine (22), and taurine (30).

EFFECTS OF PEPTIDES

Both somatomedin A (31) and somatomedin C (19) have been shown to stimulate IRS release from hypothalamic fragments. Many neuropeptides have been examined directly or indirectly for their potential ability to regulate hypothalamic IRS release. Table 2 lists those which have been tested.

SECOND MESSENGERS

The intracellular factors in hypothalamic neurons which mediate stimulatory signals are beginning to be defined. The calcium dependency of most secretogogues has been established. Richardson and Twente (33) further demonstrated that inhibition of calmodulin by various drugs interferes with IRS release subsequent to ionic depolarization. No direct effect of cyclic AMP on baseline IRS release was noted when tested directly on hypothalamic fragments (7) although Montminy et al. (34) have reported increased somatostatin secretion in response to adenylate cyclase activation by forskolin.

The role of membrane phospholipids in IRS release has been examined by Ojeda et al. (6) who found that PGE_2 and PGF_{2a} had no effect on IRS release, but that indomethacin, which blocks prostaglandin synthesis, re-

Table 2. Hypothalamic somatostatin release:
neuropeptides (references)

Peptide	Increase	Decrease	No effect
Glucagon	38,39	-	13
VIP	40	13	-
Substance P	41	-	7,13,42
Vasopressin	-	-	25
Neurotensin	7,27,41,42	-	-
Met-enkephalin	-	-	41,42,50
Beta endorphin	-	-	42,50
Somatomedins	31,32	-	-
GnRH	-	-	25
TRH	43	-	22,25,51
GRF	44,45	-	25
Somatostatin	-	25	-
CRF	46,47,48	-	25
Bombesin	49	-	-

sulted in elevated IRS secretion. This is consistent with the results of Capdevila et al. (35) who noted that a lipoxygenase inhibitor (ETYA) but not a cyclo-oxygenase inhibitor could interfere with arachidonic acid stimulated IRS release. Peterfreund and Vale (36), furthermore, reported that phorbol esters could stimulate IRS secretion from hypothalamic neurons. It is clear that several different "second messenger" systems can result in enhanced IRS release but their interaction and relative dominance remains to be defined.

REFERENCES

1. Bennett G, Edwardson J, Marcano De Cotte D, Berelowitz M, Pimstone B, Kronheim S. Release of somatostatin from rat brain synaptosomes. J Neurochem 1979; 32:1127-30.
2. Wakabayashi I, Miyazawawa H, Kanda M, et al. Stimulation of immuno-reactive somatostatin release from hypothalamic synaptosomes by high K and dopamine. Endocrinol Jpn 1977; 24:601-6.
3. Lewis B, Dieguez C, Lewis M, Hall R, Scanlon M. Hypothalamic D2 receptors mediate the preferential release of somatostatin-28 in response to dopaminergic stimulation. Endocrinology 1986 (in press).
4. Chihara K, Arimura A, Schally A. Effect of intraventricular injection of dopamine, norepinephrine, acetylcholine, and serotonin on immunoreactive somatostatin release into rat hypophyseal portal blood. Endocrinology 1979; 104:1656-62.

5. Robbins R, Leidy J, Landon R. The effects of growth hormone, prolactin, corticotropin, and thyrotropin on the production and secretion of somatostatin by hypothalamic cells in vitro. Endocrinology 1985; 117:538-43.

6. Ojeda S, Negro-Vilar A, Arimura A, McCann S. On the hypothalamic mechanism by which prostaglandin E2 stimulates growth hormone release. Neuroendocrinology 1980; 31:1-7.

7. Maeda K, Frohman L. Release of somatostatin and thyrotropin releasing hormone from rat hypothalamic fragments in vitro. Endocrinology 1980; 106:1837-42.

8. Terry L, Rorstad O, Martin J. The release of biologically and immunologically reactive somatostatin from perfused hypothalamic fragments. Endocrinology 1980; 107:794-800.

9. Epelbaum J, Tapia-Arancibia L, Kordon C. Noradrenaline stimulates somatostatin release from incubated slices of the amygdala and the hypothalamic preoptic area. Brain Res 1981; 215:393-7.

10. Negro-Vilar A, Ojeda S, Arimura A, McCann S. Dopamine and norepinephrine stimulate somatostatin release by median eminence fragments in vitro. Life Sci 1978; 23:1493-6.

11. Richardson S, Hollander C, Prasad J, Hirooka Y. Somatostatin release from rat hypothalamus in vitro: effects of melatonin and serotonin. Endocrinology 1981; 109:602-6.

12. Richardson S, Hollander C, D'Eletto R, Greenleaf P, Thaw C. Acetylcholine inhibits the release of somatostatin from rat hypothalamus in vitro. Endocrinology 1980; 107:122-9.

13. Epelbaum J, Tapia-Arancibia L, Besson J, Rotsztejn W, Kordon C. Vasoactive intestinal polypeptide inhibits release of somatostatin from hypothalamus in vitro. Eur J Pharmacol 1979; 58:493-9.

14. Gamse R, Vaccaro D, Gamse G, DiPace M, Fox T, Leeman S. Release of immunoreactive somatostatin from hypothalamic cells in culture: inhibition by gamma amino butyric acid. Proc Natl Acad Sci USA 1980; 77:5552-6.

15. Takahara J, Yunoki S, Hosogi H, Yakushiji W, Kageyama J, Tadashi O. Concomitant increases in serum growth hormone and hypothalamic somatostatin in rats after injection of GABA, amino-oxyacetic acid or gamma hydroxybutyric acid. Endocrinology 1980; 106:343-7.

16. Kanatsuka A, Makino H, Matsushima Y, Osegawa M, Yamamoto M, Kumagai S. Effect of hypophysectomy and growth hormone administration on somatostatin content in the rat hypothalamus. Neuroendocrinology 1979; 29:186-90.

17. Patel Y. Growth hormone stimulates hypothalamic somatostatin. Life Sci 1979; 24:1589-94.

18. Hoffman D, Baker B. Effect of treatment with growth hormone on somatostatin in the median eminence of hypophysectomized rats. Proc Soc Exp Biol Med 1977; 156:265-71.

19. Berelowitz M, Firestone S, Frohman L. Effects of growth hormone excess and deficiency on hypothalamic somatostatin content and release and on tissue somatostatin distribution. Endocrinology 1981; 109:714-9.

20. Chihara K, Minimata N, Kaji H, Arimura A, Fujita T. Intraventricularly injected growth hormone stimulates somatostatin release into rat hypophyseal portal blood. Endocrinology 1981; 109:2279-81.

21. Sheppard M, Kronheim S, Pimstone B. Stimulation by growth hormone of somatostatin release from the rat hypothalamus in vitro. Clin Endocrinol (Oxf) 1978; 9:583-91.

22. Berelowitz M, Kiyoshi M, Harris S, Frohman L. The effect of alterations in the pituitary-thyroid axis on hypothalamic content and in vitro release of somatostatin-like immunoreactivity. Endocrinology 1980; 107:24-9.

23. Iversen L, Iversen S, Bloom F, Douglas C, Brown M, Vale W. Calcium dependent release of somatostatin and neurotensin from rat brain in

vitro. Nature 1978; 273:161-3.

24. Berelowitz M, Kronheim S, Pimstone B, Sheppard M. Potassium stim-ulated calcium dependent release of immunoreactive somatostatin from incubated rat hypothalamus. J Neurochem 1978; 31:1537-9.

25. Richardson S, Twente S. Inhibition of rat hypothalamic somatostatin release by somatostatin: evidence for somatostatin ultrashort feedback loop. Endocrinology 1986; 118:2076-82.

26. Robbins R, Sutton R, Reichlin S. Sodium and calcium dependent somatostatin release from dissociated cerebral cortical cells in culture. Endocrinology 1982; 110:496-501.

27. Berelowitz M, Dudlak D, Frohman L. Release of somatostatin-like immunoreactivity from incubated rat hypothalamus and cerebral cortex. J Clin Invest 1982; 69:1293-1301.

28. Lengyel M, Kruseman A, Grossman A, Rees L, Besser M. Glucose-induced changes in somatostatin-14 and somatostatin-28 released from hypotha-lamic fragments in vitro. Life Sci 1984; 35:713-9.

29. Bakhit C, Koda L, Benoit R, Morrison J, Bloom F. Evidence for selective release of somatostatin-14 and -28(1-12) from rat hypothal-amus. J Neurosci 1984; 4:411-9.

30. Aguila M, McCann S. Stimulation of somatostatin release from median eminence tissue incubated in vitro by taurine and related amino acids. Endocrinology 1985; 116:1158-62.

31. Pimstone B, Sheppard M, Shapiro B, et al. Localization in and release of somatostatin from brain and gut. Fed Proc 1979; 38:2330-2.

32. Berelowitz M, Szabo M, Frohman L, Firestone S, Chu L. Somatomedin-C mediates growth hormone negative feedback by effects on both the hypothalamus and the pituitary. Science 1981; 212:1279-81.

33. Richardson S, Twente S. Mouse hypothalamic somatostatin release: roles of calcium and calmodulin. Endocrinology 1985; 117:369-75.

34. Montminy M, Lowe M, Tapia-Arancibia L, Reichlin S, Mandel G, Goodman R. Cyclic AMP regulates somatostatin mRNA accumulation in primary diencephalic cultures and in transfected fibroblast cells. J Neurosci 1986; 6:1171-6.

35. Capdevila J, Chacos N, Falck J, Manna S, Negro-Vilar A, Ojeda S. Novel hypothalamic arachidonate products stimulate somatostatin release from the median eminence. Endocrinology 1983; 113:421-3.

36. Peterfreund R, Vale W. Phorbol diesters stimulate somatostatin secretion from cultured brain cells. Endocrinology 1983; 113:200-8.

37. Charpenet G, Patel Y. Characterization of tissue and releasable molecular forms of somatostatin-28(1-12)-like immunoreactivity in rat median eminence. Endocrinology 1985; 116:1863-8.

38. Abe H, Kato T, Chiba T, Taminato T, Fujita T. Plasma immunoreactive somatostatin levels in rat hypophyseal portal blood: effects of glucagon administration. Life Sci 1978; 23:1647-54.

39. Katakami H, Kato Y, Matsushita N, Shimatsu A, Imura H. Involvement of hypothalamic somatostatin in glucagon-induced suppression of GH secretion in conscious rats. Peptides 1983; 4:849-55.

40. Tapia-Arancibia L, Reichlin S. VIP and PHI stimulate somatostatin release from cerebrocortical and diencephalic cells in culture. Brain Res 1984; 336:67-72. .

41. Sheppard M, Kronheim S, Pimstone B. Effect of Substance P, neuro-tensin, and the enkephalins on somatostatin release from the rat hypothalamus in vitro. J Neurochem 1979; 32:647-51.

42. Abe H, Chihara K, Chiba T, Masukura T, Fujita T. Effects of intra-ventricular injections of neurotensin and other various bioactive peptides on plasma immunoreactive somatostatin levels in rat hypophy-seal portal blood. Endocrinology 1981; 109:1939-43.

43. Katakami H, Arimura A, Frohman L. Hypothalamic somatostatin mediates the suppression of GH secretion by centrally administered TRH in conscious rats. Endocrinology 1985; 117:1139-45.

44. Aguila M, McCann S. Stimulation of somatostatin release in vitro by synthetic human growth hormone releasing factor by a non-dopaminergic mechanism. Endocrinology 1985; 117:762-5.
45. Katakami H, Arimura A, Frohman L. Growth hormone releasing factor stimulates hypothalamic somatostatin release: an inhibitory feedback effect on GH secretion. Endocrinology 1986; 118:1872-7.
46. Rivier C, Vale W. Involvement of CRF and somatostatin in stress-induced inhibition of GH secretion in the rat. Endocrinology 1985; 117:2478-82.
47. Peterfreund R, Vale W. Ovine CRF stimulates somatostatin secretion from cultured brain cells. Endocrinology 1982; 112:1275-83.
48. Katakami H, Arimura A, Frohman L. Involvement of hypothalamic somatostatin in the suppression of GH secretion by central CRF in conscious male rats. Neuroendocrinology 1985; 41:390-5.
49. Abe H, Chihara K, Minamitani N, et al. Stimulation by bombesin of immunoreactive somatostatin release into rat hypophyseal portal blood. Endocrinology 1981; 109:229-34.
50. Moldow R, Hollander C. Opiate peptides modulate somatostatin release from dispersed hypothalamic cells. Peptides 1981; 2:489-92.
51. Peterfreund R, Vale W. High molecular weight somatostatin secretion by cultured rat brain cells. Brain Res 1982; 239:463-78.

15

SOMATOSTATIN AND BEHAVIOR: PRECLINICAL AND CLINICAL STUDIES

Charles B. Nemeroff,*[2] Thomas J. Walsh,[3] and
Garth Bissette*

Departments of Psychiatry* and Pharmacology,[2]
Duke University Medical Center, Durham, North Carolina

Biological Sciences Research Center,[3] University of North
Carolina School of Medicine, Chapel Hill, North Carolina

INTRODUCTION

Since the discovery of the chemical identity of the hypothalamic hypophysiotropic hormones, considerable research has been conducted on their physiologic role in regulating the secretion of the adenohypophyseal hormones. Somatostatin (SRIF) has been extensively investigated in this regard and Reichlin has comprehensively discussed this literature in a recent two-part review (1,2). Study of the distribution of the hypothalamic releasing factors including thyrotropin-releasing hormone (TRH) (3), corticotropin-releasing hormone (CRF) (4) and SRIF (5) revealed that these peptides are present in substantial quantities in extrahypothalamic brain areas. The discrete localization of SRIF throughout the central nervous system (CNS) served as an impetus to study its role as a neuroregulator in the mammalian brain. A myriad of immunohistochemical (6-10) and radio-immunoassay (11-15) studies have shown SRIF to be present in high concentrations in hypothalamus, hippocampus, striatum, and cerebral cortex. In addition, the peptide is preferentially localized in the synaptosomal fraction after density gradient centrifugation (16) and is released from brain slices by depolarizing concentrations of potassium, in a calcium-dependent manner (17). Delfs et al. (18) observed SRIF biosynthesis in dissociated cell cultures from rat cerebral cortex, conclusively demonstrating that SRIF production occurs independent of the hypothalamus. Moreover, high-affinity binding sites, regarded as putative receptors, have been found by autoradiographic and biochemical (19,20) methods to be heterogeneously distributed in the mammalian CNS. Together these findings are concordant with the view that SRIF functions as a neurotransmitter or neuromodulator in the CNS. Little is known about the role of endogenous SRIF in the CNS, especially as it pertains to behavioral effects.

The purpose of the present review is to describe work conducted in our laboratories and others in two major areas: laboratory animal studies in which behavioral, neurochemical, and electrophysiological effects of SRIF have been investigated, and clinical studies in which the concentrations of SRIF (or its receptors in brain tissue) have been measured in cerebrospinal fluid (CSF) or brain tissue of patients with different neuropsychiatric disorders.

BEHAVIORAL STUDIES IN LABORATORY ANIMALS

We shall limit our discussion in this section to the effects of exogenously administered SRIF on animal behavior, electroencephalographic measures, sleep, and neurochemical indices as well as recent studies in which cysteamine, an agent which depletes SRIF, has been used in order to elucidate the role of endogenous SRIF in certain CNS structures.

In an early study, Segal and Mandell (21) reported that intracerebroventricular (ICV) infusion of SRIF significantly reduced the spontaneous locomotor activity of rats. Cohn and Cohn (22) confirmed and extended these findings. At ICV doses of 5-10 µg, SRIF markedly reduced locomotor activity. At higher doses (25-50 µg), SRIF produced "barrel rotation" in which the rats rolled in an unusual "barrel" fashion for approximately 30 minutes. In a series of studies (23-27) Rezek, Havlicek and Friesen investigated the effects of centrally administered SRIF in the rat. After ICV injection in intact or hypophysectomized rats SRIF (10 µg) produced marked behavioral excitation associated with a profound reduction of slow-wave sleep (SWS) and rapid eye movement (REM) sleep (23). The effect of SRIF was described as intense motor excitation and stereotypy, characterized by prolonged intervals of compulsive scratching and circular movements. Direct cortical application of SRIF (24) to intact and hypophysectomized rats produced behavioral effects similar to those observed after ICV administration—increases in sniffing, chewing and scratching stereotypy as well as decreased SWS and REM sleep. Difficulties in motor coordination were also observed. After intrahippocampal infusions of the tetradecapeptide (25), similar behavioral effects were observed and a dissociation of the EEG and subsequent behavior was noted. Similar behavioral excitation, stereotypy and EEG alterations were reported to occur after neostriatal and amygdaloid (27) SRIF application. In contrast to these findings, Gordin et al. (28) reported that ICV infusion of SRIF (10-600 µg) to conscious goats produced no behavioral effects.

Considerable research with SRIF has been conducted by Vecsei and his colleagues (29-31). In an early study (29), this group reported that a low ICV dose of SRIF (1 µg) increased, whereas a higher dose (5 µg) decreased the rate of electrical self-stimulation in the lateral hypothalamus. In two other studies (30,31), ICV SRIF reversed the retrograde amnesia produced by electroconvulsive shock therapy. This antiamnesic effect of $SRIF_4$ was shared by the biologically active structural analog, $D-Trp_8$, $D-Lys^{14}$-SRIF but not by the inactive congener, des-Asn^5-($D-Trp^8$, $D-Ser^{13}$)-SRIF and des $AA^{1,2,4,5,12,13}$-($D-Trp^8$)-SRIF. In addition, ICV administered SRIF also inhibited extinction of active avoidance behavior.

Based on these findings as well as the human postmortem studies (see below) that have demonstrated a reduction of SRIF in Alzheimer's disease, we have investigated the effects of hippocampal SRIF depletion induced by cysteamine on passive avoidance behavior. The impetus for these studies was provided by the discovery that parenterally administered cysteamine (2-mercaptoethylamine) depletes SRIF from peripheral tissues, e.g., gastrointestinal tract as well as the hypothalamus (32,33). Beal and Martin (34) have studied the effects of local cysteamine microinjection into the rat striatum on SRIF concentrations. They observed a dose-dependent reduction in striatal SRIF concentrations which persisted for up to 72 hours but was eventually reversible. In a preliminary study, we evaluated the effects of intrahippocampal cysteamine injection on regional brain SRIF concentrations as well as on passive avoidance behavior and locomotor activity. Rats were treated with 30 µg cysteamine HCl or vehicle (artificial CSF) bilaterally in both the dorsal and ventral hippocampus (60 µg cysteamine per hippocampus). A third group of rats was treated with cysteamine (300 mg/kg) subcutaneously. The effects of cysteamine on SRIF concentrations are shown in Table 1. The SRIF radio-immunoassay used has been previously described in detail (35,36). Systemically-administered cysteamine produced a marked reduction in hypothalamic SRIF concentrations but had no effect on SRIF concentrations in the olfactory tubercles, striatum, hippocampus, and frontal cortex. Intrahippocampal cysteamine depleted SRIF in the hippocampus by 47%; other brain areas were unaffected.

Intrahippocampal, but not subcutaneously administered, cysteamine injected 72 hours prior to training resulted in a significant impairment in the retention of the passive avoidance response (Fig. 1). Because initial step-through latencies (STL) during the training trial and sensitivity to footshock were unaffected by cysteamine, we have tentatively concluded that the retention deficits represent impairment in the acquisition or retention of the task. The rats treated with intrahippocampal cysteamine exhibited locomotor hypoactivity, which indicates that the reduced latency to respond in the passive avoidance task was not simply due to locomotor hyperactivity. These findings are concordant with the view that hippocampal SRIF-containing neurons play a role in learning and memory processes. Further work is clearly warranted.

Several investigators have studied the effects of SRIF on CNS neurochemical indices, including neurotransmitter turnover, and on electrophysiological correlates of neuronal activity. In an early study, Tan et al. (37) reported that SRIF increased uptake and inhibited release of radiolabeled calcium in guinea pig cerebral cortical synaptosomes. The effects of SRIF on monoaminergic neurotransmission has received some attention. Gothert (38) reported that SRIF inhibits the electrically-evoked release of radiolabeled norepinephrine (NE), but not dopamine or serotonin, from hypothalamic slices in vitro. Curiously, no effect on NE release from occipital cortex was observed. Using measurement of the accumulation of L-dopa and 5-hydroxytryptophan (5HTP) after inhibition of L-aromatic amino acid decarboxylase with NSD 1015 or R04-4602, Garcia-Sevilla et al. (39) reported that ICV administered SRIF enhanced both DA, NE and 5HT turnover. However, these effects occurred only after relatively large doses (10-20 μg) of the peptide. Such high doses produced profound behavioral alterations as noted above, including barrel rotation. The effect of SRIF on cyclic nucleotide concentration in the rat brain has been investigated.

Table 1. Effects of subcutaneous or intrahippocampal cysteamine on regional somatostatin concentrations.

	CSF	Cysteamine (60 μg/HPC)	Cysteamine (300 mg/kg, sc)
Olf. tubercles	450 ± 40	369 ± 98	734 ± 144
Hypothalamus	137 ± 21	110 ± 32	4 ± 13*
Striatum	43 ± 6	60 ± 9	39 + 13
Hippocampus	17 ± 2	9 ± 1*	14 ± 2
Frontal cortex	3 ± 1	4 ± 1	3 ± 1

Values represent mean (pg/mg protein ± SEM), n = > 8/group. Rats were sacrificed by decapitation 72 hours following administration of cysteamine. *P < 0.01 vs. CSF.

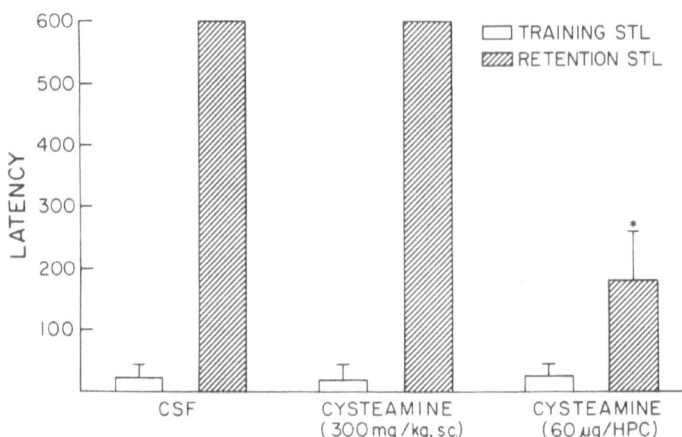

Fig. 1. The effects of cysteamine administered peripherally (300 mg/kg subcutaneously) or centrally (60 μg per hypocampus bilaterally) on responding in a passive avoidance paradigm. Although training step-through latencies (STL) are the same in each group, the rats treated with intrahippocampal cysteamine exhibit a marked and significant deficit, indicative of disruption of either acquisition or retention (n = $\geq$ 8/group).

Catalan et al. (40), using rat cerebrocortical slices, reported that SRIF increased cyclic GMP and decreased cyclic AMP concentrations; these in vitro effects were dose dependent.

Considerable research has been conducted on the electrophysiological effects of SRIF in the CNS. In an early study in anesthetized rats, Renaud and his associates (41) reported that SRIF produced inhibition of the firing rate of neurons in the hypothalamus, cerebellum and cerebral cortex. Ioffe et al. (42) refuted these findings in a study conducted in unanesthetized, habituated rabbits where microiontophoretically applied SRIF produced excitation of cortical neurons. These excitatory effects of SRIF were also observed by Dodd and Kelly (43) in a rat hippocampal slice preparation, specifically in the CA1 and CA2 pyramidal cells. Similar excitatory effects of SRIF were reported by Olpe et al. (44) in rats anesthetized with either urethane or chloral hydrate; neurons in the frontal and parietal cortex as well as in the hippocampus and striatum were excited by SRIF.

CLINICAL STUDIES

In the study of neuropeptides in psychiatric and neurological disorders, three major approaches have been taken and we have recently reviewed these data in detail (45). First, the neuropeptide in question, which in this present monograph is SRIF, or its receptors, is measured in postmortem tissue, usually brain, or in body fluids, usually CSF, from patients with one or another neuropsychiatric disorder compared to age- and sex-matched controls. The second general approach has been to treat patients with neuropeptide receptor antagonists in order to determine whether blockade of specific neuropeptide receptors has a salutary effect in a specific clinical disorder. This approach has been utilized most frequently with the opioid peptides, because of the availability of two opiate receptor antagonists, naloxone and naltrexone. Unfortunately, no specific SRIF receptor antagonists are currently available for clinical use. The third approach involves the administration of the peptide or a peptide analog that is relatively resistant to enzymatic degradation, to patients with a specific neuropsychiatric disorder. This approach is, unfortunately, highly problematic, largely for such pragmatic reasons as the very limited permeability of peptides across the blood-brain barrier. No such studies have been conducted with SRIF with the exception of case reports of intrathecally administered SRIF in the treatment of the intractable pain associated with malignant neoplasms (see below).

The neuropsychiatric disorders in which alterations in the concentration of SRIF have been reported most often are Alzheimer's disease, Huntington's chorea and major depression. Alzheimer's disease has received increasingly more attention in the past decade, and neuropeptide systems have been unequivocally demonstrated to be pathologically altered in this disorder (45,46). In their pioneering study, Davies and his associates (47) observed a marked reduction in the concentration of immunoreactive SRIF in postmortem brain tissue (hippocampus, frontal cortex, parietal cortex and superior temporal gyrus) of histologically-verified Alzheimer's disease, when compared to neurologically normal controls. They confirmed and extended these observations in a second study (48) where 7 of 8 brain regions had very substantial decreases in SRIF concentrations in the postmortem tissue of the Alzheimer's disease group. We have confirmed these findings in a study (49) of postmortem brain tissue of 10 Alzheimer's disease patients and 10 controls. Frontal and temporal cortex (Brodmann's areas 10 and 38) as well as hypothalamus exhibited significant decreases in SRIF concentrations. Other brain areas including the substantia innominata, caudate, parietal cortex and the nucleus accumbens exhibited normal SRIF concentrations. Similar results were obtained by Rossor et al. (50) and he has recently reviewed these data (51).

A significant correlation between neuropathological measures of disease severity (plaque counts and neurofibrillary tangles) and the SRIF reduction in temporal cortex was observed. SRIF concentrations were reduced in the temporal cortex but not in two other cortical areas, or in the amygdala, posterior hippocampus or putamen. Ferrier et al. (52) noted diminished concentrations of SRIF in three cortical areas and the septum in Alzheimer's disease patients while nine other brain areas exhibited relatively normal levels of the tetradecapeptide. Arai et al. (53) also confirmed the SRIF depletion in Alzheimer's disease. In a study of 21 postmortem brain regions in 7 Alzheimer's patients and 10 controls, SRIF was significantly reduced in certain cortical areas as well as hippocampus and putamen. Recently Beal and his colleagues (54) have comprehensively reviewed their own work and that of others on SRIF concentrations in neurological diseases. They measured SRIF in eight cortical regions as well as in the hippocampus and five other subcortical areas. They confirmed the reduction in the concentration of SRIF in Alzheimer's disease in all but one of the cortical areas. Candy et al. (55) have recently noted significant reductions in SRIF content of frontal and temporal cortex as well as the basal nucleus of the amygdala in Alzheimer's disease patients when compared to controls. This group also measured SRIF in the nucleus basalis of Meynert and in confirmation of our findings, reported that the concentration of this peptide is normal in this region in Alzheimer's disease. Epelbaum et al. (56) have recently shown that Parkinsonian patients with Alzheimer-like dementia exhibit marked decreases in SRIF concentrations in frontal and entorhinal cortex as well as in the hippocampus. The relationship between this presumed SRIF-containing neuronal degeneration and the well-studied cholinergic neuronal degeneration in Alzheimer's disease is not yet clear; however, colocalization of acetylcholine and SRIF has been demonstrated in cerebral cortical cells in culture by Delfs et al. (57).

The concentration of SRIF in CSF has been measured in patients with Alzheimer's disease, major depression, Huntington's chorea, and other neuropsychiatric disorders. As expected, several investigators have demonstrated reductions in CSF SRIF in patients with presumed Alzheimer's disease. The early work was conducted by Wood et al. (58) and Oram et al. (59). Recently, these findings have been confirmed and extended by several other groups including Serby et al. (60), Beal et al. (61), Raskind et al. (62) and our own group, Bissette et al. (63). Not only is SRIF in CSF reduced in patients with presumed Alzheimer's disease, but this abnormality is also observed in patients with multi-infarct dementia (61,63). Taken together, more than 100 patients with Alzheimer's disease have been studied by the research groups who have scrutinized this problem. In a recent study, our group with our Swedish collaborators (Karlsson et al., 64), have shown that Alzheimer's disease patients exposed to intensive environmental stimulation show increases in CSF SRIF concentrations when compared to Alzheimer's disease patients that receive more traditional custodial care. The specificity of the reduction in CSF SRIF in Alzheimer's disease has also been evaluated. Although patients with Huntington's chorea, normal pressure hydrocephalus and Parkinson's disease have been reported to have normal CSF concentrations of SRIF (54), certain of these findings have been refuted recently. Moreover, patients with the following diagnoses have been reported to exhibit reductions in CSF concentrations of SRIF: major depression, multiple sclerosis, and schizophrenia. Thus, although Beal et al. (54) found no reductions of SRIF in CSF from patients with either Parkinson's disease or Huntington's chorea, Dupont et al. (65) reported significant reductions in the former and Cramer et al. (66) observed similar reductions in the latter. Several investigators have reported reductions in SRIF concentrations in CSF from patients with major depression. This was first noted by Gerner and Yamada (67) in a study of 29 normal controls and 28 depressed patients. This observation has been confirmed and extended by Rubinow and his colleagues at the NIMH (68). In their study, they measured the concentration of SRIF in CSF from 39 normal healthy volunteers, 18 bipolar depressed patients, 7 unipolar depressed patients and 7 manic patients. The concentration of SRIF in CSF was significantly reduced in both the unipolar and bipolar patients compared to the controls. This same group (69) has recently reported that depressed patients that exhibit DST nonsuppression also have the lowest CSF concentrations of SRIF. Our research group has recently confirmed these findings of reduced CSF concentrations of SRIF in a study of 23 patients with major depression and 10 normal controls (63).

The concentration of SRIF has been studied in postmortem brain tissue of patients with Huntington's chorea. Our group (36) found marked elevations in the concentration of SRIF in the nucleus accumbens of patients with this neurological disorder; the nucleus caudatus also showed a significant elevation (Fig. 2). The amygdala showed no such alteration in SRIF content. These findings have been confirmed by Martin and his colleagues (Aronin et al., 70 and Beal et al., 71) who found marked increases in SRIF concentrations in the caudate, putamen and globus pallidus of patients with Huntington's disease; no such changes were noted in the amygdala, hippocampus, substantia nigra or cerebral cortex. Immunohistochemical studies have revealed a significant increase in the density of SRIF-containing fibers in the neostriatum in Huntington's disease (72). Recently, the concentration of a fragment containing the first twelve amino acids of the SRIF precursor, SRIF-28, has also been shown to be elevated in Huntington's disease (73).

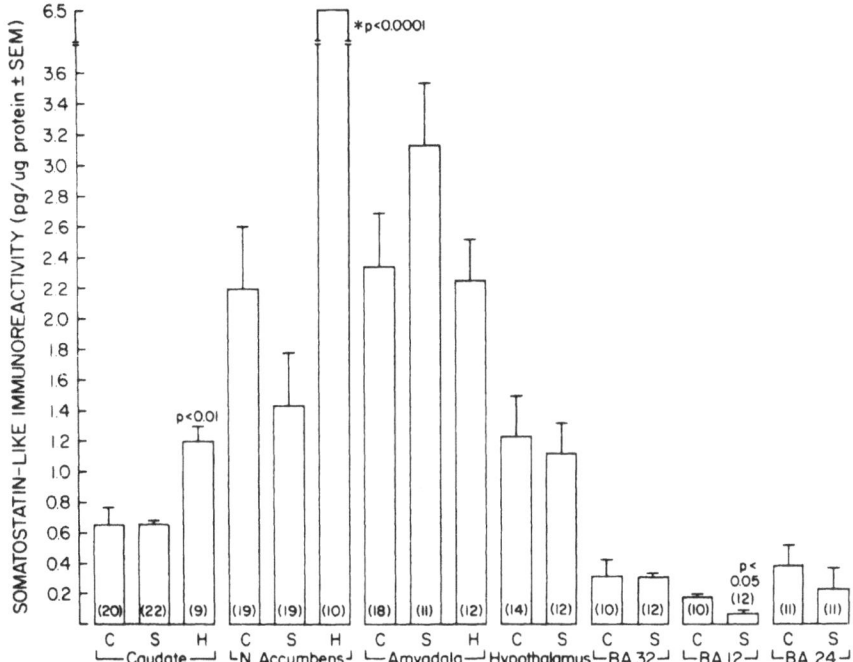

Fig. 2. Regional brain concentrations of SRIF-like immunoreactivity in normal controls (C), schizophrenics (S), and Huntington's chorea patients (H). Values are mean ± SEM; numbers in parentheses refer to the number of samples per group. Huntington's chorea patients had significantly higher concentrations of SRIF in the caudate nucleus and nucleus accumbens. The schizophrenics had lower concentrations of SRIF in one area of frontal cortex (BA 12). Modified from Nemeroff et al. (36).

Somatostatin has also been studied in schizophrenia (Fig. 2). In postmortem brain tissue, we reported that SRIF concentrations were normal in the caudate, nucleus accumbens, amygdala, hypothalamus and in two cortical areas, Brodmann's areas 12 and 24; the concentration of the peptide was significantly elevated in one area of frontal cortex, BA 32 (36). In CSF from schizophrenia patients, Rubinow and his colleagues (68,69) found normal concentrations of SRIF; our group recently reported reduced levels of the peptide in 10 schizophrenic patients (63).

CONCLUSIONS

Of the more than 40 peptides discovered thus far in mammalian brain, perhaps the best case for peptidergic involvement in neuropsychiatric disorders can be made for SRIF. It seems likely that SRIF-containing neurons degenerate in Alzheimer's disease. In addition, considerable evidence from different research groups supports the view that SRIF neurons are altered in the basal ganglia of patients with Huntington's disease. Moreover, CSF studies support the view that SRIF-containing neurons show reduced activity in several neuropsychiatric disorders including major depression, Alzheimer's disease, multiple sclerosis, schizophrenia and Parkinson's disease—all diseases with prominent cognitive dysfunction. The laboratory animal studies reviewed above, particularly those in which cysteamine was used as a tool to deplete SRIF, are also concordant with the hypothesis that hippocampal and/or cortical SRIF neurons play an important role in cognitive processes.

ACKNOWLEDGMENTS

We are grateful to Mary Lassiter and Cindy Citty for preparation of this manuscript. Supported by NIMH MH-40524, MH-40159, NIA AG-05128 and a Nanaline H. Duke Fellowship to Charles B. Nemeroff.

REFERENCES

1. Reichlin S. Somatostatin (first of two parts). N Engl J Med 1983; 309:1495.
2. Reichlin S. Somatostatin (second of two parts). N Engl J Med 1983; 309:1556.
3. Brownstein MJ, Palkovits M, Saavedra JM, Bassiri RM, Utiger RD. Thyrotropin-releasing hormone in specific nuclei of the rat brain. Science 1974; 185:267.
4. Chappell P, Smith MA, Kilts CD, et al. Alterations in corticotropin-releasing factor-like immunoreactivity in discrete rat brain regions after acute and chronic stress. J Neurosci (in press).
5. Krisch B, Leonhardt H. An intermittent somatostatin-immunoreactivity in the cortex and basal ganglia of the rat. Cell Tissue Res 1980; 205:327.
6. Hokfelt T, Efendic S, Hellerstrom C, Johansson O, Luft R, Arimura A. Cellular localization of somatostatin in endocrine-like cells and neurons of the rat with special references to the A5 cells of the pancreatic islets and to the hypothalamus. Acta Endocrinol 1975; 80(suppl 200):1.
7. Dorn A, Bernstein H-G, Hahn H-J, Kostmann G. Occurrence of somatostatin-like immunoreactivity (SLI) in the dorsal hippocampus of the sand rat (Psammomys obesus). Acta Histochem 1979; 65:276.
8. Krisch B. Differing immunoreactivities of somatostatin in the cortex and the hypothalamus of the rat. Cell Tissue Res 1980; 212:457.
9. Dalsgaard C-J, Hokfelt T, Johansson O, Elde R. Somatostatin immunoreactive cell bodie in the dorsal horn and the parasympathetic intermediolateral nucleus of the rat spinal cord. Neurosci Lett 1981; 27:336.
10. Lechen RM, Goodman RH, Rosenblatt M, Reichlin S, Habener JF. Prosomatostatin-specific antigen in rat brain: localization by immunocytochemical staining with an antiserum to an antiserum to a synthetic sequence of prepro-somatostatin. Proc Natl Acad Sci USA 1983; 80:2780.
11. Brownstein M, Arimiva A, Sato H, Kizer JS. The regional distribution of somatostatin in rat brain. Brain Res 1977; 126:584-8.
12. Epelbaum J, Tapia-Arancibia L, Kordon C, Ottesen OP, Ben-Ari Y. Regional distribution of somatostatin within the amygdaloid complex of the rat brain. Brain Res 1979; 174:172.
13. Kobayashi RM, Brown MR, Vale W. Regional distribution of neurotensin and somatostatin in rat brain. Endocrinology 1975; 96(6):1456-61.
14. Yamada T, Marshak D, Basinger S, Walsh J, Morley J, Stell W. Somatostatin-like immunoreactivity in the retina. Proc Natl Acad Sci USA 1980; 77:1691.
15. Geola FL, Yamada T, Warwick RJ, Tourtelotte WW, Hershman JM. Regional distribution of somatostatin-like immunoreactivity in the human brain. Brain Res 1981; 229:35.

16. Epelbaum J, Brazeau P, Tsang D, Brawer J, Martin JB. Subcellular distribution of radioimmunoassayable somatostatin in rat brain. Brain Res 1977; 126:309.
17. Iversen LL, Iversen SD, Bloom F, Douglas C, Brown M, Vale W. Calcium-dependent release of somatostatin and neurotensin from rat brain in vitro. Nature 1978; 273:161.
18. Delfs J, Robbins R, Connolly JL, Dichter M, Reichlin S. Somatostatin production by rat cerebral neurones in dissociated cell culture. Nature 1980; 283:676.
19. Srikant CB, Patel YC. Somatostatin receptors: identification and characterization in rat brain membranes. Proc Natl Acad Sci 1981; 78:3930.
20. Reubi JC, Rivier J, Perrin M, Brown M, Vale W. High affinity binding sites for a somatostatin-28 analog in rat brain. Life Sci 1981; 28:1049.
21. Segal DS, Mandell AJ. Differential behavioral effects of hypothalamic polypeptides. In: Prange AJ Jr, ed. The thyroid, drugs and behavior. New York: Raven Press, 1974.
22. Cohn ML, Cohn M. 'Barrel rotation' induced by somatostatin in the non-lesioned rat. Brain Res 1975; 96:138.
23. Havlicek V, Rezek M, Friesen H. Somatostatin and thyrotropin-releasing hormone: central effect on sleep and motor system. Pharmacol Biochem Behav 1976; 4:455.
24. Rezek M, Havlicek V, Hughes KR, Friesen H. Cortical administration of somatostatin (SRIF): effect on sleep and motor behavior. Pharmacol Biochem Behav 1976; 5:73.
25. Rezek M, Havlicek V, Hughes KR, Friesen H. Central site of action of somatostatin (SRIF): role of hippocampus. Neuropharmacology 1976; 15:499.
26. Rezek M, Havlicek V, Leybin L, et al. Neostriatal administration of somatostatin: differential effect of small and large doses on behavior and motor control. Can J Physiol Pharmacol 1977; 55:234.
27. Rezek M, Havlicek V, Hughes KR, Friesen H. Behavioral and motor excitation and inhibition induced by the administration of small and large doses of somatostatin into the amygdala. Neuropharmacology 1977; 16:157.
28. Gordin A, Ericksson L, Blom AK, Taskinen MR, Fyhrquist F. Lack of behavioral effects following intraventricular infusion of somatostatin in the conscious goat. Pharmacol Biochem Behav 1978; 9:255.
29. Vecsei L, Schwarzberg H, Telegdy G. The effect of somatostatin on the self-stimulation of rats. Neuroendocrinol Lett 1982; 4:37.
30. Vecsei L, Bollok I, Telegdy G. Intracerebroventricular somatostatin attenuates electroconvulsive shock-induced amnesia in rats. Peptides 1983; 4:293.
31. Vecsei L, Bollok L, Penke B, Telegdy G. Somatostatin and (D-Trp8, D-Cys14)—somatostatin delay extinction and reverse electroconvulsive shock-induced amnesia in rats. Psychoneuroendocrinology 1986; 11:111.
32. Szabo S, Reichlin S. Somatostatin in cat tissues is depleted by cysteamine administration. Endocrinology 1981; 109:2255.
33. Brown MR, Fisher LA, Sawchenko PE, Swanson LW, Vale WW. Biological effects of cysteamine: relationship to somatostatin depletion. Regul Pept 1983; 5:163.
34. Beal MF, Martin JB. Depletion of striatal somatostatin by local cysteamine injection. Brain Res 1984; 308:319.
35. Nemeroff CB, Konkol RJ, Bissette G, et al. Analysis of the disruption in hypothalamic-pituitary regulation in rats treated neonatally with monosodium L-glutamate (MSG): evidence for the involvement of tuberoinfundibular cholinergic and dopaminergic systems in neuroendocrine regulation. Endocrinology 1977; 101:613.
36. Nemeroff CB, Youngblood WW, Manberg PJ, Prange AJ Jr, Kizer JS.

Regional brain concentration of neuropeptides in Huntington's chorea and schizophrenia. Science 1983; 221:972.

37. Tan AT, Tsay D, Renaud LP, Martin JB. Effect of somatostatin on calcium transport in guinea pig cortex synaptosomes. Brain Res 1977; 123:193.

38. Gothert M. Somatostatin selectively inhibits noradrenaline release from hypothalamic neurons. Nature 1980; 287:86.

39. Garcia-Sevilla JA, Magnusson T, Carlsson A. Effect of intracerebroventricularly administered somatostatin on brain monoamine turnover. Brain Res 1978; 155:159.

40. Catalan RE, Aragones MD, Martinez AM. Somatostatin effect on cyclic AMP and cyclic GMP levels in rat brain. Biochim Biophys Acta 1979; 586:213.

41. Renaud LP, Martin JB, Brazeau P. Depressant action of TRH, LH-RH and somatostatin on activity of central neurons. Nature 1975; 255:233.

42. Ioffe S, Havlicek V, Friesen H, Chernick V. Effect of somatostatin (SRIF) and L-glutamate on neurons of the sensorimotor cortex in awake habituated rabbits. Brain Res 1978; 153:414.

43. Dodd J, Kelly JS. Is somatostatin an excitatory transmitter in the hippocampus? Nature 1978; 273:674.

44. Olpe H-R, Balcar VJ, Bittiger H, Rink H, Sieber P. Central actions of somatostatin. Eur J Pharmacol 1980; 63:127.

45. Nemeroff CB, Bissette G. Neuropeptides in psychiatric disorders. In: Berger PA, Brodie HKH, eds. American handbook of psychiatry (vol 8). Basic Books, 1986.

46. Cain ST, Nemeroff CB. Neuropeptides and neurotransmitters in Alzheimer's disease. In: Busse EW, Maddox GL, eds. Advances in gerontology and geriatrics. 13th Congress of the Intranational Association of Gerontology. New York: Springer (in press).

47. Davies P, Katzman R, Terry RD. Reduced somatostatin-like immunoreactivity in cerebral cortex from cases of Alzheimer's disease and Alzheimer senile dementia. Nature 1980; 288:279.

48. Davies P, Terry RD. Cortical somatostatin-like immunoreactivity in cases of Alzheimer's disease and senile dementia of the Alzheimer's type. Neurobiol Aging 1981; 2:9.

49. Nemeroff CB, Bissette G, Busby WH Jr, et al. Regional brain concentrations of neurotensin, thyrotropin-releasing hormone and somatostatin in Alzheimer's disease. Soc Neurosci Abst 1983; 9:1052.

50. Rossor MN, Emson PC, Mountjoy CQ, Roth M, Iversen LL. Reduced amounts of immunoreactive somatostatin in the temporal cortex in senile dementia of Alzheimer type. Neurosci Lett 1980; 20:373.

51. Rossor M, Emson P, Dawbarn D, Dockray G, Mountjoy C, Roth M. Postmortem studies in peptides in Alzheimer's disease and Huntington's disease. In: Martin JB, Barchas JD, eds. Neuropeptides in neurologic and psychiatric disease. New York: Raven Press, 1986.

52. Ferrier IN, Cross AJ, Johnson JA, et al. Neuropeptides in Alzheimer's type dementia. J Neurol Sci 1983; 62:159.

53. Arai H, Moroji T, Kosaka T. Somatostatin and vasoactive intestinal peptide in post-mortem brains from patients with Alzheimer's type dementia. Neurosci Lett 1984; 52:73.

54. Beal MF, Uhl G, Mazierek N, Kowell N, Martin JB. Somatostatin: alterations in the central nervous system in neurological diseases. In: Martin JB, Barchas JD, eds. Neuropeptides in neurologic and psychiatric disease. New York: Raven Press, 1986.

55. Candy JM, Gascoigne AD, Biggins JA, et al. Somatostatin immunoreactivity in cortical and some subcortical regions in Alzheimer's disease. J Neurol Sci 1985; 71:315.

56. Epelbaum J, Ruberg M, Mouse E, Javoy-Agid F, Dubois B, Agid Y. Somatostatin and dementia in Parkinson's disease. Brain Res 1983; 278:376.

57. Delfs JR, Zhu CH, Dichter MA. Coexistence of acetylcholinesterase

and somatostatin-immunoreactivity in neurons cultured from rat cerebrum. Science 1984; 223(4631):61-3.

58. Wood PL, Etienne P, Lal S, Gauthier S, Cajal S, Nair NPV. Reduced lumbar CSF somatostatin levels in Alzheimer's senile dementia. Life Sci 1982; 31:2073.

59. Oram JJ, Edwardson J, Millard PH. Investigation of cerebrospinal fluid neuropeptides in idiopathic senile dementia. Gerontol 1981; 27:216.

60. Serby M, Richardson SB, Twente S, Siekierski J, Rotrosen J. Somato-statin in Alzheimer's disease. Neurobiol Aging 1984; 5:187.

61. Beal MF, Growdon JH, Mazurek MF, Martin JB. CSF somatostatin-like immunoreactivity in dementia. Neurology 1986; 36:294.

62. Raskind MA, Peskink ER, Lampe JH, Risse SC, Taborsky GJ, Dorsa D. Cerebrospinal fluid vasopressin oxytocin, somatostatin, and β-endorphin in Alzheimer's disease. Arch Gen Psychiatry 1986; 43:382.

63. Bissette G, Widerlov E, Walleus H, et al. Alterations in cerebro-spinal fluid concentrations of somatostatin-like immunoreactivity in neuropsychiatric disorders. Arch Gen Psychiatry (in press).

64. Karlsson I, Widerlov E, Melin EV, et al. Changes of CSF neuropep-tides after environmental stimulation in dementia. Nordic Psychiat J 1985; 39(suppl 11):75.

65. Dupont E, Christensen SE, Hansen AP, Olivarias BF, Orskov H. Low cerebrospinal fluid somatostatin in Parkinson's disease: an irre-versible abnormality. Neurology 1982; 32:312.

66. Cramer H, Kohler J, Oeper G, Schonberg G, Schroter E. Huntington's chorea-measurements of somatostatin substance P and cyclic nucle-otides in the cerebrospinal fluid. J Neurol 1981; 225:183.

67. Gerner RH, Yamada T. Altered neuropeptide concentrations in cerebro-spinal fluid of psychiatric patients. Brain Res 1982; 238:298.

68. Rubinow DR, Gold PW, Post RM, et al. CSF somatostatin in affective illness. Arch Gen Psychiatry 1983; 40:409.

69. Doran AR, Rubinow DR, Roy A, Pickar D. CSF somatostatin and abnormal responses to dexamethasone administration in schizophrenic and depressed patients. Arch Gen Psychiatry 1986; 43:365.

70. Aronin N, Cooper PE, Lorenz LJ, et al. Somatostatin is increased in the basal ganglia in Huntington's disease. Ann Neurol 1983; 13:519.

71. Beal MF, Bird ED, Langlais PJ, Martin JB. Somatostatin is increased in the nucleus accumbers in Huntington's disease. Neurology 1984; 34:663.

72. Marshall PE, Landis DMD. Huntington's disease is accompanied by changes in the distribution of somatostatin-containing neuronal processes. Brain Res 1985; 329:71.

73. Beal MF, Benoit R, Bird ED, Martin JB. Somatostatin 28 (1-12) immunoreactivity is increased in Huntington's disease. Neurosci Lett 1985; 56:377.

16

PHYSIOLOGICAL SIGNIFICANCE OF SOMATOSTATIN IN

GROWTH HORMONE REGULATION

Gloria Shaffer Tannenbaum

Neuropeptide Physiology Laboratory, McGill University—
Montreal Children's Hospital Research Institute and the
Departments of Pediatrics, Neurology and Neurosurgery
McGill University, Montreal, Quebec H3H 1P3, Canada

INTRODUCTION

The secretion of growth hormone (GH) is pulsatile in nature in every species examined thus far. Particularly in the rat, GH secretion is characterized by a striking ultradian rhythm (1), with high-amplitude GH secretory bursts occurring at precise 3.3 hour intervals throughout a 24-hour period; in the intervening trough periods basal plasma GH levels are undetectable (Fig. 1). Current experimental evidence indicates that regulation of the secretion of GH from the pituitary gland is ultimately achieved by the interaction of two major factors produced by the hypothalamus—a stimulatory, GH-releasing factor, GRF, and an inhibitory peptide, somatostatin, which reach the adenohypophysis via the hypophyseal portal circulation. This chapter will focus on the physiological significance of somatostatin in regulation of the rhythmic secretion of GH.

ROLE OF SOMATOSTATIN IN GENERATION OF THE ULTRADIAN RHYTHM OF GH SECRETION

After the initial discovery of tetradecapeptide somatostatin (S-14) as a naturally occurring hypothalamic peptide capable of inhibiting GH secretion from cultured rat pituitary cells (2), numerous reports have confirmed a profound inhibitory effect of S-14 on GH release in response to virtually all known stimuli in a wide variety of species including man (see 3 for review).

The recent isolation and characterization of a larger molecular weight form of somatostatin containing 28 amino acids (4-6) aroused considerable interest concerning the biologic activity of this peptide. Thus, we assessed the actions of S-28, in comparison to those of S-14, on spontaneous GH secretion in unanesthetized freely-moving rats (7).

As shown in Figure 2, the subcutaneous administration of S-14 during a secretory burst caused a rapid suppression of pulsatile GH secretion; plasma GH levels remained depressed for only 30 min consistent with the known short duration of biological activity of S-14 (8). In contrast, S-28 exhibited prolonged inhibitory activity on spontaneous GH release which persisted for a significantly longer period of time (90 min), likely

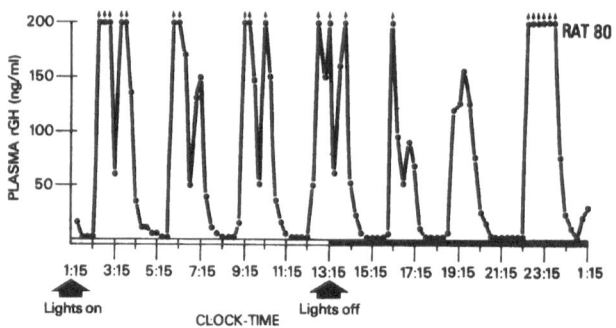

Fig. 1. Spontaneous GH secretory pattern of an individual male rat sampled over a 24-hour period.

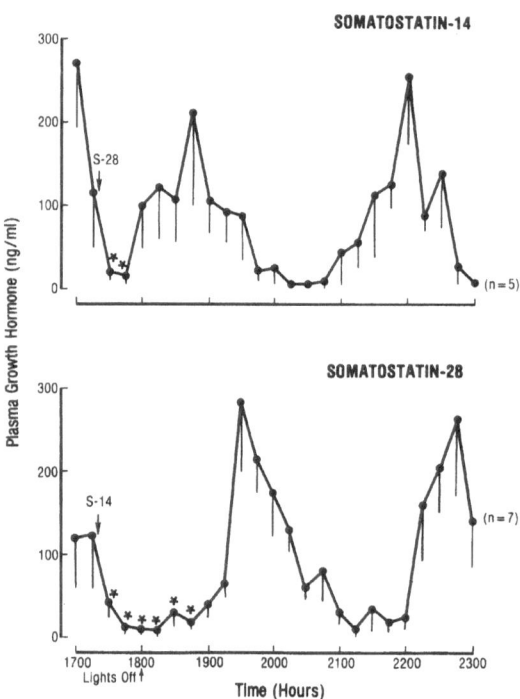

Fig. 2. Time course of effects of somatostatin-14 and somatostatin-28 on spontaneous GH secretion. The duration of significant inhibition by S-28 of mean plasma GH levels was markedly longer than that by S-14. *Significant differences of $P < 0.05$ or less compared to a control group administered normal saline.

due, at least in part, to the slower plasma degradation of S-28 compared to S-14 (9). These results demonstrated that S-28 is a potent inhibitor of spontaneous GH secretion and suggested that S-28 may not merely be a prohormone but may act as a regulatory hormone on its own to influence GH secretion.

Despite the marked GH inhibitory actions of both somatostatin peptides, the role of endogenous somatostatin in physiologic regulation of GH secretion remains to be fully elucidated. We used the technique of passive immunization to unmask the role of endogenous somatostatin in generating the normal ultradian GH rhythm. The antiserum used was directed toward the central segment of S-14, which detects S-14 and S-28 with equal affinity (10). As shown in Figure 3, administration of somatostatin antiserum during either a trough or peak period of the GH rhythm caused a rapid surge of GH secretion, likely due to postinhibitory rebound release (11), and significant elevation of subsequent GH trough levels. A similar elevation of baseline GH levels following antisomatostatin treatment has been reported in several other species (12-16). Moreover, selective lesions of the preoptic-anterior hypothalamic area, the principal cell source of somatostatinergic fibers projecting to the median eminence (17), markedly augments GH trough levels (18,19). These results suggest that endogenous circulating somatostatin is a physiologic regulator of GH trough periods and is likely released episodically into the hypophyseal portal circulation to inhibit GH release. Furthermore, since the episodic surges of GH release were not abolished by immunoneutralization with somatostatin antiserum, the findings provide support for the hypothesis that GH secretion is regulated by the interaction of at least two hypothalamic hypophysiotrophic hormones, one inhibitory, somatostatin, and the other excitatory, GRF.

SOMATOSTATIN AS A MEDIATOR OF GH RESPONSE TO NUTRITIONAL ALTERATIONS

The secretion of GH is exquisitely sensitive to changes in nutritional status. We demonstrated that the spontaneous pulses of GH release are markedly inhibited in response to prolonged food deprivation (20), insulinopenic diabetes (21,22) and intracellular glucopenia induced by 2-deoxyglucose (23). To assess the mechanism(s) mediating these GH suppression responses, we used the technique of passive immunization (24). As shown in Figure 4, administration of antisomatostatin serum to starved rats successfully restored high-amplitude GH pulses, although not the typical ultradian rhythm, suggesting that circulating somatostatin is mediating the GH suppression of starvation. Somatostatin antiserum also reversed, at least partially, the GH inhibitory reactions to diabetes (21) and glucoprivation (23) indicating a physiological role for somatostatin in these conditions. The increased somatostatin reaching the pituitary under these circumstances could originate from the hypothalamus or from peripheral tissues. The latter is more likely since alterations in pancreatic, gastrointestinal, and blood concentrations of somatostatin-like immunoreactivity (SLI) have been well documented in starvation (20,25) and various forms of diabetes (26-30). Moreover, we have recently reported a significant elevation of plasma SLI levels of starved rats (31) providing additional support for the view that the augmented somatostatin secretion originates from peripheral sites. Interestingly, the results of these studies suggest that the pattern of somatostatin secretion during starvation is converted to a tonic, rather than episodic, mode of release (31). All these findings are compatible with the hypothesis that somatostatin may be an important hormonal regulator of nutrient homeostasis (32) and suggest that blood-borne somatostatin can exert an endocrine-like action on the pituitary gland to influence GH secretion.

171

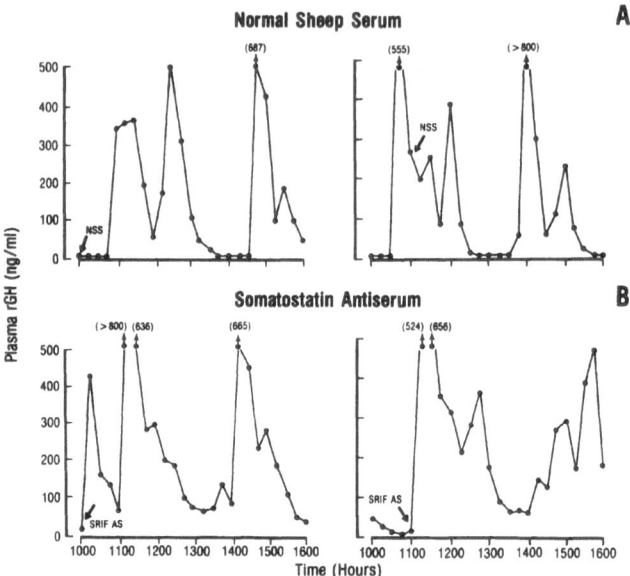

Fig. 3. Effects of passive immunization with somatostatin antiserum (SRIF AS) on the ultradian GH rhythm.
Administration of SRIF AS caused a rapid surge of GH
release and significant elevation of GH trough levels
compared to normal sheep serum (NSS)-treated controls.

Passive immunization experiments have also implicated somatostatin as
a physiological regulator of stress-induced GH suppression since pretreatment with antisomatostatin serum partially restores the GH secretory
pulses in animals subjected to stressful conditions (33,34).

INTERACTIONS OF SOMATOSTATIN AND GRF IN CONTROL OF GH SECRETION

The recent isolation and characterization of peptides with specific,
high-intrinsic GH-releasing activity from human pancreatic islet cell
carcinoma (35,36), and both human (37) and rat (38) hypothalamus, now
provide powerful probes to further delineate the physiological roles of
somatostatin and GRF, and their interrelationship, in generation of the
ultradian rhythm of GH secretion.

We used a model of GH deficiency in which rats are subjected to
electrolytic lesions of the ventromedial-arcuate (VMN-ARC) region of the
hypothalamus—a manipulation which virtually obliterates the spontaneous
GH secretory episodes (39,40; Fig. 5A). To determine whether the suppression of GH pulses is due to disruption of somatostatinergic pathways, we
administered somatostatin antiserum to VMN-ARC lesioned rats (40). As
shown in Figure 5B, antisomatostatin serum failed to restore the amplitude
of GH pulses suggesting that increased somatostatin release is not the
mechanism whereby VMN-ARC lesions cause GH suppression. In striking
contrast, administration of 3 IV boluses of a GRF analog (41) caused a
dramatic surge of GH within 5 min after each injection (Fig. 5C). These
findings suggested that the ultradian surges of GH release are dependent
on the episodic release of GRF from this region of the brain. The recent

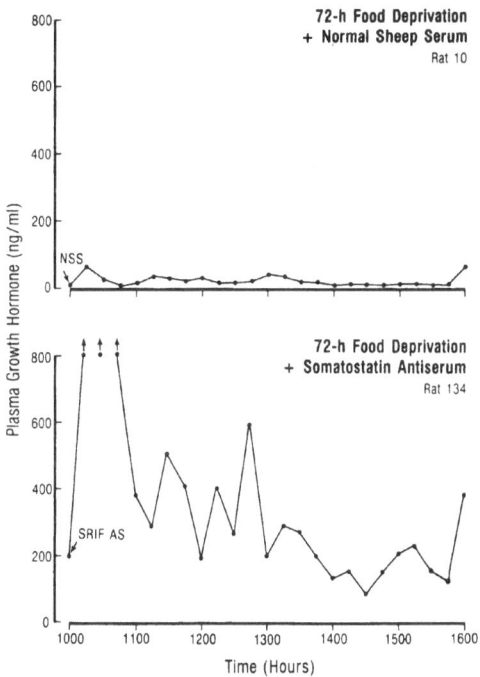

Fig. 4. Six-hour GH secretory patterns in 2
starved rats administered normal sheep serum
(NSS) or somatostatin antiserum (SRIF AS).
Immunoneutralization with SRIF AS restored
high-amplitude GH pulses, although not the
typical ultradian GH rhythm.

immunohistochemical detection of GRF immunoreactivity in both ARC and VMN
nuclei (42,43), and the demonstration that administration of monoclonal
antibodies against rat hypothalamic GRF abolished the GH pulses (44),
provide strong support for this view.

While the GRF peptides have now been shown to be powerful GH secretagogues in several species, including man (45-47), an inconsistency in
the magnitude of the response has been reported by most researchers. One
possible explanation for the variability of response may be that the
inhibitory peptide, somatostatin, was interfering with the actions of GRF.
To study the interaction between somatostatin and GRF in vivo, we administered S-14 simultaneously with GRF to VMN-ARC lesioned animals. The
concomitant administration of the two peptides resulted in a marked
inhibition of the GRF-induced GH release 5 min after injection, indicating
that somatostatin can antagonize the actions of GRF (41). This observation fits well with in vitro studies demonstrating that somatostatin
inhibits GRF-induced GH release from dispersed rat pituitary cells in
typical non-competitive antagonism (48,49). Taken together, the findings
provide support for the view that GRF and somatostatin have different
receptors on the pituitary somatotrophs.

We have continued to utilize the GRF peptides as probes to further
elucidate the interrelationship of somatostatin and GRF in GH regulation.

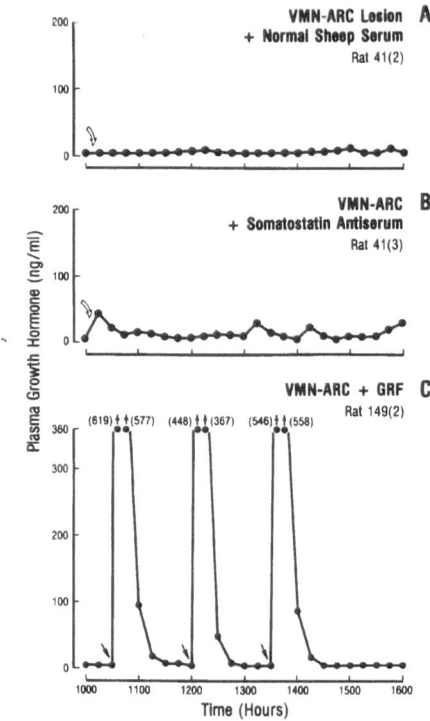

Fig. 5. Effects of administration of somatostatin antiserum and GRF on plasma GH levels in VMN-ARC lesioned rats. While antisomatostatin serum failed to significantly alter the suppressed 6-hour GH secretory profile, administration of 3 IV boluses of GRF caused a dramatic surge of GH release after each injection.

In these studies, normal, freely-moving rats were administered GRF during both peak and trough periods of the GH rhythm (50). As illustrated in Figure 6A, administration of rat (r) GRF to normal sheep serum-treated rats during a time of peak GH secretion, 1100 hours, resulted in a 2-3 fold increase in plasma GH levels. In contrast, injection of rGRF during a trough period (1300 hours) had only a minimal effect on plasma GH. Neutralization of endogenous circulating somatostatin with antisomatostatin serum eliminated the time-dependent difference and permitted a marked response to rGRF at 1300 hours (Fig. 6B), indicating that the weak GRF-induced GH release observed during trough periods is due to antagonization by endogenous somatostatin. These data provide further support for the view that the release of somatostatin from the hypothalamus into the hypophyseal portal blood is increased episodically during trough periods. It is also of interest to note that pretreatment with antisomatostatin serum significantly augmented the GH response to rGRP at 1100 hours compared to normal sheep serum controls (Fig. 6), suggesting that somatostatin may also exert a tonic inhibitory effect on GH release.

The striking time-dependent difference in the magnitude of the GH response to GRF clearly indicates that the intermittent secretion of endogenous somatostatin is an important factor which must be taken into

174

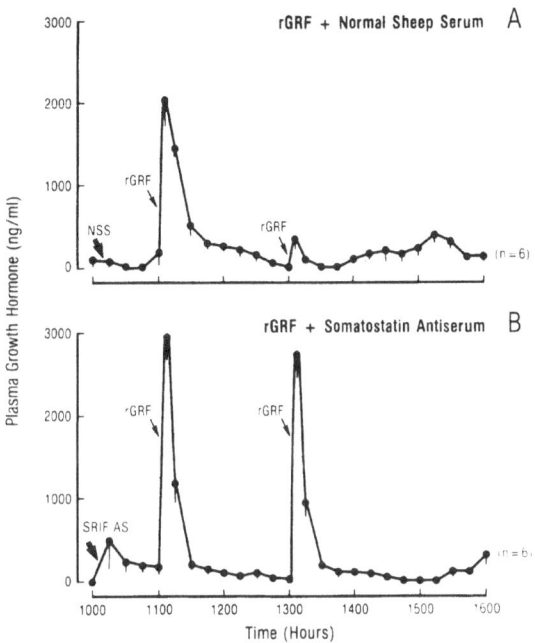

Fig. 6. Mean plasma GH response to rGRF administered during peak and trough periods of the GH rhythm to rats pretreated with either normal sheep serum (NSS) or somatostatin antiserum (SRIF AS). (A) The plasma GH response to rGRF in NSS-treated animals was significantly greater during a time of peak GH secretion (1100 hours) than during a trough period (1300 hours). (B) Immunoneutralization with SRIF AS reversed the weak response at 1300 hours (from 50, with permission).

account when assessing the in vivo biological actions of the GRF peptides, and likely explains the wide variability of response across subjects that has been reported in most clinical investigations. These results, together with the available evidence to date, lead to the hypothesis shown schematically in Figure 7 that GRF and somatostatin are secreted tonically from the hypothalamus into the hypophyseal portal blood, and that superimposed on this steady state release is an additional 3-4 hour rhythmic surge of each peptide, about 180° out of phase, providing for integration of the ultradian rhythm of GH secretion as observed in the peripheral blood. Recent experiments by Plotsky and Vale (51), in which direct measurements of immunoreactive GRF and somatostatin concentrations in rat hypophyseal portal blood were obtained, are strongly supportive of this hypothesis.

Studies by Thorner and co-workers (52) also offer support to the concept that the pulses of GH secretion in man are likely caused by a combination of enhanced GRF secretion with concomitant reduction of somatostatin secretion. In their investigations, the intrinsic pulsatile pattern of GH secretion was preserved throughout a 24-hour infusion of GRF, likely the result of the intermittent withdrawal of inhibition of GH secretion by hypothalamic somatostatin.

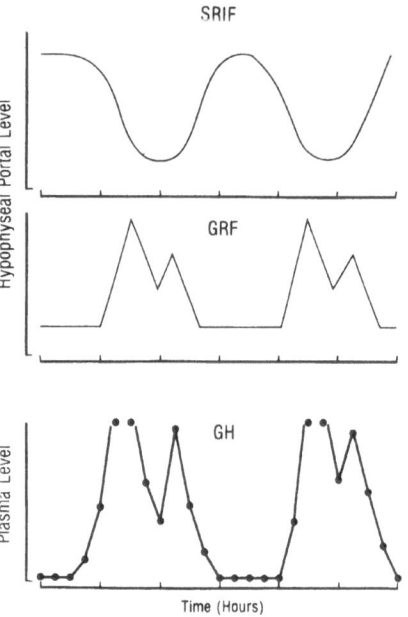

Fig. 7. Hypothetical model of the rhythmic secretion of SRIF and GRF into hypophyseal portal blood, with the net result on GH secretion, as observed in plasma (from 50, with permission).

ROLE OF SOMATOSTATIN IN FEEDBACK REGULATION OF GH SECRETION

Considerable evidence now exists to indicate that GH can regulate its own secretion via a short-loop negative feedback system. To elucidate the site of action for GH autoregulation, we injected rGH into the lateral cerebral ventricle of chronically cannulated rats (53). As shown in Figure 8B, the intracerebroventricular (icv) administration of rGH resulted in a severe suppression of spontaneous GH secretory pulses which lasted up to 6 hours. Similar results have been obtained using human GH (54). These findings provided good evidence for GH autofeedback and suggested a CNS-mediated mechanism.

Somatostatin appears to play a role in GH autoregulation at the hypothalamic level. Somatostatin concentrations in the hypothalamus are altered in response to GH perturbations in vivo (55-57), and in vitro administration of GH results in a dose-dependent stimulation of somatostatin release from incubated rat hypothalami (58,59). Furthermore, icv administration of rGH in doses similar to that used in our study has been shown to provoke an increase in somatostatin release in the hypophyseal portal blood (60). To assess the physiological significance of GH-induced somatostatin secretion, we examined the effects of passive immunization with antisomatostatin serum in animals receiving GH centrally. The results provided support for only a partial role for endogenous somatostatin in mediating GH autofeedback (61). More recent studies suggest that the mechanism whereby GH inhibits its own secretion likely involves decreased output of hypothalamic GRF concomitant with increased release of somatostatin (62).

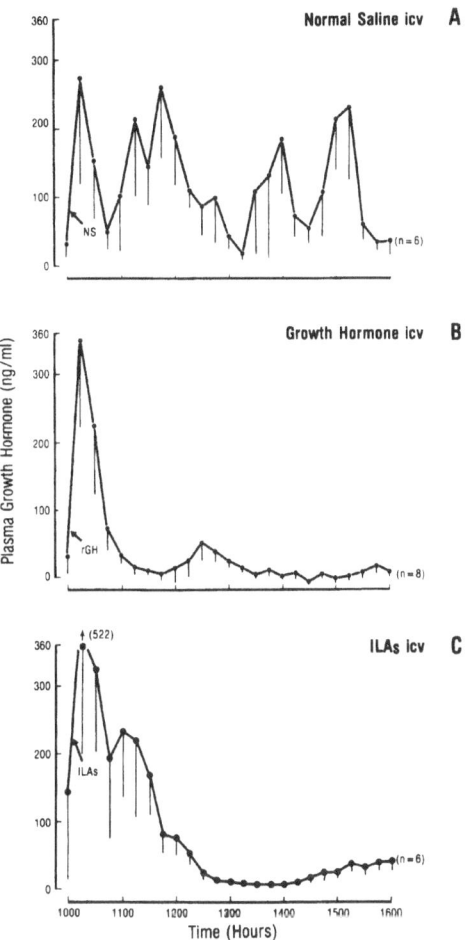

Fig. 8. Effects of intracerebroventricular administration of normal saline (A), rat GH (B), and ILAs (C) on pulsatile GH secretion. Central injection of rGH and ILAs caused a severe suppression in amplitude of spontaneous GH surges after an interval of 1 and 2 hours, respectively, compared to normal saline controls.

The somatomedins/insulin-like growth factors (IGFs) constitute a family of peptides, under GH control, that exhibits growth-promoting and insulin-like activities on several tissues (63). We assessed the possible involvement, at a CNS level, of ILAs, a preparation enriched in IGFs, in feedback regulation of pulsatile GH secretion (64). As illustrated in Figure 8C, icv injection of ILAs caused a marked suppression in amplitude of spontaneous GH pulses, which was a specific effect of the somatomedin-enriched preparation. Similar results were obtained using a purified preparation of somatomedin-C (54), suggesting that the somatomedin/IGFs may participate in long-loop feedback regulation of GH secretion.

Evidence for a role for somatostatin in mediating this response comes from studies by Berelowitz et al. (65) which demonstrate that somatomedin-C stimulates somatostatin release from rat hypothalamic fragments in vitro. Thus, the somatomedins may participate in a long-loop GH negative feedback system via the mechanism of increased hypothalamic somatostatin release. However, the possibility that the IGFs have a simultaneous inhibitory effect on hypothalamic GRF release requires further exploration.

Finally, the results of several recent studies suggest that both somatostatin and GRF may be capable of regulating their own secretion, and consequently modifying pituitary GH release, possibly through an ultra-short-loop negative feedback mechanism. Lumpkin et al. (66) demonstrated that icv administration of somatostatin caused a paradoxical stimulation of GH release and postulated that hypothalamic somatostatin may self-regulate. There is also some in vitro evidence for autoregulation of somatostatin secretion by cultured fetal hypothalamic cells (67). However, we recently demonstrated significant leakage of the somatostatin peptides from the cerebrospinal fluid into the systemic circulation following icv injection (68). Thus, it is possible that the increased GH release observed in vivo is due, at least in part, to somatostatin-induced postsuppression rebound at the level of the pituitary gland, a phenomenon well documented for S-14 (11). Further experimentation will be necessary to adequately address this question. In the case of GRF, icv GRF at low doses causes GH suppression, suggesting autoregulation (69,70). However, the possibility that icv GRF suppresses GH release by stimulation of hypothalamic somatostatin cannot be ruled out in view of recent in vitro reports demonstrating that GRF directly stimulates somatostatin release from hypothalamic (71) and median eminence fragments (72). In addition, recent immunohistochemical studies have revealed possible synaptic inter-actions between GRF and somatostatin neurons (73). Taken together, these latter findings suggest the possibility of reciprocal regulation between GRF and somatostatin neurons and underscore the complexity of the physio-logical control mechanisms involved in the regulation of GH secretion.

ACKNOWLEDGMENTS

This work was supported by grants from the Medical Research Council of Canada. The author is a Senior Scholar of the Ponds de la recherche en sante du Quebec. I thank Wendy Gurd and Martine Lapointe for invaluable technical assistance and Julie Temko for excellent secretarial help. The generous supply of rGH RIA materials from the NIADDK is gratefully acknowledged.

REFERENCES

1. Tannenbaum GS, Martin JB. Evidence for an endogenous ultradian rhythm governing growth hormone secretion in the rat. Endocrinology 1976; 98:562.
2. Brazeau P, Vale W, Burgus N, et al. Hypothalamic peptide that inhibits the secretion of immunoreactive pituitary growth hormone. Science 1973; 179:77.
3. Martin JB, Brazeau P, Tannenbaum GS, et al. Neuroendocrine organi-zation of growth hormone regulation. In: Reichlin S, Baldessarini R, Martin JB, eds. The hypothalamus. New York: Raven Press, 1978.
4. Pradayrol L, Jornvall H, Matt V, Ribert A. N-terminally extended somatostatin: the primary structure of somatostatin-28. FEBS Lett 1980; 109:55.
5. Esch F, Bohlen P, Ling N, Benoit R, Brazeau P, Guillemin R. Primary structure of ovine hypothalamic somatostatin-28 and somatostatin-25.

Proc Natl Acad Sci USA 1980; 77:6827.

6. Schally AV, Huang W-Y, Chang RCC, et al. Isolation and structure of prosomatostatin: a putative somatostatin precursor from pig hypothalamus. Proc Natl Acad Sci USA 1980; 77:4489.

7. Tannenbaum GS, Ling N, Brazeau P. Somatostatin-28 is longer acting and more selective than somatostatin-14 on pituitary and pancreatic hormone release. Endocrinology 1982; 111:101.

8. Brazeau P, Vale W, Rivier J, Guillemin R. Acylated des (Ala[1]-Gly[2])-somatostatin analogs: prolonged inhibition of growth hormone secretion. Biochem Biophys Res Commun 1974; 60:1202.

9. Patel YC, Wheatley T. In vivo and in vitro plasma disappearance and metabolism of somatostatin-28 and somatostatin-14 in the rat. Endocrinology 1983; 112:220.

10. Rorstad OP, Epelbaum P, Brazeau P, Martin JB. Chromatographic and biological properties of immunoreactive somatostatin in hypothalamic and extrahypothalamic brain regions of the rat. Endocrinology 1979; 105:1083.

11. Stachura ME. Influence of synthetic somatostatin on growth hormone release from perifused rat pituitaries. Endocrinology 1976; 99:678.

12. Ferland L, Labrie F, Jobin M, Arimura A, Schally AV. Physiological role of somatostatin in the control of growth hormone and thyrotropin secretion. Biochem Biophys Res Commun 1976; 68:149.

13. Steiner RA, Stewart JK, Barber J, et al. Somatostatin: a physiological role in the adolescent male baboon. Endocrinology 1978; 102:1587.

14. Schusdziarra V, Rouiller D, Arimura A, Unger RH. Antisomatostatin serum increases levels of hormones from the pituitary and gut, but not from the pancreas. Endocrinology 1978; 103:1956.

15. Varner MA, Davis SL, Reeves JJ. Temporal serum concentrations of growth hormone, thyrotropin, insulin, and glucagon in sheep immunized against somatostatin. Endocrinology 1980; 106:1027.

16. Terry LC, Martin JB. The effects of lateral hypothalamic-medial forebrain stimulation and somatostatin antiserum on pulsatile growth hormone secretion in freely behaving rats: evidence for a dual regulatory mechanism. Endocrinology 1981; 109:622.

17. Alpert LC, Brawer JR, Patel YC, Reichlin S. Somatostatinergic neurons in anterior hypothalamus: immunohistochemical localization. Endocrinology 1976; 98:255.

18. Rice RW, Critchlow V. Extrahypothalamic control of stress-induced inhibition of growth hormone secretion in the rat. Endocrinology 1976; 99:970.

19. Willoughby JO, Martin JB. Pulsatile growth hormone secretion: inhibitory role of medial preoptic area. Brain Res 1978; 148:240.

20. Tannenbaum GS, Rorstad O, Brazeau P. Effects of prolonged food deprivation on the ultradian growth hormone rhythm and immunoreactive somatostatin tissue levels in the rat. Endocrinology 1979; 104:1733.

21. Tannenbaum GS. Growth hormone secretory dynamics in streptozotocin diabetes: evidence of a role for endogenous circulating somatostatin. Endocrinology 1981; 108:76.

22. Tannenbaum GS, Colle E, Gurd W, Wanamaker L. Dynamic time-course studies of the spontaneously diabetic BB Wistar rat. I. Longitudinal profiles of plasma growth hormone, insulin, and glucose. Endocrinology 1981; 109:1872.

23. Painson JC, Tannenbaum GS. Effects of intracellular glucopenia on pulsatile growth hormone secretion: mediation in part by somatostatin. Endocrinology 1985; 117:1132.

24. Tannenbaum GS, Epelbaum J, Colle E, Brazeau P, Martin JB. Antiserum to somatostatin reserves starvation-induced inhibition of growth hormone but not insulin secretion. Endocrinology 1978; 102:1909.

25. Shapiro B, Berelowitz M, Pimstone BL, Kronheim S, Sheppard M. Tissue and serum somatostatin-like immunoreactivity in fed, 15-h fasted, and

72-h-fasted rats. Diabetes 1979; 28:182.

26. Petersson B, Elde R, Efendic S, et al. Somatostatin in the pancreas, stomach and hypothalamus of the diabetic Chinese hamster. Diabetologia 1977; 13:463.

27. Patel YC, Cameron DP, Bankier A, et al. Changes in somatostatin concentration in pancreas and other tissues of streptozotocin diabetic rats. Endocrinology 1978; 103:917.

28. Berelowitz M, Shapiro B, Kronheim S. Growth hormone release inhibitory hormone-like immunoreactivity in pancreas and gut in streptozotocin diabetes in the rat and response to insulin administration. Clin Endocrinol (Oxf) 1979; 10:195.

29. Patel YC, Wheatley T, Malaisse-Lagae F, Orci L. Elevated portal and peripheral blood concentration of immunoreactive somatostatin in spontaneously diabetic (BBL) Wistar rats. Diabetes 1980; 29:757.

30. Tannenbaum GS, Colle E, Wanamaker L, Gurd W, Goldman H, Seemayer T. Dynamic time-course studies of the spontaneously diabetic BB Wistar rat. II. Insulin-, glucagon-, and somatostatin-reactive cells in the pancreas. Endocrinology 1981; 109:1880.

31. Painson J-C, Brazeau P, Lengyel AM, Tannenbaum GS. Interactions of somatostatin and growth hormone-releasing factor (GRF) in starvation [Abstract]. International Conference on Somatostatin, Washington, DC, May 6-8, 1986.

32. Schusdziarra V. Role of somatostatin in nutrient regulation. In: Patel YC, Tannenbaum GS, eds. Somatostatin. New York: Plenum Press, 1985.

33. Terry LC, Willoughby JO, Brazeau P, Martin JB, Patel Y. Antiserum to somatostatin prevents stress-induced inhibition of growth hormone secretion in the rat. Science 1976; 192:565.

34. Arimura A, Smith WD, Schally AV. Blockade of the stress-induced decrease in blood GH by anti-somatostatin serum in rats. Endocrinology 1976; 98:540.

35. Guillemin R, Brazeau P, Bohlen P, Esch F, Ling N, Wehrenberg WB. Growth hormone-releasing factor from a human pancreatic tumor that caused acromegaly. Science 1982; 218:585.

36. Rivier J, Spiess J, Thorner M, Vale W. Characterization of a growth hormone-releasing factor from a human pancreatic islet tumour. Nature 1982; 300:276.

37. Ling N, Esch F, Bohlen P, Brazeau P, Wehrenberg WB, Guillemin R. Isolation, primary structure, and synthesis of human hypothalamic somatocrinin: growth hormone-releasing factor. Proc Natl Acad Sci USA 1984; 81:4302.

38. Spiess J, Rivier J, Vale W. Characterization of rat hypothalamic growth hormone-releasing factor. Nature 1983; 303:532.

39. Martin JB, Renaud LP, Brazeau P. Pulsatile growth hormone secretion: suppression by hypothalamic ventromedial lesions and by long-acting somatostatin. Science 1974; 186:538.

40. Eikelboom R, Tannenbaum GS. Effects of obesity-inducing ventromedial hypothalamic lesions on pulsatile growth hormone and insulin secretion: evidence for the existence of a growth hormone-releasing factor. Endocrinology 1983; 112:212.

41. Tannenbaum GS, Eikelboom R, Ling N. Human pancreas GH-releasing factor analog restores high-amplitude GH pulses in CNS lesion-induced GH deficiency. Endocrinology 1983; 113:1173.

42. Bloch B, Brazeau P, Ling N, et al. Immunohistochemical detection of growth hormone-releasing factor in brain. Nature 1983; 301:607.

43. Merchenthaler I, Vigh S, Schally AV, Petrusz P. Immunocytochemical localization of growth hormone-releasing factor in the rat hypothalamus. Endocrinology 1984; 114:1082.

44. Wehrenberg WB, Brazeau P, Luben R, Bohlen P, Guillemin R. Inhibition of the pulsatile secretion of growth hormone by monoclonal antibodies to the hypothalamic growth hormone releasing factor (GRF). Endo-

crinology 1982; 111:2147.

45. Wehrenberg WB, Ling N, Brazeau P, et al. Somatocrinin, growth hormone releasing factor, stimulates secretion of growth hormone in anesthetized rats. Biochem Biophys Res Commun 1982; 109:382.

46. Chihara K, Minamitani N, Kaji H, Kodama H, Kita T, Fujita T. Human pancreatic growth hormone-releasing factor stimulates release of growth hormone in conscious unrestrained male rabbits. Endocrinology 1983; 113:2081.

47. Thorner MO, Rivier J, Spiess J, et al. Human pancreatic growth hormone-releasing factor selectively stimulates growth hormone secretion in man. Lancet 1983; 1:24.

48. Brazeau P, Ling N, Bohlen P, Esch F, Ying S-Y, Guillemin R. Growth hormone releasing factor, somatocrinin, releases pituitary growth hormone in vitro. Proc Natl Acad Sci USA 1982; 79:7909.

49. Vale W, Vaughan J, Yamamoto G, Spiess J, Rivier J. Effects of synthetic human pancreatic (tumor) GH releasing factor and somatostatin, triiodothyronine and dexamethasone on GH secretion in vitro. Endocrinology 1983; 112:1553.

50. Tannenbaum GS, Ling N. The interrelationship of growth hormone (GH)-releasing factor and somatostatin in generation of the ultradian rhythm of GH secretion. Endocrinology 1984; 115:1952.

51. Plotsky PM, Vale W. Patterns of growth hormone-releasing factor and somatostatin secretion into the hypophysial portal circulation of the rat. Science 1985 230:461.

52. Vance ML, Kaiser DL, Evans WS, et al. Pulsatile growth hormone secretion in normal man during a continuous 24-hour infusion of human growth hormone releasing factor (1-40). J Clin Invest 1985; 75:1584.

53. Tannenbaum, GS. Evidence for autoregulation of growth hormone secretion via the central nervous system. Endocrinology 1980; 107:2117.

54. Abe H, Molitch ME, Van Wyk JJ, Underwood LE. Human growth hormone and somatomedin C suppress the spontaneous release of growth hormone in unanesthetized rats. Endocrinology 1983; 113:1319.

55. Wakabayashi I, Demura R, Kanda M, Demura H, Shizume K. Effect of hypophysectomy on hypothalamic somatostatin content in rats. Endocrinol Jpn 1976; 23:439.

56. Hoffman DL, Baker BL. Effect of treatment with growth hormone on somatostatin in the median eminence of hypophysectomized rats. Proc Soc Exp Biol Med 1977; 156:265.

57. Patel YC. Growth hormone stimulates hypothalamic somatostatin. Life Sci 1979; 24:1589.

58. Sheppard MC, Kronheim S, Pimstone BL. Stimulation by growth hormone of somatostatin release from the rat hypothalamus in vitro. Clin Endocrinol 1978; 9:583.

59. Berelowitz M, Firestone SL, Frohman LA. Effects of growth hormone excess and deficiency on hypothalamic somatostatin content and release and on tissue somatostatin distribution. Endocrinology 1981; 109:714.

60. Chihara K, Minamitani N, Kaji H, Arimura A, Fujita T. Intraventricularly injected growth hormone stimulates somatostatin release into rat hypophysial portal blood. Endocrinology 1981; 109:2279.

61. Tannenbaum GS. Studies on the mechanism for "short-loop" feedback control of growth hormone secretion. In: Raptis S, Gerich JE, eds. Proceedings of the second international symposium on somatostatin. West Germany: University Press Tubingen, 1985.

62. Tannenbaum GS. Physiological role of somatostatin in regulation of pulsatile growth hormone secretion. In: Patel YC, Tannenbaum GS, eds. Somatostatin. New York: Plenum Publishing, 1985.

63. Phillips LS, Vassilopoulou-Sellin R. Somatomedins. New Engl J Med 1980; 302:371, 438.

64. Tannenbaum GS, Guyda HJ, Posner BI. Insulin-like growth factors: a

role in growth hormone negative feedback and body weight regulation via brain. Science 1983; 220:77.

65. Berelowitz M, Szabo M, Frohman LA, Firestone S, Chu L, Hintz RL. Somatomedin-C mediates growth hormone negative feedback by effects on both the hypothalamus and the pituitary. Science 1981; 212:1279.

66. Lumpkin MD, Negro-Vilar A, McCann SM. Paradoxical elevation of growth hormone by intraventricular somatostatin: possible ultra-short-loop feedback. Science 1981; 211:1072.

67. Peterfreund RA, Vale WW. Somatostatin analogs inhibit somatostatin secretion from cultured hypothalamus cells. Neuroendocrinology 1984; 39:397.

68. Tannenbaum GS, Patel YC. On the fate of centrally administered somatostatin in the rat: massive hypersomatostatinemia resulting from leakage into the peripheral circulation has effects on growth hormone secretion and glucoregulation. Endocrinology 1986; 118:2137.

69. Lumpkin MD, Samson WK, McCann SM. Effects of intraventricular growth hormone-releasing factor on growth hormone release: further evidence for ultrashort-loop feedback. Endocrinology 1985; 116:2070.

70. Katakami H, Arimura A, Frohman LA. Growth hormone (GH)-releasing factor stimulates hypothalamic somatostatin release: an inhibitory feedback effect on GH secretion. Endocrinology 1986; 118:1872.

71. Iwasaki K, Arimura A. The stimulation of somatostatin (SS) release by hpGRF44 from rat hypothalamic cells and fragments in vitro [Abstract 963]. Program of the Seventh International Congress of Endocrinology, Quebec City, Quebec, Canada, 1984.

72. Aguila MC, McCann SM. Stimulation of somatostatin release in vitro by synthetic human growth hormone-releasing factor by a nondopaminergic mechanism. Endocrinology 1985; 117:762.

73. Sawchenko PE, Swanson LW, Rivier J, Vale WW. The distribution of growth hormone-releasing factor (GRF) immunoreactivity in the central nervous system of the rat: an immunohistochemical study using antisera directed against rat hypothalamic GRF. J Comp Neurol 1985; 237:100.

17

SOMATOSTATIN AND DEPRESSION

David R. Rubinow, Robert M. Post, Candace Davis, Allen Doran

National Institute of Mental Health
9000 Rockville Pike
Bethesda, Maryland 20892

INTRODUCTION

Much evidence supports a role for somatostatin as a modulator of central nervous system (CNS) activity and indirectly suggests the relevance of somatostatin to several neuropsychiatric disorders, particularly depression. First, in addition to localization of somatostatin and somatostatin receptors throughout the CNS (1-4), somatostatin displays neurophysiologic effects (5,6) and regulatory interactions with brain neurotransmitters and peptides (7). Thus, somatostatin appears to act in the CNS as a neuromodulator or neurotransmitter (8). Second, following intracerebroventricular (ICV) or intracerebral administration, somatostatin has been observed to alter many behaviors that are disturbed in depression. For example, depression is characterized by decreased total and slow wave sleep and shortened REM latency (9), increases or decreases in appetite and/or locomotor activity, decreased pain sensitivity (10) and impaired cognition (11). Central somatostatin administration has been observed to produce decreased total, slow wave and REM sleep (12,13), dose-related biphasic (increase or decrease) alterations in eating (14-16) and locomotor activity (17), analgesia (18,19), and enhancement of learning and reversal of induced learning deficits (20,21). Altered levels of brain and CSF somatostatin have been described in several neuropsychiatric disorders including depression. Increases in CSF somatostatin have been observed in certain types of inflammatory or destructive CNS disorders (22) and reduced levels have been reported in patients with senile dementia (23), Parkinson's disease (24,25), Alzheimer's disease (26,27) and multiple sclerosis during relapse (28,29). As described elsewhere in this volume, decreased brain and CSF somatostatin levels in Alzheimer's disease are widely replicated findings; the clinical relevance of these findings is further suggested by reports of correlations between cognitive impairment and the degree of reduction of somatostatin levels in brain (30) and CSF (31), by observation of the colocalization of somatostatin neurons with neurofibrillary tangles and plaques (32,33), and by demonstration that the brain areas showing the greatest reduction of somatostatin are those that are most markedly hypometabolic as determined by PET scan (34).

CSF somatostatin concentrations have been measured in several psychiatric populations. Gerner and Yamada (35) and Rubinow et al. (36) reported significant decreases in CSF somatostatin in depressed patients compared with normal controls. These findings have been confirmed in several subsequent studies. Black et al. (37) described lower ventricular CSF somatostatin levels in depressed patients studied prior to cingulotomy compared with hydrocephalic patients; values in depressed patients were also significantly lower than those seen in the lumbar CSF of 12 normal controls. Agren and Lundqvist (38) reported that somatostatin levels in a group of depressed patients studied during their worst week of depression were significantly lower than those observed in a group of depressed patients studied more than two months following their most depressed week. Bissette et al. (39) observed significantly lower CSF somatostatin values in depressed patients compared with normal volunteers; significantly lower levels were also observed in groups of patients with dementia or schizophrenia. Sunderland et al. (unpublished manuscript) have observed decreased CSF somatostatin in elderly depressed patients and patients with Alzheimer's disease compared with age-matched controls. Reports of increased somatostatin levels during mania (35) and decreased levels in schizophrenics (39) and anorectic patients (35) have not been confirmed (36,40; Kaye et al., unpublished manuscript). Postmortem studies of brain somatostatin concentrations in depressed patients have not been reported to date. No consistent alterations in brain somatostatin in schizophrenic patients have been observed, although reductions in somatostatin concentration in the frontal cortex (41) and in the hippocampus in a subgroup of patients (42) have been described. Postmortem studies may be complicated by the relatively rapid reduction in brain somatostatin that has been reported to occur within the first six hours following death (43).

CSF SOMATOSTATIN IN AFFECTIVE ILLNESS

Low Levels in Depression

We performed lumbar punctures between 8:00 and 9:00 a.m. under medication-free conditions on inpatient subjects who met DSM-III criteria (44) for major affective disorder (n = 81), schizophrenia (n = 44), or dysthymic disorder (n = 5) and on 47 inpatient normal volunteers who were carefully screened to rule out the presence of medical or psychiatric illness. Among the patients with major affective disorder, 49 (23 unipolar, 26 bipolar) were depressed, 23 euthymic or improved, and 9 manic. As shown in Figure 1, significant intergroup differences were observed (ANOVA F = 3.90, df = 5, P < 0.005). Significantly lower levels of CSF somatostatin were observed in depressed patients (42.3 ± 3.2 pg/ml) compared with normal volunteers (62.1 ± 5.4 pg/ml) (t = 3.10, P < 0.01), patients with affective illness in the improved state (61.3 ± 5.4 pg/ml) (t = 3.08, P < 0.01), or schizophrenics (65.2 ± 4.2 pg/ml) (t = 4.38, P < 0.001) (45). No other significant intergroup differences were noted. Somatostatin levels did not appear related to the severity of the depression nor to the age or sex of the patients. Depression-related decreases in CSF somatostatin were also observed in 9 patients who underwent lumbar punctures under medication-free conditions during both depressed and improved or manic states; i.e., the values obtained during depression were significantly lower than those obtained during the other states (paired t = 3.24, P < 0.02). One possible explanation for differences between depressed and normal individuals was a difference in circadian patterns of CFS somatostatin. To test this hypothesis, paired lumbar punctures performed between 8:00 and 9:00 a.m. and 8:00 and 9:00 p.m. in 8 depressed patients and 8 normal volunteers under medication-free conditions revealed no consistent circadian change; however, the nonsignificant decrease in the volunteers' somatostatin in the evening and the increase in the patients' evening values resulted in very similar mean somatostatin values during the evening in patients and volunteers (49.46 ± 8.42 pg/ml and 47.74 ± 4.02 pg/ml, respectively).

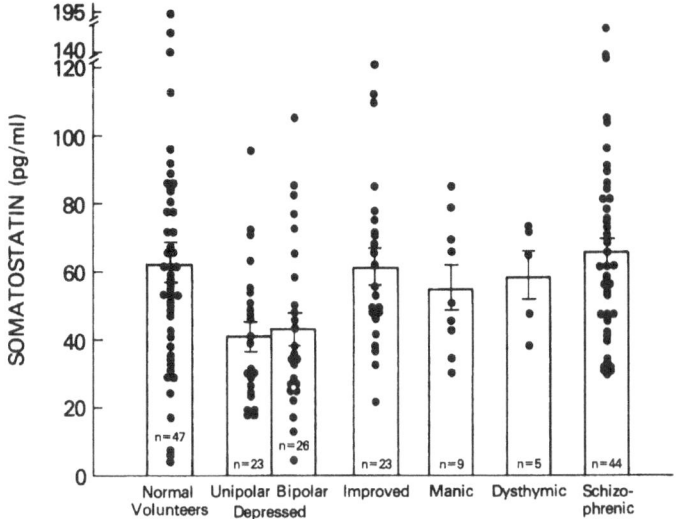

Fig. 1. CSF somatostatin is significantly lower in bipolar and unipolar depressed patients as compared with normal volunteers, schizophrenic patients, and patients with affective illness during the improved state (45).

While the meaning of depression state-related decreases in CSF somatostatin is presently unclear, a body of indirect evidence reviewed elsewhere (7,45). suggests that CSF somatostatin in large part reflects brain secretion, with somatostatin entering the CSF through nerve terminals located adjacent to the third ventricle (46) or in the periventricular organs (47) and by cellular diffusion via the Virchow-Robins spaces of the brain. Although the changes in CSF somatostatin seen in depression may represent alterations in brain secretion, the existence of several neuropsychiatric disorders that are characterized by decreased CSF somatostatin suggests that a central etiologic role for somatostatin dysregulation in depression is unlikely. It is more probable that the CSF alterations in somatostatin reflect central neurotransmitter or neuropeptide abnormalities. Additionally, it is also possible that the changes in CSF somatostatin observed are epiphenomenal to depression-related circadian abnormalities (48), with the lumbar puncture possibly coincident with the trough of a disturbed circadian rhythm. A circadian rhythm has been described for CSF somatostatin in monkeys, with highest values at night (49,50). While we observed no significant circadian effect on CSF somatostatin in depressed patients or volunteers who underwent both morning and evening lumbar punctures, highly similar evening somatostatin values were noted in both patient and normal volunteer groups. Thus, detection of decreased CSF somatostatin levels in depressed patients relative to normals appears dependent on the time of day at which the samples are obtained and therefore may represent disturbed circadian rather than total somatostatin secretion. Finally, it may be that diminished CSF somatostatin, in the neuropsychiatric disorders characterized by this abnormality, reflects a common central neuroregulatory disturbance or mediates a common manifestation of these disorders. For example, recent animal studies suggest that somatostatin may facilitate learning and memory (delay extinction of a learned avoidance response and reverse electroshock-induced learning impairment), with diminished performance observed following administration of a somatostatin depleting agent (cysteamine) (20,21,51). It is, therefore, noteworthy that cognitive impairment is a feature of those neuropsychiatric disorders associated with decreased CSF somatostatin and that reductions in CSF somatostatin have been correlated with the degree of cognitive impairment in patients with Alzheimer's disease (30,31) or Parkinson's disease (25).

Endocrine Correlates of Low Somatostatin in Depression

The most commonly reported biological abnormality in depression is the disinhibition of the hypothalamic-pituitary-adrenal (HPA) axis, evidenced by resistance to or early escape from dexamethasone suppression (52), disinhibition of nocturnal cortisol secretion, loss or blunting of circadian variation of cortisol secretion (53), cortisol hypersecretion (54) and increased urinary-free cortisol excretion (55). Heisler et al. (56) observed the ability of somatostatin to inhibit the secretion of ACTH from mouse pituitary tumor cells (AtT-20/D16-16) following stimulation with a variety of secretagogues including corticotropin releasing factor (CRF), isoproterenol and vasoactive intestinal polypeptide. Further, Brown et al. (57) described the inhibition of stress-induced CRF release by somatostatin in vivo. We therefore questioned whether the decreased CSF somatostatin in depression might reflect decreased central somatostatin activity and therefore be associated with HPA axis disinhibition. Figure 2 illustrates the relationship between CSF somatostatin and a measure of HPA axis activity, the dexamethasone suppression test (DST), in medication-free depressed and schizophrenic patients. Two-way ANOVA revealed a main effect for response to DST (suppression/nonsuppression) ($F = 5.05$, $P < 0.05$), with no main effect of or interaction with diagnosis; i.e., irrespective of diagnosis, patients who escaped from dexamethasone suppression displayed lower levels of CSF somatostatin (40). A significant inverse relationship between CSF somatostatin levels and maximum postdexamethasone plasma cortisol was also observed in depressed patients but not in schizophrenics. This relationship was not attributable to differences in the age or clinical severity of the patients.

While it is tempting to speculate that decreases in CSF somatostatin may be paralleled by reductions in cortical and/or hypothalamic somatostatin which might permit disinhibition of stimulated ACTH and cortisol hypersecretion following dexamethasone, evidence for diminished hypothalamic somatostatin in association with decreased CSF somatostatin is currently lacking. Thus, the replicability as well as the significance of the inverse relationship between plasma cortisol following dexamethasone and CSF somatostatin remain to be determined. Nemeroff et al. (personal communication, 1985) have preliminary evidence of a similar relationship in normal volunteers but not in depressed patients, while Agren and Lundqvist (38) did not observe this relationship in a study in which they employed a variant of the conventional DST. However, Serby et al. (58) have reported a remarkably similar significant negative relationship between CSF somatostatin and response to dexamethasone administration in patients with Alzheimer's disease. Additionally, other evidence suggests that the relationship between the somatostatin and HPA axis systems may be physiologically important and may offer a means for investigating disorders characterized by regulatory disturbances of these systems. This evidence includes reports of CRF stimulation of somatostatin secretion in vitro and in vivo (59-61) as well as observations of a significant positive relationship between CSF CRF and somatostatin in several psychiatric populations including affective disorder patients during the euthymic state (Berrettini et al., unpublished manuscript), anorexics and bulimics (Kaye et al., unpublished manuscript) and schizophrenics (Doran et al., unpublished manuscript). Further, Kling et al. (unpublished manuscript) have recently observed decreased CSF somatostatin in patients with ACTH-dependent Cushing's syndrome, while Wolkowitz et al. (62) reported prednisone-induced reductions in CSF somatostatin levels in normal volunteers. These findings, in combination with the similarity of CSF somatostatin levels in depressed and schizophrenic patients when grouped according to response to dexamethasone, offer the possibility that lower levels of somatostatin observed in depression may be the product rather than the source of the HPA axis dysregulation observed in this disorder.

Effects of Psychopharmacologic Agents

If alterations in somatostatin may play a role in some of the clinical or biochemical abnormalities observed in depression, drug-induced changes in somatostatin may constitute important mechanisms of actions for psychopharmacologic agents. Administration of carbamazepine, an anticonvulsant that is also effective in the acute and prophylactic treatment of manic depressive illness (63), was associated with a significant decrease in CSF somatostatin (64). The changes in CSF somatostatin observed were not due to changes in mood state, as each patient studied had comparable

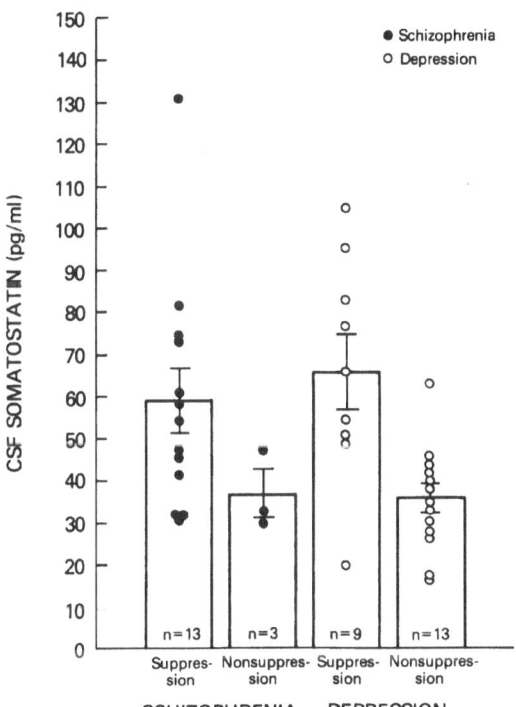

Fig. 2. CSF somatostatin values were significantly reduced in schizophrenic and depressed patients who show nonsuppression following dexamethasone administration (45).

depression ratings at the time of both lumbar punctures. No significant effects were seen with several other psychopharmacologic agents employed (lithium carbonate, desmethylimipramine, piribedil), although a significant increase in CSF somatostatin was observed in a small group of patients during treatment with zimelidine (64). A significant reduction in CSF somatostatin concentration has also been observed in schizophrenic patients during treatment with the neuroleptic fluphenazine (Doran et al., unpublished manuscript), consistent with reports of neuroleptic-induced reductions in somatostatin-like immunoreactivity in several brain regions, including striatum, amygdala, hypothalamus, and nucleus accumbens (65). However, a recently published study observed an increase in CSF somatostatin in schizophrenic patients treated with haloperidol (66). Thus, the in vivo effect of neuroleptics on CSF somatostatin is currently uncertain.

No mechanism for carbamazepine-induced reductions of CSF somatostatin has been identified, although alterations of central neurotransmitter or neuropeptide activity by this medication appears most likely. The relevance of this effect is nonetheless suggested by other reported observations of relationships between carbamazepine and somatostatin. Blunting of kindled elevations in brain somatostatin in rats by carbamazepine has been reported (67), although an absence of effect on basal somatostatin in various brain regions has also been observed (Weiss et al., unpublished data). Other evidence linking changes in brain somatostatin to the development and treatment of seizures includes reports of long-term increases in somatostatin in brain regions (amygdala and sensorimotor, piriform, and entorhinal cortex) following kindling (68), kindling-related down regulation of somatostatin receptors in the hippocampus (69), precipitation of seizures following ICV or intracerebral injection of somatostatin (70,71), and inhibition of kindled seizures following administration of somatostatin depleting agents (72).

CONCLUSIONS

We have observed decreases in CSF somatostatin in depressed patients, a significant inverse relationship between CSF somatostatin and postdexamethasone plasma cortisol (a major neuroendocrine abnormality in depression) and a significant decrease in CSF somatostatin following treatment with carbamazepine, an anticonvulsant effective in the treatment of manic depressive illness. Syndromal alterations in depression were not observed when evening lumbar punctures were performed in small groups of depressed patients and normal volunteers. Finally, while reduced levels of brain and CSF somatostatin concentrations in Alzheimer's disease are part of an irreversible, degenerative neurologic process, the somatostatin dysregulation in depression, like that seen in multiple sclerosis, is transient and reversible and thus appears to be a consequence of functional alterations in somatostatin secretion and/or metabolism.

REFERENCES

1. Brownstein M, Arimura A, Stao H, Schally AV, Kizer JS. The regional distribution of somatostatin in the rat brain. Endocrinology 1975; 96:1456-61.
2. Johannson O, Hokfelt T. Thyrotropin releasing hormone, somatostatin and enkephalin: distribution studies using immunohistochemical techniques. J Histochem Cytochem 1980; 28:364-6.
3. Srikant CB, Patel YC. Somatostatin receptors. Adv Exp Med Biol 1985; 188:291-304.
4. Leroux P, Quirion R, Pelletier G. Localization and characterization of brain somatostatin receptors as studied with somatostatin-14 and

somatostatin-28 receptor radioautography. Brain Res 1985; 347:74-84.

5. Renaud LP, Martin JB, Brazeau P. Depressant action of TRH, LH-RH and somatostatin on activity of central neurons. Nature 1975; 255:233-5.

6. Delfs JR, Dichter MA. Effects of somatostatin on mammalian cortical neurons in culture: physiological actions and unusual dose response characteristics. J Neurosci 1983; 3:1176-88.

7. Reichlin S. Systems for the study of regulation of neuropeptide secretion. In: Martin JB, Reichlin S, Bick KL, eds. Neurosecretion and brain peptides. New York: Raven Press, 1981.

8. Reichlin S. Somatostatin in the nervous system. In: Schmitt FO, Bird SJ, Blood FE, eds. Molecular genetic neuroscience. New York: Raven Press, 1982.

9. Gillin JC, Sitaram N, Wehr T, et al. Sleep and affective illness. In: Post RM, Ballenger JC, eds. Neurobiology of mood disorders. Baltimore: Williams & Wilkins, 1983.

10. Davis GC, Buchsbaum MS, Naber D, et al. Altered pain perception and CSF endorphins in psychiatric illness. Ann NY Acad Sci 1982; 398:36-373.

11. Weingartner H, Silberman EK. Cognitive changes in depression. In: Post RM, Ballenger JC, eds. Neurobiology of mood disorders. Baltimore: Williams & Wilkins, 1983.

12. Rezek M, Havlicek V, Hughes KR, Friesen H. Cortical administration of somatostatin (SRIF): effect on sleep and motor behavior. Pharmacol Biochem Behav 1976; 5:73-7.

13. Havlicek V, Rezek M, Friesen H. Somatostatin and thyrotropin releasing hormone: central effect on sleep and motor system. Pharmacol Biochem Behav 1976; 4:455-9.

14. Aponte G, Leung P, Gross D, Yamada T. Effects of somatostatin on food intake in rats. Life Sci 1984; 35:741-6.

15. Lotter EC, Woods SC. Somatostatin decreases food intake. Diabetes 1977; 26(suppl 1):358.

16. Rezek M, Havlicek V, Hughes KR, Friesen H. Central site of action of somatostatin (SRIF): role of hippocampus. Neuropharmacology 1976; 15:499-504.

17. Rezek M, Havlicek V, Hughes KR, Friesen H. Behavioural and motor excitation and inhibition induced by the administration of small and large doses of somatostatin into the amygdala. Neuropharmacology 1977; 16;157-62.

18. Havlicek V, Rezek M, Leybin L, Friesen H. Analgesic effect of cerebral ventricular administration of somatostatin (SRIF). Fed Proc 1977; 36:363.

19. Meynadier J, Chrubasik J, Dubar M, Wunsch E. Intrathecal somatostatin in terminally ill patients. A report of two cases. Pain 1985; 23:9-12.

20. Vecsei L, Kiraly C, Bollok I, et al. Comparative studies with somatostatin and cysteamine in different behavior tests on rats. Pharmacol Biochem Behav 1984; 21:833-7.

21. Walsh TJ, Emerich DF, Winokur A, Banki C, Bissette G, Nemeroff CB. Intrahippocampal injection of cysteamine depletes somatostatin and produces cognitive impairments in the rat. Soc Neuroscience Abstr 1985; 11:621.

22. Patel YC, Rao K, Reichlin S. Somatostatin in human cerebrospinal fluid. N Engl J Med 1977; 296:529-33.

23. Oram JJ, Edwardson J, Millard PH. Investigation of cerebrospinal fluid neuropeptides in idiopathic senile dementia. Gerontology 1981; 27:216-23.

24. Dupont E, Christensen SE, Hansen AP, Olivarius B deF, Orskov H. Low cerebrospinal fluid somatostatin in Parkinson's disease: an irreversible abnormality. Neurology 1982; 32:312-4.

25. Epelbaum J, Ruberg M, Moyse E, Javoy-Agid F, Dubois B, Agid Y. Somatostatin and dementia in Parkinson's disease. Brain Res 1983;

278:376-9.

26. Wood PL, Etienne P, Lal S, Gauthier S, Cajal S, Nair NPV. Reduced lumbar CSF somatostatin in Alzheimer's disease. Life Sci 1982; 31:2073-9.

27. Serby M, Richardson SB, Twente S, Siekierski J, Corwin J, Rotrosen J. CSF somatostatin in Alzheimer's disease. Neurobiol Aging 1984; 5:187-9.

28. Sorensen KV, Christensen SE, Dupont E, Hansen AP, Pedersen E, Orskov H. Low somatostatin content in cerebrospinal fluid in multiple sclerosis. Acta Neurol Scand 1980; 61:186-91.

29. Beal MF, Mazurek MF, Black PMcL, Martin JB. Human cerebrospinal somatostatin in neurologic disease. J Neurol Sci 1985;71:91-104.

30. Davies P. Neurotransmitters in Alzheimer's disease. Read before the International Study Group on the Pharmacology of Memory Disorders Associated with Aging, Zurich, April 1, 1981.

31. Soininen HS, Jolkkonen JT, Reinikainen KJ, Halonen TO, Riekkinen PJ. Reduced cholinesterase activity and somatostatin-like immunoreactivity in the cerebrospinal fluid of patients with dementia of the Alzheimer type. J Neurol Sci 1984; 63:167-72.

32. Morrison JH, Rogers J, Scherr S, Benoit R, Bloom FE. Somatostatin immunoreactivity in neuritic plaques of Alzheimer's patients. Nature 1985; 314:90-2.

33. Roberts GW, Crow TJ, Polak JM. Localization of neuronal tangles in somatostatin neurones in Alzheimer's disease. Nature 1985; 314:92-4.

34. Tamminga CA, Foster NL, Chase TN. Reduced brain somatostatin levels in Alzheimer's disease. N Engl J Med 1985; 313(20):1294-5.

35. Gerner RH, Yamada T. Altered neuropeptide concentrations in cerebrospinal fluid of psychiatric patients. Brain Res 1982; 238:298-302.

36. Rubinow DR, Gold PW, Post RM, et al. CSF somatostatin in affective illness. Arch Gen Psychiatry 1983; 40:409-12.

37. Black PM, Ballantine HT, Carr DB, Beal MF, Martin JB. Beta-endorphin and somatostatin concentrations in the cerebrospinal fluid of patients with depressive disorder [Abstract]. 39th Annual Convention of the Society of Biological Psychiatry, 1984; 135:177.

38. Agren H, Lundqvist G. Low levels of somatostatin in human CSF mark depressive episodes. Psychoneuroendocrinology 1984; 9:233-48.

39. Bissette G, Walleus H, Widerlov E, et al. Reductions of cerebrospinal fluid concentrations of somatostatin-like immunoreactivity (SRIF-LI) in dementia, major depression and schizophrenia [Abstract]. Abstracts of the 14th Annual Meeting of the Society for Neuroscience, vol 10 (part 2), 1984; 11:1093.

40. Doran A, Rubinow D, Roy A, Pickar D. CSF somatostatin and abnormal response to dexamethasone administration in schizophrenic and depressed patients. Arch Gen Psychiatry 1986; 43:365-9.

41. Nemeroff CB, Youngblood WW, Manberg PJ, Prange AJ, Kizer JS. Regional brain concentrations of neuropeptides in Huntington's chorea and schizophrenia. Science 1983; 221:972-5.

42. Ferrier IN, Cross AJ, Johnson JA, et al. Neuropeptides in Alzheimer type dementia. J Neurol Sci 1983; 62:159-70.

43. Sorensen KV. Rapid post-mortem decomposition of the somatostatin cells in human brain. An immunohistochemical examination. Biomed Pharmacother 1984; 38:458-61.

44. American Psychiatric Association. Diagnostic and statistical manual of mental disorders, 3rd ed. Washington, DC: APA, 1981.

45. Rubinow DR. Cerebrospinal fluid somatostatin and psychiatric illness. Biol Psychiatry 1986; 21:341-65.

46. Knigge KM, Bennett-Clarke C, Burchanowski B, Joseph SA, Romagnano MA, Sternberger LA. Relationships of some releasing-hormone-producing neuron systems to the ventricles of the brain. In: Motta M, ed. Endocrine functions of the brain. New York: Raven Press, 1980.

47. Weindl A, Sofroniew MB. Relation of neuropeptides to mammalian

circumventricular organs. In: Martin JB, Reichlin S, Bick KL, eds. Advances in biochemical psychopharmacology. New York: Raven Press, 1982.

48. Wehr TA. Biological rhythms and manic-depressive illness. In: Post RM, Ballenger JC, eds. Neurobiology of mood disorders, vol 1. Baltimore: Williams and Wilkins, 1984.

49. Berelowitz M, Perlow MJ, Hoffman HJ, Frohman LA. The diurnal variation of immunoreactive thyrotropin-releasing hormone and somatostatin in the cerebrospinal fluid of the rhesus monkey. Endocrinology 1981; 109:2102-9.

50. Arnold MA, Reppert SM, Rorstad OP, et al. Temporal patterns of somatostatin in the cerebrospinal fluid of the rhesus monkey: effect of environmental lighting. J Neurosci 1982; 2:674-80.

51. Vecsei L, Bollok I, Telegdy G. Intracerebroventricular somatostatin attenuates electroconvulsive shock-induced amnesia in rats. Peptides 1983; 4:293-5.

52. Carroll BJ, Curtis GC, Mendels J. Neuroendocrine regulation in depression. I. Limbic system-adrenocortical dysfunction. Arch Gen Psychiatry 1976; 33:1039-44.

53. Sachar EJ, Hellman L, Roffwarg HP, Halpern FS, Fukushima DK, Gallagher TF. Disrupted 24-hour patterns of cortisol secretion in psychotic depression. Arch Gen Psychiatry 1973; 28:19-24.

54. Gibbons JL. Cortisol secretion rates in depressive illness. Arch Gen Psychiatry 1964; 10:572-5.

55. Carroll BJ, Curtis GC, Davies BM, Mendels J, Sugerman AA. Urinary free cortisol excretion in depression. J Psychol Med 1976; 6:43-50.

56. Heisler S, Reisine T, Hook V, Axelrod J. Somatostatin inhibits multireceptor stimulation of cyclic AMP formation and adrenocorticotropin secretion in mouse pituitary tumor cells. Proc Natl Acad Sci USA 1982; 79:6502-7.

57. Brown MR, Rivier C, Vale W. Central nervous system regulation of adrenocorticotropin secretion: role of somatostatins. Endocrinology, 1984; 114:1546-9.

58. Serby M, Richardson SB, Rypma B, Twente S, Rotrosen JP. Somatostatin regulation of the CRF-ACTH-cortisol axis. Biol Psychiatry 1986 (in press).

59. Aguila MC, McCann SM. The influence of hGRF, CRF, TRH and LHRH on SRIF release from median eminence fragments. Brain Res 1985; 348: 180-2.

60. Katakami H, Arimura A, Frohman LA. Involvement of hypothalamic somatostatin in the suppression of growth hormone secretion by central corticotropin-releasing factor in conscious male rats. Neuroendocrinology 1985; 41:390-3.

61. Rivier C, Vale W. Involvement of corticotropin-releasing factor and somatostatin in stress-induced inhibition of growth hormone secretion in the rat. Endocrinology 1985; 117:2478-82.

62. Wolkowitz OM, Rubinow DR, Breier A, Doran AR, Pickar D. Steroid effects in normals: a prospective study. 139th Annual Meeting of the American Psychiatric Association, Washington, DC, 1986.

63. Post RM, Ballenger JC, Uhde TW, Bunney WE. Efficacy of carbamazepine in manic-depressive illness: implications for underlying mechanisms. In: Neurobiology of mood disorders, vol 1. Baltimore: Williams and Wilkins, 1984.

64. Rubinow DR, Post RM, Gold PW, Ballenger JC, Reichlin S. Effect of carbamazepine on cerebrospinal fluid somatostatin. Psychopharmacology 1985; 85:210-3.

65. Beal MF, Martin JB. Effects of neuroleptic drugs on brain somatostatin-like-immunoreactivity, Neurosci Lett 1984;47:125-30.

66. Gattaz WF, Rissler K, Gattaz D, Cramer H. Effects of Haloperidol on somatostatin-like immunoreactivity in the CSF of schizophrenic patients. Psychiatry Res 1986; 17:1-6.

67. Higuchi T. Neuropeptides and amygdaloid kindling. In: Wada JA, ed. Kindling III. New York: Raven Press, 1985.

68. Kato N, Higuchi T, Friesen HG, Wada JA. Changes of immunoreactive somatostatin and B-endorphin content in rat brain after amygdaloid kindling. Life Sci 1983; 32:2415-22.

69. Higuchi T, Kokubu T, Sikand GS, Wada JA, Friesen HG. A study of somatostatin receptors in amygdaloid-kindled rat brain. J Neurochem 1984; 43:1271-6.

70. Havlicek V, Friesen HG. Comparison of behavioural effects of SRIF and B-endorphin in animals. In: Collu R, Barbeau A, Rochefort JG, Ducharm JR, eds. Central nervous system effects of hypothalamic hormones and other peptides. New York: Raven Press, 1979.

71. Iofee S, Havlicek V, Friesen HG, Chernick V. Effect of iontophoretically applied somatostatin (SRIF) on cortical neurons in awake unanesthetized animals. Fed Proc Abstrc 1977; 36:364.

72. Higuchi T, Sikand GS, Kato N, Wada JA, Friesen HG. Profound suppression of kindled seizures by cysteamine: possible role of somatostatin to kindled seizures. Brain Res 1983; 288:359-62.

18

CYTOPROTECTION BY SOMATOSTATINS

K. H. Usadel, H. Kessler*, G. Rohr, K. Kusterer,
K. D. Palitzsch, and U. Schwedes

II. Medizinische Klinik, Klinikum Mannheim
University of Heidelberg and *Institut fur Organische
Chemie, University of Frankfurt, FRG

Several compounds, i.e., ethanol, acids, bases, histamine and others which are completely different in their chemical structures have the ability to injure gastric mucosa following oral administration in experimental animals and in humans (1). Histological changes include hemorrhagic lesions and necrosis of the epithelium. Prostaglandins, H2-receptor blockers, sulfhydryls, somatostatin and some analogs of somatostatin will protect gastric and duodenal mucosa in such experimental ulcer models (1-8). This protective effect which is independent of acid secretion and may be produced by several compounds was called "Cytoprotection." This term very recently was redefined by experts in 1986 (9) as "Organ specific reduction or prevention of vulnerability of cells and tissues against injury for cell preservation in vitro and in vivo." A number of findings suggest that somatostatin exerts cytoprotective action. Several clinical indications for treatment with somatostatin are based on its abilities to inhibit specific secretions of the gastrointestinal (GI) tract (19).

Somatostatin has a favorable effect on the course of experimental acute pancreatitis, gastric ulcers, and erosions as well as of duodenal ulcers (6). Mortality rates are also reduced by somatostatin. But suppression of GI secretion may not be the only mechanism by which somatostatin protects tissues from damage. Beneficial effects were seen in lung lesions after cysteamine, α-amanitin and diphtheria toxin, in adrenal necrosis after diphtheria toxin and cysteamine, in liver necrosis after phalloidin and galactosamine, and in other experimental shock models, e.g., Escherichia coli endotoxin, and antitumor drug indications (7). All these experimentally induced injuries were ameliorated by somatostatin pretreatment, and it has been suggested, therefore, that somatostatin exerts a local cytoprotective effect.

The cytoprotective effort may be exerted only if administered in advance of toxin exposure. Somatostatin is thought to be an efficient therapeutic tool for preventing acute pancreatitis after ERCP (11), but treatment of patients with acute pancreatitis in a multicenter double blind trial (APTS-study [Acute pancreatitis therapy with somatostatin]) has not shown a significant difference between continuous IV treatment over 6 days with somatostatin versus placebo (12). Pancreatitis was already present when patients were admitted to hospitals, and possibly cytoprotection could not be achieved.

Therapy in upper gastric-intestinal bleeding, i.e., gastric erosions, gastric and duodenal ulcerations of somatostatin must be different. Several double blind trials have proven the efficacy of the compounds (13,14,15,16) but the mechanism of its action is not fully understood. It has been postulated that somatostatin protects non-damaged mucosal cells, and promotes regeneration of the mucosa. Furthermore several additional mechanisms may be involved such as inhibition of acid secretion and reduction of splanchnic blood flow. Our own experience using various experimental models which lead to parenchymal lesions (7) have additionally shown that only pretreatment or very early treatment with somatostatin exerts cytoprotection. This is especially true for gastric and hepatic lesions (8).

Of importance in determining the mechanism of somatostatin effect is the structure/activity of the compound. Analogs of somatostatin with increased potency for the inhibition of hormone secretion have been synthesized (17,18,19,20) effective in acromegaly, several hormone-producing GI tumors, and in the Dawn phenomenon.

Since somatostatin-14 exerts at least two principally different modes of action, namely inhibition of hormonal secretion and cytoprotection, we have raised the question whether these actions of somatostatin analogs can be dissociated.

An important effect of somatostatin and some analogs was described by Ziegler et al. (22). Synthesis and conformation studies of analogs used were described by Kessler et al. (23,24). It could be demonstrated that cyclic somatostatin-14 inhibits the uptake of phallotoxins and of cholic acids in isolated liver cells in a concentration dependent manner. Some cyclic hexapeptide analogs inhibited very strongly both kinds of transport. The most potent compound was the analog no. 7 (Fig. 1). The inhibition of transport of cholate uptake was thought unlikely to be a hormonal effect of somatostatin, because concentrations needed were about 1,000-fold higher than circulating levels.

This finding indicates the existence of non-endocrine receptor-mediated but cell-membrane located effects which might be responsible for cytoprotection. Rao et al. (25) demonstrated that bleb formation of rat hepatocytes in vitro occurs after addition of various toxins especially phalloidin. Dose dependent cytoprotection could be achieved either by somatostatin-14 or by various analogs. Investigations by Ziegler et al. (22) demonstrate corresponding results. It could be shown that an increase of activity of the analogs occurred in both experimental models.

Figure 1 represents the relationship between the cytoprotective and the endocrine effect of various minianalogs of somatostatin. The 50% cytoprotective dose (CD 50) was evaluated in rat hepatocytes in vitro by Rao et al. (25). The endocrine effect is expressed by the relative dose for inhibition of growth hormone release. These experiments were done by Dr. Reichlin (Boston) by using a very sensitive pituitary cell culture assay (26). Analogous inhibition of growth hormone with the same relative dose could also be demonstrated in whole rats by Dr. J. Sandow (Hoechst AG, Frankfurt, FRG).

In comparison to somatostatin-14, the analogs 2-7 (Fig. 1) show increased cytoprotection and a corresponding decrease of endocrine activity. It is important to note that analog 6 which has no endocrine effect and a high cytoprotective effect differs in comparison to analog 5 only by a retroinverse sequence of amino acids. This change of conformation must be responsible for this change in efficacy. The part of the molecule which might be responsible for the cytoprotection of analog no. 7 (Fig. 1)

		CYTOPROTECTION CD50 (μMOL)	RELATIVE DOSE FOR GH-RELEASE INHIBITION
1	SOMATOSTATIN	109	≈ 1
2	H-D-PHE-CYS-PHE-D-TRP-LYS-THR-CYS-THR-ol	50	0.33
3	CYCLO(-PRO-PHE-D-TRP-LYS-THR-PHE-)	28	0.59
4	CYCLO(-PHE-PHE-TRP-LYS-THR-D-PHE-)	14	NO EFFECT
5	CYCLO(-PHE-PHE-D-TRP-LYS-THR-PHE-)	5.7	3.7
6	CYCLO(-PHE-THR-LYS-D-TRP-PHE-PHE-)	5.1	NO EFFECT
7	CYCLO(-PHE-THR-LYS-TRP-PHE-D-PRO-)	3.4	NO EFFECT

Fig. 1. Relationship of cytoprotective and endocrine potency of somatostatin (no. 1) and some of its analogs (no. 2, Ref. 17; no. 3, Ref. 18; no. 4, Ref. 23; no. 5, Ref. 23; no. 6 + 7, Ref. 23, CD 50 = dose for 50% of total cytoprotection (Ref. 25).

is shown in Figure 2. It also becomes more clear that the amino acid sequence -Phe-D-Trp-Lys-Thr- is responsible for the endocrine activity of somatostatins (Fig. 3). This sequence is also present in the analogs of somatostatin which are endocrinologically very active, i.e., analog Sandoz (= no. 2, Fig. 1) and analog MSD (no. 3, Fig. 1).

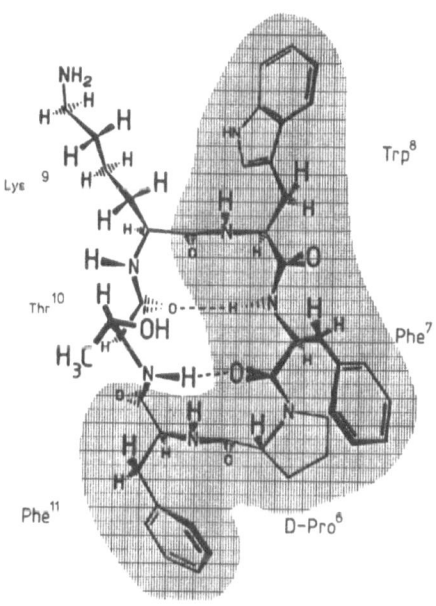

Fig. 2. Somatostatin analog 008 (= no. 7, Fig. 1). The part of the molecule supposed to be responsible for cytoprotection is indicated.

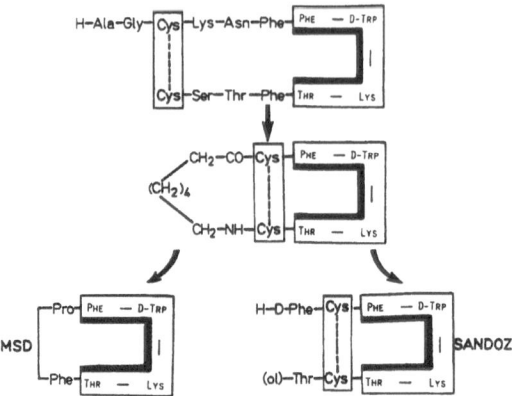

Fig. 3. The amino acid sequence -Phe-D-Trp-Lys-Thr- and cyclic conformation is responsible for the endocrine activity of somatostatin and its endocrine-superactive minianalogs, i.e., the octapeptide synthesized by Sandoz, Switzerland (= no. 2, Fig. 1) and the hexapeptide of MSD, Sharp & Dohme, USA (= no. 3, Fig. 1) respectively.

From these data we draw the following conclusions: (A) Somatostatins are biologically active in a cyclic confirmation. (B) For the endocrine effect, the amino acid sequence -Phe-D-Trp-Lys-Thr- of the molecule is essential. Conformation is essential for cytoprotection. The molecule may contain total amino acid sequence of B, but this is not essential for cytoprotection.

Our preliminary findings indicate that analogs of somatostatin reveal cytoprotective properties also under 4 experimental in vivo conditions:

1. Pancreatitis associated protein (PAP) reported by Keim et al. (27) could be reduced significantly by analog 008 (= analog no. 7, Fig. 1) in cerulein induced pancreatitis in the rat, as compared to equimolar doses of regular somatostatin (Fig. 4) which itself would also exert cytoprotection in a higher dose.

2. Using comparable doses of somatostatins as in experiment 1, analog 008 significantly increased survival rate analogously in rats after taurocholate induced pancreatitis (Fig. 5) according to the method of Lankisch et al. (28).

3. Somatostatin-14 and its analog 008 (no. 7, Fig. 1) prevented gastric hemorrhagic erosions in rats caused by ethanol. Somatostatin (10-250 μg) or the analog (equimolar to 50 μg) were given IP followed 10 min later by 1 ml of 75% ethanol p.o. in groups of 10 rats each. Hemorrhagic mucosal lesions (measured by computerized planimetry 1 hour later) involved 18.1 ± 3.2% of the glandular stomach while after somatostatin (10^{-7} mol/rat) 6.3 ± 1.1%. The analog at 10^{-7}, 10^{-8} or 10^{-9} mol/rat decreased the area of erosions to 4.9 ± 1.8% (P < 0.05), 2.0 ± 0.7% (P < 0.005) or 2.9 ± 0.9% (P < 0.005). This demonstrates that this endocrinologically not active analog exerts prominent gastric cytoprotection.

196

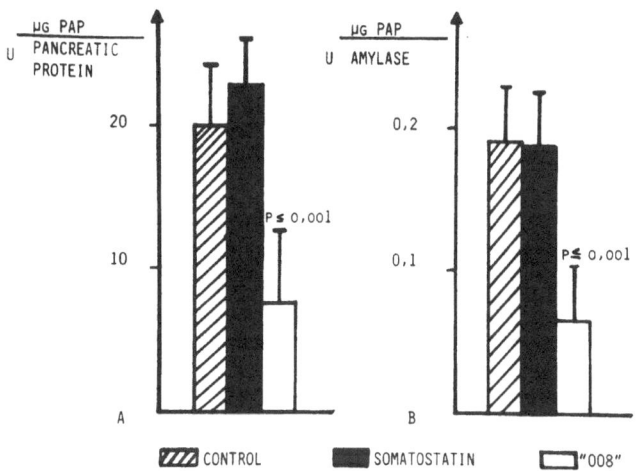

Fig. 4. Infusion of cerulein 5×10^{-6} g/kg x hour in rats for 6 hours (control). Simultaneous infusion of somatostatin (5×10^{-6} g/kg x hour) for 6 hours (somatostatin) or somatostatin analog 008, equimolar somatostatin for 6 hours ("008" = no. 7 in Fig. 1). Content of pancreatitis associated protein (PAP) in pancreatic tissue after 24 hours. Each group: n = 15. Vertical bars represent the mean ± SEM.

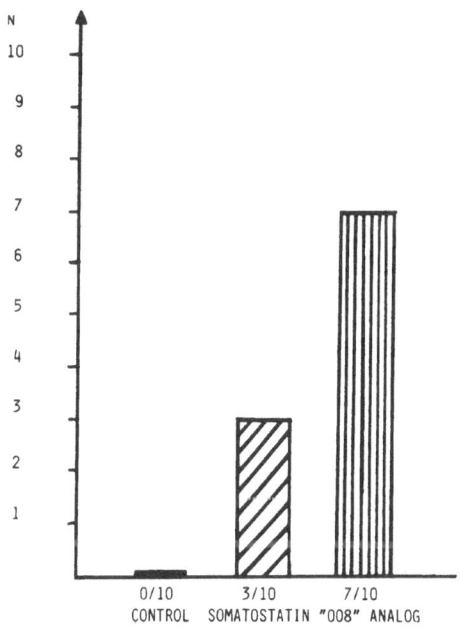

Fig. 5. Survival rate of rats in taurocholate-induced pancreatitis (29), A = control, B = treatment with somatostatin, C = treatment with analog "008" (= no. 7 in Fig. 1).

4. Somatostatin exerts a cytoprotective effect also on cysteamine-induced duodenal ulcerations in rats when high doses of the peptide were used. After 24 hours fasting 60 male Wistar rats (220-280 g) were given 28 mg/100 g body weight of cysteamine-HCl by oral tube, three times within 8 hours. Half of the rats served as controls, the others were injected sc with 50 μg of the analog SMS 201-995 (no. 2, Fig. 1) 25% of the dose which was used for regular somatostatin (6,7) 4 times in intervals of 12 hours, starting 1 hour prior to the first administration of cysteamine. Survivors were killed on the third day. All rats underwent autopsy and the stomach and duodenum were examined for ulcerations. The intensity of the lesion was rated on a scale (0—no lesion; 1—erosions; 2—deep ulcers; 3—penetrating or perforating ulcers). Fifteen of the controls but only 6 of the treated rats died within 48 hours. The incidence of cysteamine-induced duodenal ulceration was diminished by SMS treatment from 27/30 (incidence/total) in controls to 9/30. The median (range) intensity of duodenal ulcerations decreased from 3 (0-3) in the controls to 0 (0-1) in the treated group. Those results demonstrate that this endocrine active analog exerts even in a lower dose the same cytoprotective effect on cysteamine-induced ulcers as the mother compound.

Concerning the molecular size and biological activities of somatostatins, the following hypothesis can be postulated (Fig. 6). In the development of somatostatin analogs an increase of biological activities could be achieved in two ways: If endocrine activity is potentiated, the cytoprotective activity is potentiated as well. In analogs with superactive cytoprotection the endocrine activity is lost. In both, molecular size is smaller (hexa-, octapeptides) in comparison to regular somatostatin which contains 14 amino acids.

Whether the stimulation of phagocytosis in reticuloendothelial cells as reported by Szabo (29) is also due to the cytoprotective action of somatostatins is still unclear but "stabilization" of cell membranes as a result of cytoprotection might also be responsible for this effect. More investigations are needed to clarify the question whether cytoprotection of somatostatins is important for clinical use.

CONCLUSIONS

1. Somatostatin-14 exerts endocrine and cytoprotective effects.

2. In analogs of somatostatin with increased activity cytoprotective effect is also increased.

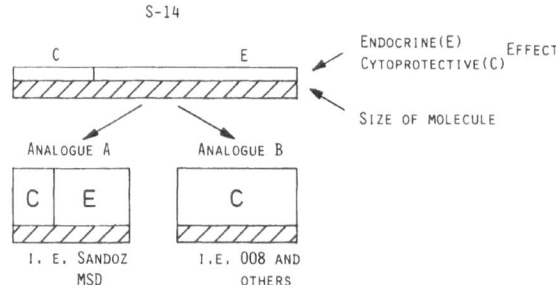

Fig. 6. Molecular size and biological activities of somatostatins, Sandoz = no. 2, MSD = no. 3, 008 = no. 7 (Fig. 1).

3. Cytoprotective effects of somatostatin can be dissociated from its endocrine effects, suggesting that different mechanisms are involved in cytoprotection and secretory cell inhibition.

REFERENCES

1. Robert A, Nezamis JE, Lancaster C, Hanchar AJ. Cytoprotection by prostaglandins in rats: prevention of gastric necrosis produced by alcohol, HCL, NaOH, hypertonic NaCL and thermal injury. Gastroenterology 1979; 77:433.
2. Miller TA. Protective effects of prostaglandins against gastric mucosal damage: current knowledge and proposed mechanisms. Am J Physiol 1983; 245:G601.
3. Robert A. Cytoprotection by prostaglandins. Gastroenterology 1979; 77:761.
4. Lacy ER, Ito S. Microscopic analysis of ethanol damage to rat gastric mucosa after treatment with a prostaglandin. Gastroenterology 1982; 83:619.
5. Szabo S, Trier JS, Frankel PW. Sulfhydryl compounds may mediate gastric cytoprotection. Science 1981; 214:200.
6. Schwedes U, Usadel KH, Szabo S. Cysteamine-induced duodenal ulcer: prevention by somatostatin (SRIF). Eur J Pharmacol 1975; 44:195.
7. Usadel KH, Schwedes U, Wdowinski JM. Pharmacol effects of somatostatin in acute organ lesion. Inn Med 1982; 9:204.
8. Szabo S, Usadel KH. Cytoprotection—organoprotection by somatostatin: gastric and hepatic lesions. Experientia 1982; 38:245.
9. Usadel KH, Schwedes U, eds. Proceedings of the international symposium: Mechanisms of cell injury, cytoprotection—organoprotection. Klin Wochenschr, 1986 (in press).
10. Reichlin S. Somatostatin. N Engl J Med 1983; 309:1495 and 1556.
11. Cicero GF, Laugier R, Sahel J, Manganaro M, Sarles H. Effects of somatostatin on clinical, biochemical and morphological changes following ERCP. Ital J Gastroenterol 1985; 17:265.
12. Usadel KH, Uberla KK, Leuschner U. Treatment of acute pancreatitis with somatostatin: results of the multicenter double-blind trial (APTS-Study). Dig Dis Sci 1985; 30:992.
13. Kayasseh L, Gyr K, Keller U, Stalder GA. Somatostatin and cimetidine in peptic-ulcer haemorrhage. Lancet 1980; I:844.
14. Coraggio F, Scarpato P, Spina M, Lombardi S. Somatostatin and ranitidine in the control of iatrogenic haemorrhage of the upper gastrointestinal tract. Br Med J 1984; 289:224.
15. Magnusson I, Ihre T, Johansson C, Selingson U, Torngren S, Uvnas-Moberg K. Randomised double-blind trial of somatostatin in the treatment of massive upper gastrointestinal haemorrhage. Gut 1985; 26:221.
16. Antonioli A, Gandolfo M, Rigo GP, et al. Somatostatin and cimetidine in the control of acute upper gastrointestinal bleeding, a controlled multicenter study. Hepatogastroenterology 1986; 33:71.
17. Bauer W, Briner U, Doepfner W, et al. SMS 201-995: a very potent and selective octapeptide analogue of somatostatin with prolonged action. Life Sci 1982; 31:1133.
18. Veber DF, Freidinger RM, Schwenk Perlow D, et al. A potent cycle hexapeptide analogue of somatostatin. Nature 1981; 292:55.
19. Lamberts SWJ, Oosterom R, Neufeld M, del Pozo E. The somatostatin analogue SMS 201-995 induces long-acting inhibition of growth hormone secretion without rebound hypersecretion in acromegalic patients. J Clin Endocrinol Metab 1985; 60:1161.
20. Plewe G, Schrezenmeir J, Nolken G, et al. Long-term treatment of acromegaly with the somatostatin analogue SMS 201-995 over 6 months. Klin Wochenschr 1986; 64:389.

21. Del Pozo E, Neufeld M, Schluter K, et al. Endocrine profile of a long-acting somatostatin derivative SMS 201-995, study in normal volunteers following subcutaneous administration. Acta Endocrinol (Copenh) 1986; 111:433.

22. Ziegler K, Frimmer M, Kessler H, et al. Modified somatostatin as inhibitors of a multispecific transport system for bile acids and phallotoxins in isolated hepatocytes. Biochim Biophys Acta 1985; 845:86.

23. Kessler H, Bernd M, Damm I. Peptide confirmations, NMR investigations of cyclic hexapeptides containing the active sequence of somatostatin. Tetrahedron Letters 1982; 23:4685.

24. Kessler H, Eiermann V. Peptide confirmations, hormone and heteronuclear 2 D NMR spectroscopy of cyclic pentapeptides containing the active sequence of somatostatin. Tetrahedron Letters 1982; 23:4689.

25. Rao GS, Lemoch H, Kessler H, Damm I, Knoll S, Usadel KH. Cytoprotection by novel synthetic analogues of somatostatin. Acta Endocrinol (Copenh) 1984; 105(suppl 264):96.

26. Heimann ML, Nekola MV, Murphy WA, Lance VA, Coy DH. An extremely sensitive in vitro model for elucidating structure-activity relationships of growth hormone-releasing factor analogs. Endocrinology 1985; 116:410.

27. Keim V, Rohr G, Stockert HG, Haberich FJ. An additional secretory protein in the rat pancreas. Digestion 1984; 29:242.

28. Lankisch PG, Winckler K, Bohrmann M, Schmidt H, Creutzfeldt W. The influence of glucagon on acute experimental pancreatitis in the rat. Scand J Gastroenterol 1974; 9:725.

29. Szabo S. Somatostatin stimulates clearance and hepatic uptake of colloidal carbon in the rat. Life Sci 1983; 3:1975.

19

EVIDENCE FOR PARACRINE FUNCTION OF SOMATOSTATIN

Werner Creutzfeldt

Division of Gastroenterology and Metabolism
Department of Medicine
University of Gottingen, FRG

The title of this debate, "Somatostatin is a hormone," and my task to question this thesis implies that I have proof against this proposition. There are numerous data supporting the hormonal role of somatostatin and I suppose that they will be presented in the next lecture. However, there are also data available which suggest that somatostatin is a local chemical transmitter. It is more difficult to prove such a function. This puts me in the position of representing the speculative part of this debate, simply because the methodology of measuring paracrine function is not as simple as the methodology in classical endocrinology.

I strongly believe that the discussion of hypothetical or semantic questions is of little value for the understanding of physiology or pathophysiology. Therefore, such discussions should not be led with the fervor of a medieval religious debate. Rather, they should be an intellectual exercise and a stimulus to design better methods and experiments.

THE PARACRINE CONCEPT

How did it all start? Incidently, at the Georg-August University of Gottingen where I am working since more than 20 years the first experimental proof for an endocrine function has been established nearly 140 years ago, but here also the concept of paracrine secretion has been developed nearly 40 years ago. Therefore, I am not arguing out of chauvinistic reasons for either of the two theories.

In 1849 Arnold A. Berthold, Professor of Comparative Anatomy, published his classical experiments about the transplantation of the testis in castrated cockerels and concluded that his finding must be due to a secretion via the blood (1). In 1953 Friedrich Feyrter, Chairman of the Department of Pathology at the University of Gottingen, published a monograph with the title "On the peripheral endocrine (paracrine) glands of man" in which he introduced the concept of paracrine secretion as an important function of the "disseminated endocrine organs" (2). As a major part of these he had described the "clear cells" ("Helle Zellen") in the epithelium of many organs. Feyrter was a pure morphologist and histochemist. He had no proof that the clear cells in the mucosa of many organs were hormone-producing cells and never referred to the classical work of physiologists such as Bayliss and Starling or Edkins. He formulated his hypothesis by looking at the localization and structure of the clear cells and speculated on a <u>local</u> effect of their hormonal products, designating this function as "<u>paracrine</u>." Figure 1 demonstrates schematically the different modes of secretion in the gut epithelium as suggested by Feyrter. A. G. E. Pearse recognized later that his APUD-cell series was identical with the clear cell system and gave Feyrter full credit for his work (3).

SOMATOSTATIN PLASMA LEVELS

When the field of gastrointestinal endocrinology rapidly expanded in the sixties, gut peptides were regarded as hormones, secreted by the peptide and amine producing cells of the gastrointestinal mucosa. The physiological role could be approached by measuring circulating hormone levels after endogenous release or exogenous administration. A prerequisite was reliable methods for estimation of hormone plasma levels and their different molecular forms. These are not always available or their validity disputed as in the case of somatostatin. Table 1 gives a list of varying fasting and meal-stimulated plasma levels of somatostatin published in recent years. This indicates the uncertain ground on which we are moving if a so-called physiological amount of an infused peptide is defined by peptide levels measured by an unreliable radioimmunoassay. The problems of the radioimmunoassay of somatostatin are discussed in several recent papers (4,5). Noteworthy is also the fact that the rise after a meal was usually only twofold or less while other gastrointestinal hormones such as gastrin, GIP, insulin or pancreatic polypeptide increase three- to six-fold after a meal.

A major problem arises if several molecular forms of a peptide with different biological but similar immunological potency are circulating in the blood, as in the case of somatostatin. Recent work has revealed that

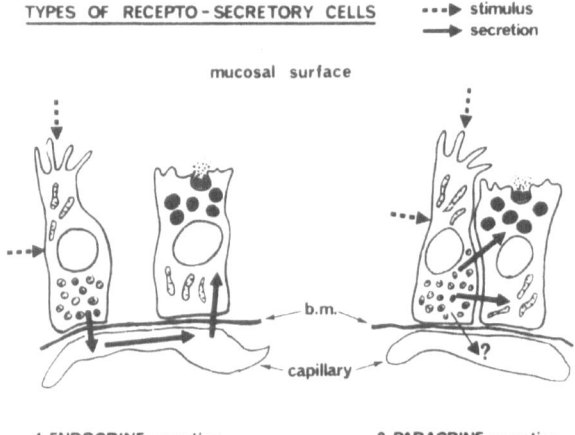

Fig. 1. Schematic drawing of two types of recepto-secretory cells producing gastrointestinal hormones. The endocrine cell type secretes its product into the blood stream and affects distant cells; the paracrine cell type secretes its product into the intracellular space where it acts locally.

Table 1. Fasting and meal-stimulated SLI serum concentrations.

Reference	Year	Method of extraction	Mean basal concentrations (pg/ml)	Rise following mixed-meal (pg/ml)
Wass et al. (25)	1980	Vycor glass	28	29
Penman et al. (26)	1981	Vycor glass	29	51
Tsuda et al. (27)	1981	Affinity chromatography	9	6
Zyznar et al. (28	1981	Gel filtration	8	12
Vinik et al. (29)	1981	None	174	130
Polonsky et al. (5a)	1983	Gel filtration	33	18
Conlon et al. (5)	1983	PEG	20	6
Colturi et al. (30)	1984	C-18-silicate	6	7
Schusdziarra et al. (25)	1985	None	120	45
Lucey et al. (32)	1985	Vycor glass	18; 50	30; 60

in man the circulating somatostatin-like immunoreactivity (SLI) is mainly somatostatin 28 (SS-28) (5a). On a molar infusion basis, SS-14 and SS-28 appear to be equipotent regarding their biological effect. However, when acid inhibitory effect was compared against increment in plasma concentrations produced by peptide infusion, SS-14 was roughly tenfold more potent than SS-28 (5b). In other words: infusion rates of SS-14 aiming to achieve postprandial SLI plasma levels measured by RIA in man, where mainly SS-28 is circulating, will be one order of magnitude beyond the physiological range of postprandial SS-14 levels. This fact indicates that most, if not all, SS-14 infusion studies in man performed up to now are pharmacological studies and do not prove an endocrine role of somatostatin.

Furthermore, one has to remember that circulating hormone concentrations are meaningless in case of neurotransmission or local secretion of the chemical transmitter. Many gut hormones have been found both in epithelial cells and in nerves, some only in epithelial cells and some in nerves. VIP is an example of a pure neuropeptide. Estimation of VIP plasma levels is meaningless if one wants to study its physiological role: since transmission occurs via the synaptic cleft, plasma levels do not reflect physiological events but are merely an overspill of unused and sometimes even degraded material. The same holds true if a transmitter is secreted into a local portal system or into the intercellular space nearby or directly brought to the target cells by cell to cell contact via gap junctions (with or without processes).

D-CELL MORPHOLOGY

Somatostatin-producing D-cells are unique in exhibiting long cytoplasmatic processes extending into the neighborhood, especially in the gastric mucosa and the pancreatic islets. It has been suggested that these processes, which end with small bulbous expansions, directly deliver somatostatin onto the membranes of their putative effector cells (6, 7).

Such cells have even been considered to represent intermediates between (neurosecretory) neurons and endocrine cells (6). Furthermore, it has been demonstrated that gastric somatostatin cells transport their secretory products in a proximo-distal direction in these paracrine processes (8). This polar orientation of the D-cell in the gastric antral mucosa can also be demonstrated ultrastructurally and quantified by morphometric analysis of subcellular organelle distribution. We have recently observed that the volume density of D-cell secretory granules in the cytoplasmatic processes increases in the activated state (intragastric HCl infusion) and decreases in the resting state (vagotomy). However, until now the mode of secretion of antral D-cells has not yet been defined. Recent work by Grube and Bohn and by Aponte et al. has concentrated on the D-cells of the pancreatic islets of man (9) and rat (10). There, the long processes of the D-cells mostly extend to the capillaries. This has been interpreted as indicative for an endocrine function of pancreatic D-cells. However, the same authors report that only 50% of the insulin-secreting B-cells reach the capillaries. This observation indicates that extension of a cell to a capillary does not necessarily mean an endocrine function and vice versa. The capillary process could serve as a sensor by which the D-cell receives information on the concentration of hormones or metabolites, i.e., stimulators for somatostatin secretion. Hormone release could take place along the whole surface of these cell processes. In this context it is of interest that 100% of pancreatic D-cells have cell to cell contact to B-cells, 37% to A-cells and 67% to other D-cells (11).

CONTRIBUTION OF DIFFERENT ORGANS TO PLASMA SOMATOSTATIN

The widespread distribution of somatostatin in the gastrointestinal tract raises the question whether different organs equally contribute to somatostatin plasma levels. This has been investigated by several authors. According to Taborsky and Ensinck (12), 97% of circulating somatostatin originates from the gastrointestinal tract while the pancreas contributes less than 3%. The discrepancy of these figures to earlier investigations is explained by the fact that in these studies organ blood flow has not been measured. The authors conclude that pancreatic somatostatin regulates insulin and glucagon secretion in a paracrine fashion or via a portal system. In addition, the same authors have shown that the pancreas extracts significant quantities of somatostatin (13). This may be important for the degradation of locally secreted somatostatin. For somatostatin to act as a paracrine substance implies that there must be an efficient system for inactivation within the organ of synthesis which will serve to limit the release of the peptide into the general circulation. It has recently been shown that the gut possesses such a proteolytic inactivation system (14).

Also of interest is the observation that somatostatin is present in epithelial cells of the intestinal mucosa mainly as somatostatin 28 (15). It has even been suggested by Baskin and Ensinck that intestinal D-cells lack enzymes for further cleavage of the SS-28 molecule analogous to the processing of glicentin in the intestinal compared to pancreatic A-cells. Therefore, the small intestine may be the source of circulating SS-28 like peptides which have been shown to increase in plasma after a meal by Polonsky et al. (5a) and also at this meeting by Ensinck.

EXCLUSION OF D-CELL FUNCTION

More direct evidence for a paracrine function of somatostatin, especially its restraining effect on secretory processes, stems from experiments aiming at the exclusion of D-cell function. Thus, Taniguchi

204

et al. (16) showed with isolated rat islets that pre-incubation for one hour with somatostatin antiserum significantly increased insulin release at low glucose concentrations. This has been confirmed by Itoh et al. (17). It has also been demonstrated by Saffouri et al. (18) in the isolated vascularly perfused rat stomach that the infusion of somatostatin antiserum increases gastrin release. Similar results have been reported by Short et al. (19). Also with antral mucosa in tissue culture an enhanced gastrin release could be shown during incubation with somatostatin antiserum by Wolfe et al. (20).

It has been argued that similar effects can be achieved in vivo with antibody infusion. Since γ-globulins do not readily leave the vascular bed these experiments seem to prove an endocrine function of somatostatin. This argument is applicable only for acute effects of antibody infusion. Otherwise antireceptor antibody-related diseases (such as Grave's disease or myasthenia gravis) would not exist and could not be experimentally reproduced. But also acute effects of circulating antibodies on paracrine signal transmission should be possible if one assumes the existence of an equilibrium between the concentration of peptides in the intercellular space and the vascular bed. In this case also peptides secreted in a paracrine fashion will be drained into the circulation by the antibody. The existence of such an equilibrium follows from the above mentioned in vitro experiments with perfused organs or incubated tissue.

More recently, cysteamine has been used in order to eliminate D-cell function. This substance is believed to modify the somatostatin molecule and, by this, rendering it biologically and immunologically unreactive. Isolated islets from cysteamine-pretreated rats released more insulin in response to glucose (21). Similar results were reported by Patel et al. who studied the addition of cysteamine in monolayer cultures of neonatal rat islets (22). These authors investigated also the effect of somatostatin antiserum alone and in combination with cysteamine. Also the 12-fold increase of gastrin secretion from the isolated perfused rat stomach during addition of 10 mM cysteamine to the perfusate as demonstrated by McIntosh et al. (23) clearly shows the restraining role of the antral D-cells on the G-cells. The authors have interpreted their results differently because at that time the mode of action of cysteamine on the somatostatin molecule had not yet been elucidated.

Finally, Taborsky (24) studied the effect of a non-immunoreactive somatostatin analogue, which inhibits somatostatin release in dogs, on glucagon and insulin release. He demonstrated a several-fold increase of glucagon and a 60% increase of insulin secretion parallel to somatostatin decrease.

CONCLUSION

It is difficult not to conclude from these experiments that somatostatin locally restrains hormone release from antral mucosa and pancreatic islets. On the other hand, these findings do not exclude the possibility that somatostatin also has systemic effects and may act as endocrine transmitter. However, the ability of somatostatin to inhibit numerous functions of the gastrointestinal tract and its extremely short half-life time in plasma is in favor of paracrine rather than systemic action at least of SS-14. Otherwise the restraining or dampening effect of this peptide is difficult to envisage. The complex secretory pathways of somatostatin in the gastrointestinal tract as discussed today are schematically summarized in Figure 2. This scheme offers a more differentiated approach to the question whether somatostatin does act as a hormone or a paracrine transmitter and is, of course, open for modification.

SUMMARY

Forty years ago, F. Feyrter postulated on purely morphological
grounds that the "clear cells" in the mucosa of the gut and the bronchial
system produce substances which are secreted into the neighboring tissue
and by this regulate the function of the gut and the bronchi. He called
this function "paracrine," i.e., something between endocrine and exocrine
secretion. This hypothesis has been widely accepted in modern gastrointestinal endocrinology, especially for somatostatin-secreting cells.
However, direct proof for this mode of secretion or action is difficult to
provide. At present, two lines of evidence support the idea of paracrine
action of somatostatin: (1) Immunocytochemical and ultrastructural
studies have demonstrated organelles responsible for signal transmission
into the neighborhood of D-cells in different organs, especially in the
stomach; (2) In vitro studies have shown that perfusion of isolated organs
or incubation of tissues with somatostatin antibodies or cysteamine
increase the secretion of gut and pancreatic hormones from these tissues.
This suggests that somatostatin restrains locally hormone release.

Last but not least, logical thinking deduces localized rather than
systemic effects of somatostatin with its multiple inhibitory potency.

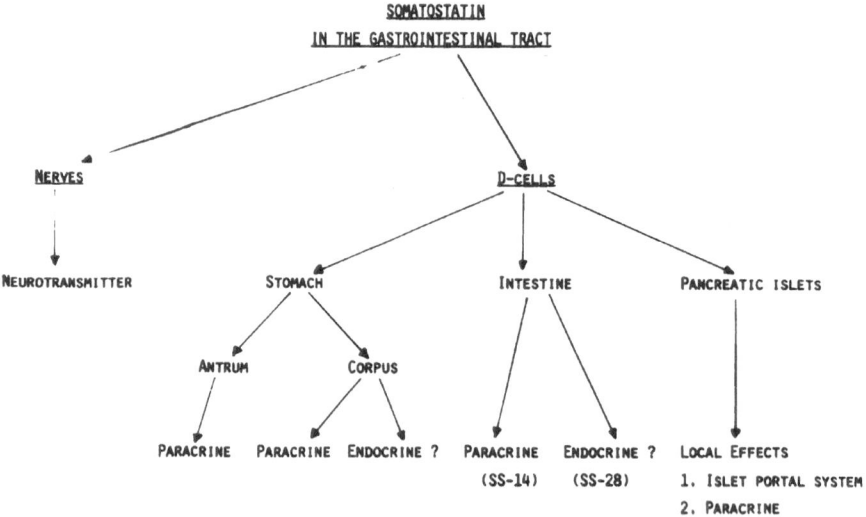

Figure 2.

REFERENCES

1. Berthold A. Transplantation der Hoden. Arch Anat Physiol u wiss Med 1849; 42-6.
2. Feyrter F. "Uber die peripheren endokrinen (parakrinen Drusen des Menschen." Wien: Maudrich, 1953.
3. Pearse AGE. The endocrine cells of the GI tract: origins, morphology and functional relationships in health and disease. Clin Gastroenterol 1974; 3:491-510.
4. Conlon JM, Bridgeman M, Alberti KGMM. The nature of big plasma somatostatin: implications for the measurement of somatostatin-like immunoreactivity in human plasma. Analyt Biochem 1982; 125:243-52.
5. Conlon JM, McCulloch AJ, Alberti KGMM. Circulating somatostatin concentrations in healthy and non-insulin-dependent (type II) diabetic subjects. Diabetes 1983; 32:723-9.
5a. Polonsky KS, Shoelson SM, Docherty HM. Plasma somatostatin-28 increases in response to feeding in man. J Clin Invest 1983; 71:1514-8.
5b. Seal A, Yamada T, Debas H, Hollinshead J, Osadchey B, Aponte G, Walsh J. Somatostatin-14 and -28: clearance and potency on gastric function in dogs. Am J Physiol 1982; 243:G97-102.
6. Larsson LI, Goltermann N, de Magistris L, Rehfeld JF, Schwartz TW. Somatostatin cell processes as pathways for paracrine secretion, Science 1979; 205:1393-5.
7. Alumets J, Ekelund M, El Munshid HA, Hakanson R, Loren I, Sundler F. Topography of somatostatin cells in the stomach of the rat: possible functional significance. Cell Tissue Res 1979; 202:177-88.
8. Larsson L-I. Evidence for anterograde transport of secretory granules in processes of gastric paracrine (somatostatin) cells. Histochemistry 1984; 80:323-6.
9. Grube D, Bohn R. The microanatomy of human islets of Langerhans, with special reference to somatostatin (D-) cells. Arch Histol Jpn 1983; 46:327-53.
10. Aponte G, Gross D, Yamada T. Capillary orientation of rat pancreatic D-cell processes: evidence for endocrine release of somatostatin. Am J Physiol 1985; 249:G599-606.
11. Grube D, Eckert I, Speck PT, Wagner H-J. Immunohistochemistry and microanatomy of the islets of Langerhans. Biomed Res 1983; 4(suppl): 25-36.
12. Taborsky GT, Ensinck JW. Contribution of the pancreas to circulating somatostatin-like immunoreactivity in the normal dog. J Clin Invest 1984; 73:216-23.
13. Taborsky GT, Ensinck JW. Extraction of somatostatin by the pancreas. Endocrinology 1983; 112:303-7.
14. Weber M, Cole T, Conlon JM. Specific binding and degradation of somatostatin by membrane vesicles from pig gut. Am J Physiol (in press).
15. Baskin DG, Ensinck JW. Somatostatin in epithelial cells of intestinal mucosa is present primarily as somatostatin 28. Peptides 1984; 5:615-21 (1984).
16. Taniguchi H, Utsumi M, Hasegawa M, et al. Physiologic role of somatostatin. Insulin release from rat islets treated by somatostatin antiserum. Diabetes 1977; 26:700-2.
17. Itoh M, Mandarino L, Gerich JE. Antisomatostatin gamma globulin augments secretion of both insulin and glucagon in vitro. Evidence for a physiologic role for endogenous somatostatin in the regulation of pancreatic A- and B-cell function. Diabetes 1980; 29:693-6.
18. Saffouri B, Weir G, Bitar K, Makhlouf G. Stimulation of gastrin secretion from the perfused rat stomach by somatostatin antiserum. Life Sci 1979; 25:1749-54.
19. Short GM, Doyle W, Wolfe MM. Effect of antibodies to somatostatin on

acid secretion and gastrin release by the isolated perfused rat stomach. Gastroenterology 1985; 88:984-8.

20. Wolfe MM, Jain DK, Reel GM, McGuigan JE. Effects of carbachol on gastrin and somatostatin release in rat antral tissue culture. Gastroenterology 1984; 87:86-93.

21. Kanatsuka A, Makino H, Osegawa M, Kasanuki J, Suzuki T, Yoshida S, Horie H. Is somatostatin a true local inhibitory regulator of insulin secretion? Diabetes 1984; 33:510-5.

22. Patel YC, Pierzchala I, Amherdt M, Orci L. Effects of cysteamine and antibody to somatostatin on islet cell function in vitro. J Clin Invest 1985; 75:1249-55.

23. McIntosh C, Bakich V, Trotter T, Kwok YN, Nishimura E, Pederson R, Brown J. Effect of cysteamine on secretion of gastrin and somato- statin from the rat stomach. Gastroenterology 1984; 86:834-8.

24. Taborsky GJ. Evidence of a paracrine role for pancreatic somato- statin in vivo. Am J Physiol 1983; 245:E598-603.

25. Wass JAH, Penman E, Dryburgh JR, et al. Circulating somatostatin after food and glucose in man. Clin Endocrinol 1980; 12:569-74.

26. Penman E, Wass JAH, Medbak S, Morgan L, Lewis JM, Besser GM, Rees LH. Response of circulating immunoreactive somatostatin to nutritional stimuli in normal subjects. Gastroenterology 1981; 81:692-9.

27. Tsuda K, Sakurai H, Seino Y, Seino S, Tanigawa K, Kuzuya H, Imura H. Somatostatin-like immunoreactivity in human peripheral plasma measur- ed by radioimmunoassay following affinity chromatography. Diabetes 1981; 30:471-4.

28. Zyznar ES, Pietri AO, Harris V, Unger RH. Evidence for the hormonal status of somatostatin in man. Diabetes 1981; 30:883-6.

29. Vinik AI, Levitt NS, Pimstone BL, Wagner L. Peripheral plasma somatostatin-like immunoreactive responses to insulin hypoglycemia and a mixed meal in healthy subjects and in noninsulin-dependent maturity-onset diabetics. J Clin Endocrinol Metab 1981; 52:330-7.

30. Colturi TJ, Unger RH, Feldman M. Role of circulating somatostatin in regulation of gastric acid secretion, gastrin release, and islet cell function. J Clin Invest 1984; 74:417-23.

31. Schusdziarra V, Lawecki J, Ditschuneit HH, Lukas B, Maier V, Pfeiffer EF. Effect of low-dose somatostatin infusion on pancreatic and gastric endocrine function in lean and obese nondiabetic human subjects. Diabetes 1985; 34:595-601.

32. Lucey MR, Wass JAH, Fairclough P, Webb J, Webb S, Medbak S, Rees LH. Autonomic regulation of postprandial plasma somatostatin, gastrin, and insulin. Gut 1985; 26:683-8.

20

EVIDENCE FOR THE ENDOCRINE ROLE OF SOMATOSTATIN

Volker Schusdziarra

Department of Internal Medicine II

Technical University of Munich, Germany

INTRODUCTION

Somatostatin-like immunoreactivity has been demonstrated to be present in D-cells which are located in the fundic and antral region of the stomach, in the islets of Langerhans of the pancreas, and in the small intestine (1-7). The powerful inhibitory effect of somatostatin when infused in high pharmacological doses on the secretory function of those cells that are located in close proximity to D-cells has led to the assumption of a local or paracrine action of somatostatin (8-10). Thus, somatostatin released from fundic D-cells could have an effect on acid secretion, antral D-cell somatostatin could inhibit gastrin release and within the islets of Langerhans locally released somatostatin could reduce insulin and glucagon secretion (11-14).

The development of a specific radioimmunoassay for the measurement of somatostatin-like immunoreactivity (SLI) in vitro and in vivo (15) has provided the basis for determinations of SLI release into the vascular space and, subsequently, this has led to the hypothesis of R. H. Unger et al. (16) that somatostatin might be a true endocrine factor in addition to any paracrine mode of action. If somatostatin is indeed an endocrine or hormonal factor, the following criteria should be fulfilled: (1) SLI from the stomach and pancreas has to be released into the circulation under physiological conditions such as the ingestion of a meal. (2) The infusion of synthetic somatostatin at a physiological dose that raises plasma SLI levels comparable to those observed after the ingestion of a meal should exert an inhibitory effect on one or more target organs. (3) Somatostatin deficiency should result in an augmented response of the potential target organs of circulating SLI and, if possible, this increased biological responsiveness should be corrected by replacement of somatostatin to normal concentrations.

RELEASE OF SOMATOSTATIN INTO THE CIRCULATION

Basal peripheral plasma SLI levels are maintained substantially by SLI secretion from the splanchnic organs. As shown in dogs, there is a substantial portal vein—inferior vena cava and also arterial—peripheral vein gradient. Similar data have been obtained in rats and, to a certain extent, in humans (17-20). The peripheral arteriovenous gradient which by

far exceeds that of insulin and glucagon and which increases with augmented SLI secretion could reflect a high rate of uptake by tissues and/or
rapid destruction in the circulation (18). Since in most studies SLI
measurements are performed in peripheral venous plasma these determinations could result in an underestimation of the actual changes of SLI
levels reaching the respective target organs via the arterial circulation.

The ingestion of a mixed meal elicits a significant stimulation of
peripheral SLI levels in dogs and man (21-25). In rats, a postprandial
increase of SLI levels has been observed in the portal vein but not in
peripheral plasma (19,30). As shown in Table 1, the increments of plasma
SLI levels following the ingestion of meals are in a range between 10 and
90 pg/ml. This might be due to the various extraction procedures employed
in the various studies.

Stimulation of SLI secretion occurs during the gastric and intestinal
phase of a meal, and absorbed and circulating nutrients might contribute
to pancreatic but not gastric SLI release (31-36).

Sham-feeding-induced activation of the cephalic phase elicits an
increase of peripheral SLI levels in dogs (37) but not in humans (38).

Postprandial stimulation of SLI levels is the result of the nutrient
content of a meal. The volume of the test meal has no significant effect
on peripheral SLI levels suggesting that gastrointestinal distention is a
rather unimportant mechanism for SLI secretion in contrast to its effect
on gastrin secretion in dogs and man (39-42).

This leaves the nutrients as major stimuli for splanchnic SLI secretion (17). The best stimulus in dogs is a protein-rich test meal (39,42)
whereas in humans a fat-rich meal is more efficient (25,41,42). The
smallest SLI response in both species is observed after carbohydrate-rich
test meals (25,41,42). This might be due to the inhibitory effect of
insulin on SLI secretion. Furthermore, circulating glucose stimulates
only pancreatic but not gastric SLI release and prestimulated gastric SLI
secretion is even inhibited by elevated glucose levels (31-34, 43). The

Table 1. Postprandial increase of SLI levels
in peripheral venous plasma.

Schusdziarra et al. 1978 (21)	dog	50 pg/ml
Chayvialle et al. 1980 (22)	dog	60 pg/ml
Wass et al. 1980 (23)	man	40 pg/ml
Vinik et al. 1981 (24)	man	90 pg/ml
Zyznar et al. 1981 (26)	man	12 pg/ml
Conlon et al. 1983 (27)	man	7 pg/ml
Polonsky et al. 1983 (28)	man	25 pg/ml
O'Shaughnessy et al. 1985 (25)	man	16 pg/ml
Schusdziarra et al. 1985 (29)	man	45 pg/ml

role of intragastric acid as a stimulus of SLI release is unequivocal in dogs (17,44) while in humans acid may not be of similar importance (45). In rats acidification of the stomach does not affect SLI release in vivo and in vitro (39,46), suggesting considerable species differences with regard to the contribution of acid to postprandial SLI secretion.

BIOLOGICAL SIGNIFICANCE OF POSTPRANDIALLY-ELEVATED PLASMA SLI LEVELS

Infusion Studies

The infusion of somatostatin at high pharmacological doses has been shown to have a potent inhibitory effect upon virtually all gastrointestinal and pancreatic exo- and endocrine functions as well as gastrointestinal motor activity (see 47-50 for review).

The studies demonstrate the potential target organs for endogenously released somatostatin. While some target organs could be influenced by locally released somatostatin via paracrine mechanisms, other functions would have to be regulated via circulating somatostatin (i.e., gallbladder contraction) due to the lack of somatostatin containing D-cells in these organs. In addition, it is conceivable that paracrine and endocrine effects of somatostatin might act synergistically on a given target cell.

In vitro studies in the isolated dog pancreas have shown that low doses of somatostatin inhibit insulin and glucagon secretion (52). These data in the perfused pancreas indicate that A- and B-cells have a receptor population which is very sensitive towards low concentrations of somatostatin. Since receptor binding studies have shown that downregulation of somatostatin receptors occurs during exposure to high concentrations of somatostatin-14 and conversely depletion of endogenous somatostatin results in upregulation of somatostatin-receptors (51), these sites cannot be exposed to the high concentrations of locally released somatostatin. It is very likely that tight junctions which have been demonstrated in the islets of Langerhans provide the basis for the separation of a somatostatin-rich compartment which comprises the locally or paracrine acting somatostatin from a somatostatin-poor compartment which permits biological effects of the much lower concentrations of circulating somatostatin (52).

In analogy to these experiments, studies in the isolated rat stomach have shown that low doses of somatostatin inhibit gastrin release (53). These in vitro studies strongly support the concept of an endocrine action of somatostatin in addition to a paracrine mode of action even on the same target cells.

In vivo the infusion of synthetic somatostatin-14 at physiological rates, giving a rise of plasma somatostatin levels comparable to that observed after the ingestion of a meal, elicits inhibitory effects on several gastrointestinal functions as summarized in Table 2. These data support the concept of an endocrine action of postprandially released somatostatin. These infusion studies have been performed with somatostatin-14. Since in the postprandial state both molecular forms—somatostatin-14 and somatostatin-28—are secreted into the circulation (28,29, 55,63), it will be necessary to examine the biological effect of physiological doses of somatostatin-28. Studies in dogs suggest that physiological doses of somatostatin-28 inhibit gastric and pancreatic exocrine functions (55,63). However, in these studies the total postprandial increment of plasma SLI levels has been reproduced with somatostatin-28. It will be necessary to give both peptides together reproducing the relative contribution of each peptide to the total rise of postprandial plasma SLI levels. This might be of considerable interest because somato-

Table 2. Effect of physiological infusion rates of synthetic
somatostatin-14 on gastrointestinal and pancreatic
exocrine and endocrine functions.

Schusdziarra et al. 1979 (54)	2.5 ng/kg min	Triglyceride and xylose uptake	dog
Vaysse et al. 1981 (55)	4.5 ng/kg min	Pancreatic volume, bicar- bonate and enzyme secretion	dog
Uvnas-Wallensten et al. 1981 (44)	4.0 ng/kg min	Gastric acid secretion	dog
Aizawa et al. 1981 (56)	1.5 ng/kg min	Delay of gastric interdigestive contractions	dog
Nakabayashi et al. 1981 (57)	2.5 ng/kg min	Triglyceride absorption	dog
Johansson et al. 1981 (58,59)	0.7 ng/kg min	Gallbladder emptying Pancreatic enzyme secretion Glucose absorption Gastric emptying	man
Zyznar et al. 1981 (26)	0.5 ng/kg min	Insulin Glucagon	man
Feurle et al. 1982 (60)	1.5 ng/kg min	Insulin	dog
Schusdziarra et al. 1982 (30)	1.0 ng/kg min	Insulin	rat
Souquet et al. 1983 (61)	2.0 ng/kg min	Basal insulin, glucagon	man
Colturi et al. 1983 (62)	2.0 ng/kg min	Acid and gastrin secretion	man
O'Shaughnessy et al. 1985 (25)	1.3 ng/kg min	Insulin, GIP, PP	man

statin-28 is degraded much slower in plasma; on the other hand, however, its potency on the basis of identical plasma levels is considerably less compared to somatostatin-14 (63).

Somatostatin Deficiency

In dogs the injection of an antisomatostatin serum neutralizes acutely the endogenous circulating somatostatin. The antibody did not leave the circulation suggesting that the observed effects are the result of an acute deficiency of circulating plasma somatostatin while the locally acting somatostatin in the interstitial space was unaffected. Such an acute reduction of plasma SLI levels elicits an increase of basal growth hormone and enteroglucagon levels and augments the postprandial rise of plasma gastrin, insulin, pancreatic polypeptide and enteroglucagon while there is no effect on plasma GIP, glucagon and motilin levels (64,65). In addition the postprandial rise of triglyceride levels is accelerated in this state of acute hyposomatostatinemia. These data strongly support the concept that circulating somatostatin attenuates the postprandial secretion of certain gastrointestinal hormones and retards the rate at which nutrients enter the circulation. Such an action of somatostatin as a "shock-absorber" would prevent an exaggerated and overshooting response of various secretory and/or motor functions in the gastrointestinal tract, thereby reducing perturbations of nutrient influx and facilitating the maintenance of nutrient homeostasis.

In the isolated rat stomach model the injection of antisomatostatin serum elicits an increase of basal gastrin secretion (66). This effect reflects a paracrine mode of action of somatostatin, because there is no recirculating hormone in this model. It suggests that somatostatin exerts an inhibitory tone on basal gastrin secretion via a paracrine pathway which would be in agreement with the antibody studies in the conscious dog. The injection of antisomatostatin serum into the circulation could result in an increased flux of somatostatin from the interstitial space into the circulation and even though the antiserum does not leave the vascular space, the observed changes could reflect a paracrine action of somatostatin due to the reduction of interstitially located somatostatin. If so, one might expect in dogs an effect on basal as well as on postprandial gastrin levels. This, however, has not been observed (65) and, therefore, an increased somatostatin flux from the interstitial space to the circulation in states of plasma somatostatin deficiency seems to be highly unlikely.

Somatostatin deficiency in humans can be observed in obese subjects with hyperinsulinism and normal glucose tolerance (29). Reduced basal and postprandial plasma somatostatin levels are associated with increased basal and postprandial plasma insulin and gastrin levels. The infusion of somatostatin-14 restores in part reduced circulating somatostatin in these obese subjects and decreases basal insulin and postprandial insulin and gastrin levels (29). Furthermore the attenuated postprandial response of pancreatic polypeptide levels in the obese subjects is reduced even further during low dose somatostatin infusion. These data demonstrate that deficiency of plasma somatostatin as observed in this group of obese subjects results in an increased sensitivity to infused somatostatin-14 indicating the possibility of an upregulation of somatostatin receptors as shown already in different models (51). This is supportive evidence that in humans plasma somatostatin in the peripheral circulation is of biological importance.

In conclusion, several lines of evidence support the view that somatostatin is, apart from any paracrine effect, a true endocrine substance affecting its target cells via the circulation. The ingestion of a meal elicits an increase of peripheral circulating plasma somatostatin levels which can attenuate several gastrointestinal and pancreatic exo- and endocrine functions and which retards the rate of nutrient entry.

Thus, locally released somatostatin might affect one or the other individual function in the gastrointestinal tract via a paracrine mode of action, while circulating somatostatin is an important factor of the regulation of nutrient influx and maintains, together with insulin and glucagon secretion from the islets of Langerhans, nutrient homeostasis.

REFERENCES

1. Hokfelt T, Efendic S, Hellerstrom C, Johansson O, Luft R, Arimura A. Cellular localization of somatostatin in endocrine-like cells and neurons of the rat with special references to the A-cells of the pancreatic islets and to hypothalamus. Acta Endocrinol 1975; 80 (suppl 200):5.
2. Orci L, Baetens D, Dubois MP, Rufener C. Evidence for the D-cell of the pancreas secreting somatostatin. Horm Metab Res 1975; 7:400.
3. Polak JM, Grimelius L, Pearse AGE, Bloom SR, Arimura A. Growth hormone release inhibiting hormone in gastrointestinal and pancreatic D-cells. Lancet 1975; 1:1220.
4. Luft R, Efendic S, Hokfelt T, Johansson O, Arimura A. Immunohisto-chemical evidence for the localization of somatostatin-like immunore-activity in a cell population of the pancreatic islets. Med Biol 1974; 52:428.
5. Dubois MP. Immunoreactive somatostatin is present in discrete cells of the endocrine pancreas. Proc Natl Acad Sci USA 1975; 72:1340.
6. Pelletier G, Leclerc R, Arimura A, Schally AV. Immunohistochemical localization of somatostatin in the rat pancreas. J Histochem Cytochem 1975; 23:699.
7. Alumets J, Sundler F, Hakanson R. Distribution, ontogeny and ultra-structure of somatostatin immunoreactive cells in the pancreas and gut. Cell Tissue Res 1977; 185:465.
8. Orci L, Unger RH. Hypothesis: functional subdivisions of islets of Langerhans and possible role of D-cells. Lancet 1975; II:1243-4.
9. Creutzfeldt W. Effects of gastrointestinal hormones—physiological or pharmacological? In: Case RM, Goebell H, eds. Stimulus-secretion coupling in the gastrointestinal tract. Lancaster: MTP, 1976:415-28.
10. Pearse AGE, Polak JM, Bloom SR. The newer gut hormones. Cellular sources, physiology, pathology and clinical aspects. Gastroenterol-ogy 1977; 72:746-61.
11. Bloom SR, Mortimer CH, Thorner MO, et al. Inhibition of gastrin and gastric acid secretion by growth hormone release inhibiting hormone. Lancet 1974; I:1106-9.
12. Alberti KGMM, Christensen NJ, Christensen SE, et al. Inhibition of insulin secretion by somatostatin. Lancet 1973; II:1299-301.
13. Gerich JE, Lorenzi M, Schneider V, et al. Inhibition of pancreatic glucagon response to arginine by somatostatin in normal man and in insulin-dependent diabetics. Diabetes 1974; 23:870-80.
14. Koerker DJ, Ruch W, Chidechel E, et al. Somatostatin: hypothalamic inhibitor of the endocrine pancreas. Science 1974; 184:482-3.
15. Harris V, Conlon JM, Srikant CB, et al. Measurements of somato-statin-like immunoreactivity in plasma. Clin Chim Acta 1978; 87:275-83.
16. Unger RH, Ipp E, Schusdziarra V, Orci L. Hypothesis: physiologic role of pancreatic somatostatin and the contribution of D-cell disorder to diabetes mellitus. Life Sci 1977; 20:2081.
17. Schusdziarra V, Harris V, Conlon JM, Arimura A, Unger RH. Pancreatic and gastric somatostatin release in response to intragastric and intraduodenal nutrients and HCl in the dog. J Clin Invest 1978; 62:509.
18. Schusdziarra V, Zyznar E, Rouiller D, Harris V, Unger RH. Free somatostatin in the circulation: amounts and molecular sizes of somatostatin-like immunoreactivity in portal, aortic and vena caval plasma of fasting and meal-stimulated dogs. Endocrinology 1980; 107:1572.
19. Berelowitz M, Kronheim S, Pimstone B, Shapiro B. Somatostatin-like immunoreactivity in rat blood. J Clin Invest 1978; 61:1410.
20. Vinik AJ, Shapiro B, Glaser B, Wagner L. Circulating somatostatin in

primates. In: Bloom SR, Polak JM, eds. Gut Hormones. Edinburgh: Churchill Livingstone, 1981:371.

21. Schusdziarra V, Rouiller D, Harris V, Conlon JM, Unger RH. The response of plasma somatostatin-like immunoreactivity to nutrients in normal and alloxan diabetic dogs. Endocrinology 1978; 103:2264.

22. Chayvialle JA, Myata M, Rayford PL, Thompson JC. Effects of test meal, intragastric nutrients, and intraduodenal bile on plasma intestinal peptide in dogs. Gastroenterology 1980; 79:844.

23. Wass JAH, Penman E, Dryburgh JR, et al. Circulating somatostatin after food and glucose in man. Clin Endocrinol 1980; 12:569.

24. Vinik AJ, Levitt NS, Pimstone B, Wagner L. Peripheral plasma somato-statin-like immunoreactivity response to insulin hypoglycemia and a mixed meal in healthy subjects and in non-insulin-dependent maturity-onset diabetics. J Clin Endocrinol Metab 1981; 52:330.

25. O'Shaughnessy DJ, Long RG, Adrian TE, et al. Somatostatin-14 mod-ulates postprandial glucose levels and release of gastrointestinal and pancreatic hormones. Digestion 1985; 31:234-42.

26. Zyznar E, Pietri A, Harris V, Unger RH. Evidence for the hormonal status of somatostatin in man. Diabetes 1981; 30:883.

27. Conlon JM, McCulloch AJ, Alberti KGMM. Circulating somatostatin concentrations in healthy and non-insulin-dependent (type II) diabet-ic subjects. Diabetes 1983; 32:723-9.

28. Polonsky KS, Shoelson SE, Docherty HM. Plasma somatostatin-28 increase in response to feeding in man. J Clin Invest 1983; 71:1514-8.

29. Schusdziarra V, Lawecki J, Ditschuneit HH, Lukas B, Maier V, Pfeiffer EF. Effect of low-dose somatostatin infusion on pancreatic and gastric endocrine function in lean and obese nondiabetic human subjects. Diabetes 1985; 34:595-601.

30. Schusdziarra V, Bender H, Torres A, Pfeiffer EF. Dose-dependent inhibitory and non-inhibitory action of somatostatin on insulin release in rats. Regul Pept 1982; 4:147.

31. Schusdziarra V, Dobbs RE, Harris V, Unger RH. Immunoreactive somato-statin levels in plasma of normal and alloxan diabetic dogs. FEBS Lett 1977; 81:69.

32. Schauder P, McIntosh C, Arends G, Arnold R, Frerichs H, Creutz-feldt W. Somatostatin and insulin release from isolated rat pan-creatic islets stimulated by glucose. FEBS Lett 1976; 68:25.

33. Ipp E, Dobbs RE, Arimura A, Vale W, Harris V, Unger RH. Release of immunoreactive somatostatin from the pancreas in response to glucose, amino acids, pancreozymin-cholecystokinin and tolbutamide. J Clin Invest 1977; 60:760.

34. Schusdziarra V, Schmid R. Physiological and pathophysiological aspects of somatostatin. Scand J Gastroenterol 1986 (in press).

35. Schusdziarra V, Rouiller D, Pietri A, et al. Pancreatic and gastric release of somatostatin-like immunoreactivity during the intestinal phase of meal. Am J Physiol 1979; 273:555.

36. Schusdziarra V, Rouiller D, Harris V, Unger RH. Gastric and pan-creatic release of somatostatin-like immunoreactivity during the gastric phase of a meal. Effects of truncal vagotomy and atropine in the anesthetized dog. Diabetes 1979; 28:658.

37. De Graef J, Woussen-Colle MC. Effects of sham feeding, bethanechol, and bombesin on somatostatin release in dogs. Am J Physiol 1985; 248:61-7.

38. Feldman M, Unger RH, Walsh JH. Effect of atropine on plasma gastrin and somatostatin concentrations during sham feeding in man. Regul Pept 1985; 12:345-52.

39. Schusdziarra V. Role of somatostatin in nutrient regulation. In: Patel YC, Tannenbaum GS, eds. Somatostatin. New York: Plenum Press, 1985:425-36.

40. Schusdziarra V, Holland A, Maier V, Pfeiffer EF. Effect of naloxone

on pancreatic and gastric endocrine function in response to carbohydrate and fat-rich test meals. Peptides 1984; 5:65.

41. Penman E, Wass JAH, Medbak S, Morgan L, Lewis JM, Rees GM. Response of circulating immunoreactive somatostatin to nutritional stimuli in normal subjects. Gastroenterology 1981; 81:692.

42. Schusdziarra V, Rewes B, Lenz N, Maier V, Pfeiffer EF. Evidence for a role of endogenous opiates in postprandial somatostatin release. Regul Pept 1983; 6:355.

43. Schusdziarra V, Schmid R, Eberl TH. Peptidergic stimulation of gastric somatostatin release is modulated by insulin and glucose. Acta Endocrinol 1986; 111(suppl 274):30.

44. Uvnas-Wallensten K, Efendic S, Johansson C, Sjodin L, Cranwell PD. Effect of intra-antra and intrabulbar pH on somatostatin-like immunoreactivity in peripheral venous blood of conscious dogs. The possible function of somatostatin as an inhibitory hormone of gastric acid secretion and its possible identity with bulbogastrone and antral chalone. Acta Physiol Scand 1981; 111:397.

45. Lucey MR, Fairclough PD, Wass JAH, Penman E, Besser GM, Rees LH. Is gastric acid a factor in post-prandial plasma somatostatin release in man? Gastroenterology 1983; 84:61.

46. Schusdziarra V, Bender H, Pfeiffer A, Pfeiffer EF. Modulation of acetylcholine-induced secretion of gastric bombesin-like immunoreactivity by cholinergic and histamine H_2-receptors, somatostatin and intragastric pH. Regul Pept 1984; 8:189.

47. Schusdziarra V. Somatostatin—a regulatory modulator connecting nutrient entry and metabolism. Horm Metab Res 1980; 12:563.

48. McIntosh C, Arnold R. The radioimmunoassay and physiology of somatostatin in the pancreas and gastrointestinal tract. Z Gastroenterol 1978; 16:330.

49. Patel YC, Zingg HH, Fitzpatrick D, Srikant CB. Somatostatin: some aspects of its physiology and pathophysiology. In: Bloom SR, Polak JM, eds. Gut hormones. Edinburgh: Churchill Livingstone, 1981:339.

50. Arimura A, Fishback JB. Regulation of somatostatin secretion. Neuroendocrinology 1981; 33:246.

51. Srikant CB, Patel YC. Somatostatin receptors. In: Patel YC, Tannenbaum GS, eds. Somatostatin. New York: Plenum Press, 1985: 291-304.

52. Kawai K, Ipp E, Orci L, Perrelet A, Unger RH. Circulating somatostatin acts on the islets of Langerhans by way of somatostatin-poor compartment. Science 1982; 218:477.

53. Koop H, Bothe E, Dyonisius J, Arnold R. Gastric somatostatin: paracrine or endocrine mode of action? Dig Dis Sci 1984; 29:44.

54. Schusdziarra V, Harris V, Arimura A, Unger RH. Evidence for a role of splanchnic somatostatin in the homeostasis of ingested nutrients. Endocrinology 1979; 104:1705.

55. Vaysse N, Chayvialle JA, Pradayrol L, et al. Somatostatin-28: comparison with somatostatin-14 for plasma kinetics and low-dose effects on the exocrine pancreas in dogs. Gastroenterology 1981; 81:700.

56. Aizawa I, Itoh Z, Harris V, Unger RH. Plasma somatostatin-like immunoreactivity during the interdigestive period in the dog. J Clin Invest 1981; 68:206.

57. Nakabayashi H, Sagara H, Usukara N, et al. Effect of somatostatin on flow rate and triglyceride levels of thoracic duct lymph in normal and vagotomized dogs. Diabetes 1981; 30:440.

58. Johansson C, Kollberg B, Efendic S, Uvnas-Wallensten K. Effects of graded doses of somatostatin on gallbladder emptying and pancreatic enzyme output after oral glucose in man. Digestion 1981; 22:24.

59. Johansson C, Visen O, Efendic S, Uvnas-Wallensten K. Effect of somatostatin on gastrointestinal propagation and absorption of oral

glucose in man. Digestion 1981; 22:126.

60. Feurle GE, Spoleanschi P, Stander M, Klempa I. Dose-response study of somatostatin on meal-stimulated levels of pancreatic polypeptide and insulin in the dog. Digestion 1982; 23:119.

61. Souquet JC, Rambliere R, Riou JP, et al. Hormonal and metabolic effects of near physiological increase of plasma immunoreactive somatostatin-14. J Clin Endocrinol Metab 1983; 56:1076.

62. Colturi RJ, Unger RH, Peters M, Feldman M. Physiologic role for circulating somatostatin in gastric secretion in man. Gastroenterology 1983; 84:60.

63. Seal A, Yamada T, Debas H, et al. Somatostatin-14 and -28: clearance and potency on gastric function in dogs. Am J Physiol 1982; 243:G97-102.

64. Schusdziarra V, Rouiller D, Arimura A, Unger RH. Antisomatostatin serum increase levels of hormones from the pituitary and gut but not from the pancreas. Endocrinology 1979; 103:1956.

65. Schusdziarra V, Zyznar E, Rouiller D, et al. Splanchnic somatostatin: a hormonal regulator of nutrient homeostasis. Science 1980; 207:530.

66. Saffouri B, Weir G, Bitar K, Makhlouf G. Stimulation of gastrin secretion from the perfused rat stomach by somatostatin antiserum. Life Sci 1979; 25:1749-54.

IV. SOMATOSTATIN IN GASTROINTESTINAL FUNCTION

21

GUT SOMATOSTATIN

Tadataka Yamada

Department of Internal Medicine
University of Michigan Medical School
Ann Arbor, MI

Although somatostatin was initially isolated from sheep hypothalami in 1973 (1), Fujita and Kobayashi predicted the presence of an inhibitor of gastric acid secretion in characteristic endocrine cells of the gastric mucosa on the basis of histological studies as early as 1971 (2). Subsequently, the development of antisera against somatostatin by Arimura et al. (3) permitted the demonstration of somatostatin-like immunoreactivity (SLI) in a variety of sites throughout the gastroenteropancreatic system using radioimmunoassay and immunohistochemical techniques (4-8). SLI has been demonstrated not only in endocrine-like cells in the mucosa but also in intrinsic and extrinsic neurons in the submucosal and muscle layers throughout the gut (7-15). Of particular note is the unusual morphological appearance of D-cells in the mucosa of the gastric antrum and fundus. As depicted in Figure 1, they are characterized by long cytoplasmic processes that end with button-like swellings on nearby target cells (12,13,16) suggesting some direct contact between D-cells and their targets within the gastric mucosa. Such histological observations have given rise to the concept of paracrine or local regulatory actions for somatostatin in the gut, the topic of a subsequent chapter by Makhlouf. Moreover, D-cells in the antral mucosa appear to be of the "open" type; thus, in addition to the more traditional routes of stimulation, it is possible that some D-cells are sensitive to intraluminal stimuli such as acid or nutrients through receptors on their luminal surfaces.

The special properties of SLI-containing cells and their ubiquitous presence throughout the gut provide somatostatin with the unique potential of influencing a wide variety of gastrointestinal functions. Indeed, as depicted on Table 1, somatostatin has been shown to exert many biological actions in the gut. The challenge presented to the investigator has been to characterize the mechanisms and target cells for somatostatin action, as well as to sort out the differences between physiological and pharmacological effects. These questions are addressed in a subsequent chapter by Mogard et al.

In vivo studies have been complicated by the difficulties in assaying somatostatin in plasma. Various techniques of extraction (18-25) and assay buffer manipulation (26,27) have been employed in order to minimize the effect of factors in the plasma that interfere with the radioimmunoassay. Nevertheless, substantial controversy exists as to the accuracy of SLI measurements in plasma.

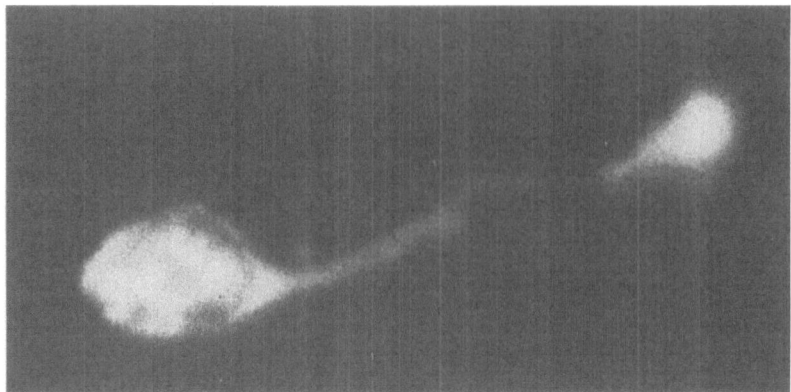

Fig. 1. Immunohistochemically stained D-cells in rat fundic mucosa. The cell is characterized by a long cytoplasmic process ending in a bulbous swelling, presumably at its junction with a target cell. (Courtesy of Dr. Wilfred Weinstein, University of California, Los Angeles.)

Many of the physiological functions of the gut such as absorption, secretion, and motility are highly integrated, thus they are difficult to study in in vitro systems. Nevertheless, recent development of techniques for isolating various targets for gut somatostatin have facilitated the investigation of the peptide's mechanism of action. Studies using systems for examining isolated organs (perfused stomachs, intestinal muscle strips, pancreatic lobules, and intestinal mucosal sheets) and their corresponding isolated cells (parietal cells, smooth muscle cells, pancreatic acinar cells, and intestinal epithelial cell lines) are described in the following chapters by Owyang and Wiley, Soll, Dharmsathaphorn, and Solomon. They shed light on the direct actions of somatostatin on its targets, by whatever means the peptide reaches its site of action, and provide useful models for elucidating the subsequent intracellular signal transduction events (Fig. 2).

Some of the same difficulties encountered in studying somatostatin action are encountered in studying SLI release because of the wide distribution and unique anatomy of somatostatin-containing cells in the gut. Since D-cells may receive stimulatory and inhibitory inputs from the gut lumen, the circulation, local neurons, and possible paracrine effectors, it has been difficult for investigators to sort out the direct versus indirect regulatory mechanisms governing SLI secretion. The wide variety of stimulants and inhibitors of gastric SLI secretion obtained from in vivo studies or isolated perfused stomach preparations are listed on Table 2 (28). Despite extensive efforts to localize the exact site of somatostatin secretion using selective venous cannulation and isolated suborgan culture techniques, the dispersion of D-cells throughout the gastric mucosa has made the confirmation of direct regulatory mechanisms virtually impossible. Recently, techniques have been developed to disperse D-cells from the canine fundus and enrich them by counterflow elutriation to a purity approaching 70% (29-33). These studies, reviewed in the following chapter by Chiba et al., have provided the first opportunity to examine D-cells directly and the results obtained form the basis for a hypothesis on the intracellular mechanisms of gastric SLI release (Fig. 3). Undoubtedly this hypothesis will be tested extensively in the future.

Table 1. Biological actions of somatostatin in the gut.

1. Inhibition of exocrine secretion
   a) Stomach
      acid
      pepsinogen
   b) Pancreas
      digestive enzymes
      bicarbonate
   c) Liver
      bile acid-independent bile flow
      ductular secretion
   d) Salivary gland
      amylase

2. Inhibition of neuroendocrine secretion
   a) Gastrointestinal tract—gastrin, CCK, secretin, VIP, GIP, motilin, gut glucagon, EGF, acetylcholine
   b) Pancreas—insulin, glucagon, pancreatic polypeptide

3. Motility
   a) Inhibition
      late phase of gastric emptying
      gastric MMCs
      gallbladder contraction
      ileal longitudinal muscle contraction
   b) Stimulation
      early phase of gastric emptying
      intestinal MMCs

4. Intestinal transport
   a) Inhibition
      secretion of fluid and bicarbonate
      absorption of calcium, glucose, glucatose, glycerol, fructose, xylose, lactose, amino acids, triglycerides

5. Miscellaneous
   a) Inhibition of splanchnic blood flow
   b) Inhibition of tissue growth and proliferation
   c) Food intake
      stimulation in fasted animals
      inhibition in fed animals

This brief introduction to the frontiers of research in gut somatostatin provides only a glimpse of the extensive work ongoing in many laboratories. The development of useful models for the study of somatostatin release and action has opened the gastrointestinal tract to research questions that were answered more easily in other organs. This is a fortuitous circumstance because the many potential effects and widespread localization of somatostatin in the gut indicate a principal role for the peptide in regulating the physiology of the gastrointestinal tract in health and disease.

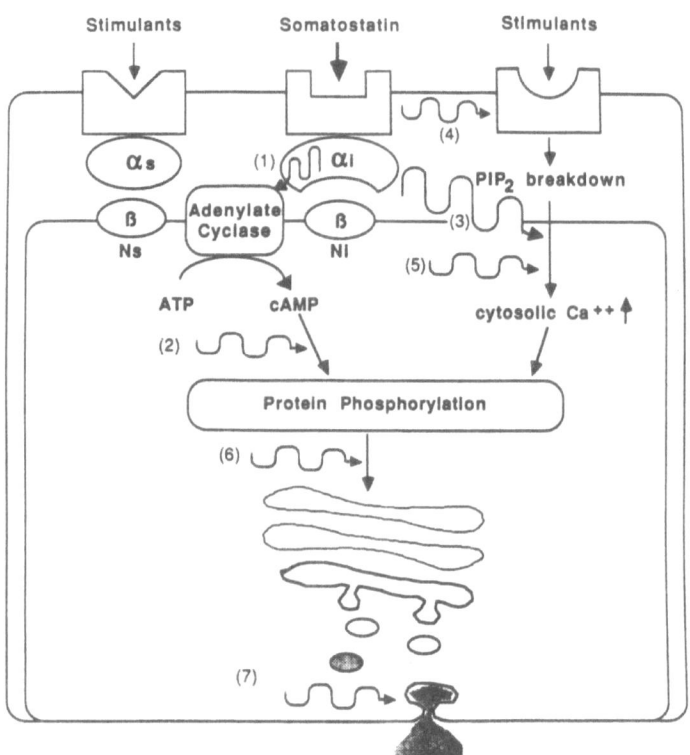

Fig. 2. Postulated sites of action of somatostatin on its target cell: (1) Ni-mediated inhibition of adenylate cyclase, (2) inhibition of cAMP action, (3) Ni-mediated inhibition of non-cAMP dependent pathways, (4) dephosphorylation of receptors, (5) inhibition of cytosolic Ca^{++} accumulation, (6) dephosphorylation of proteins via phosphoprotein phosphatases, and (7) inhibition of exocytosis.

Table 2. Agents which influence gastric somatostatin release.

	Stimulants	Inhibitors
A.	Luminal factors	
	HCl	NaHCO$_3$
	Mechanical	Peptone
	Casein	
	Fat	
	Glucose	
B.	Circulating nutrients	
	Free fatty acid	
C.	Peptides	
	Glucagon	Substance P
	Secretin	Met-enkephalin
	VIP	Dermorphin
	GIP	Insulin
	Calcitonin	PP
	CGRP	GRP
	Gastrin	
	CCK	
	Bombesin	
D.	Neurotransmitters and amines	
	Epinephrine	Acetylcholine
	Norepinephrine	GABA
	Dopamine	Serotonin
E.	Nucleotides and prostaglandins	
	Cyclic AMP	
	Prostaglandin E$_2$	
F.	Drugs	
	Theophylline	
	Tolbutamine	
	TPA	
	Diacylglyceride	
	Dimethylphenyliperazinium	

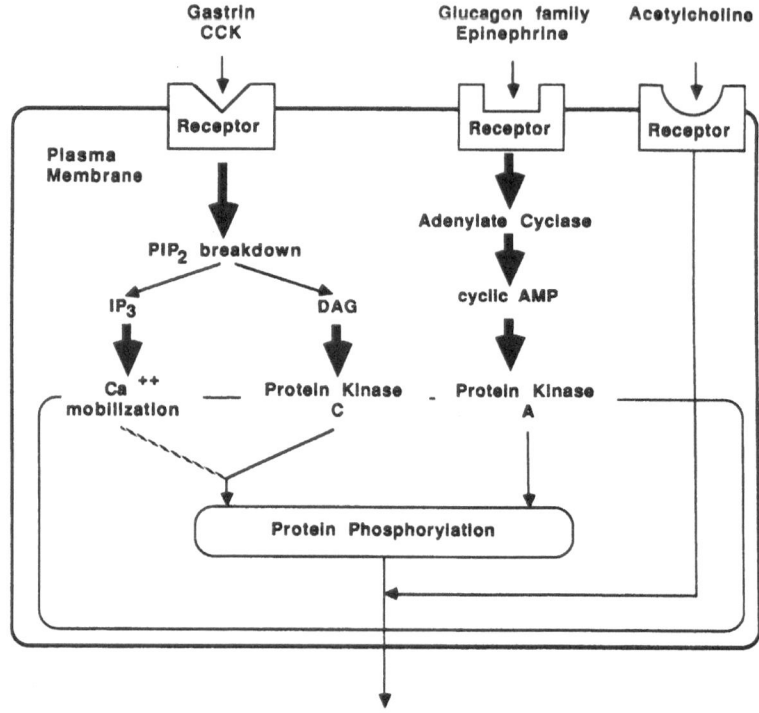

Fig. 3. Intracellular mechanisms governing somatostatin release.

REFERENCES

1. Brazeau P, Vale W, Burgus R, et al. Hypothalamic polypeptide that
   inhibits the secretion of immunoreactive pituitary growth hormone.
   Science 1973; 179:77-9.
2. Fujita T, Kobayashi S. Experimentally induced granule release in the
   endocrine cells of dog pyloric antrum. Z Zellforsch 1971; 116:52-60.
3. Arimura A, Sato H, Dupont A, Nishi N, Schally A. Somatostatin:
   abundance of immunoreactive hormone in rat stomach and pancreas.
   Science 1975; 189:1007-9.
4. Hokfelt T, Efendic S, Hellerstrom C, Johansson O, Luft R, Arimura A.
   Cellular localization of somatostatin in endocrine-like cells and
   neurons of the rat with special references to the A1 cells of the
   pancreatic islets and to the hypothalamus. Acta Endocrinol (Copenh)
   1975; 80(suppl 200):5-41.
5. Kronheim S, Berelowitz M, Pimstone BL. A radioimmunoassay for growth
   hormone release-inhibiting hormone: method and quantitative tissue
   distribution. Clin Endocrinol (Oxf) 1976; 5:619-30.
6. Vale W, Ling N, Rivier J, et al. Somatostatin: anatomic and phylogenetic distribution of somatostatin. Metabolism 1976; 25(suppl 1):
   1491-4.
7. Rufener C, Dubois MP, Malaisse-Lagae F, Orci L. Immunofluorescent
   reactivity to anti-somatostatin in the gastrointestinal mucosa of the
   dog. Diabetologia 1975; 11:321-4.

8. Polak J, Pearse AGE, Grimelius L, Bloom S, Arimura A. Growth hormone release-inhibiting hormone in gastrointestinal and pancreatic D cells. Lancet 1975; 1:1220-2.

9. Baskin DG, Ensinck JW. Somatostatin in epithelial cells of intestinal mucosa is present primarily as somatostatin-28. Peptides 1984; 5:615-21.

10. Costa M, Furness JB. Somatostatin is present in a subpopulation of noradrenergic nerve fibers supplying the intestine. Neuroscience 1984; 13:911-9.

11. Jakobs KH, Aktories K, Schultz G. A nucleotide regulatory site for somatostatin inhibition of adenylate cyclase in S49 lymphoma cells. Nature 1983; 303:177-8.

12. Kusumoto Y, Iwanaga T, Ito S, Fujita T. Juxtaposition of somatostatin cell and parietal cell in the dog stomach. Arch Histol Jpn 1979; 42:459-65.

13. Larsson LI, Goltermann N, Demagistris L, Rehfeld JF, Schwartz TW. Somatostatin cell processes as pathways for paracrine secretion. Science 1979; 205:1393-5.

14. Lehy T, Peranzi G, Cristina ML. Correlative immunocytochemical and electron microscopic studies: identification of (entero)glucagon-somatostatin- and pancreatic polypeptide-like-containing cells in the human colon. Histochemistry 1981; 71:67-80.

15. Schultzberg M, Dreyfus CF, Gershon MD, et al. VIP-, enkephalin-, substance P-and somatostatin-like immunoreactivity in neurons intrinsic to the intestine: immunohistochemical evidence from organotypic tissue cultures. Brain Res 1978; 155:239-48.

16. Larsson LI. Distribution and morphology of somatostatin cells. In: Patel YC, Tannenbaum GS, eds. Somatostatin. New York: Plenum Press, 1985:383-402.

17. Fujita T, Kobayashi S. The cells and hormones of the GEP endocrine system—the current of studies. In: Fujita T, ed. Gastro-entero-pancreatic endocrine system. A cell-biological approach. Tokyo: Igaku Shoin, 1973:1-16.

18. Arimura A, Lundqvist G, Rothman J, et al. Radioimmunoassay of somatostatin. Metabolism 1978; 27:1139-44.

19. Etzrodt H, Rosenthal HJ, Schroder KE, Pfeiffer EF. Radioimmunoassay of somatostatin in human plasma. Clin Chim Acta 1983; 1343:241-51.

20. Hilsted L, Holst JJ. On the accuracy of radioimmunological determination of somatostatin in plasma. Regul Pept 1982; 4:13-31.

21. Uvnas-Moberg K, Andersson B, Posloncec B. Plasma levels of somatostatin following a test meal in dogs. Acta Physiol Scand 1982; 114:253-9.

22. Patel Y, Wheatley T, Fitz-Patrick D, Brock G. A sensitive radioimmunoassay for immunoreactive somatostatin in extracted plasma: measurement and characterization of portal and peripheral plasma in the rat. Endocrinology 1980; 107:306-13.

23. Penman E, Wass JAH, Medbak S, et al. Response of circulating immunoreactive somatostatin to nutritional stimuli in normal subjects. Gastroenterology 1981; 81:692-9.

24. Tsuda K, Sakurai H, Seino Y, et al. Somatostatin-like immunoreactivity in human peripheral plasma measured by radioimmunoassay following affinity chromatography. Diabetes 1981; 30:471-4.

25. Vasquez B, Harris V, Unger R. Extraction of somatostatin from human plasma on octadecylsilyl silica. J Clin Endocrinol Metab 1982; 55:807-9.

26. Vinik AI, Levitt NS, Pimstone BL, Wagner L. Peripheral plasma somatostatin-like immunoreactive responses to insulin hypoglycemia with a mixed meal in healthy subjects and in noninsulin-dependent maturity-onset diabetes. J Clin Endocrinol Metab 1981; 52:330-7.

27. Seal A, Yamada T, Debas H, et al. Somatostatin-14 and -28: clearance and potency on gastric function in dogs. Am J Physiol 1982;

243:G97–102.

28. Yamada T, Chiba T. Somatostatin. In: Makhlouf GM, ed. Handbook of physiology: neuroendocrinology of the gut. Washington, DC: American Physiological Society, 1986 (in press).

29. Soll AH, Yamada T, Park J, Thomas LP. Release of somatostatin-like immunoreactivity by canine fundic mucosal cells in primary culture. Am J Physiol 1984; 247:G558–66.

30. Yamada T, Soll AH, Park J, Elashoff J. Autonomic regulation of somatostatin release: studies with primary cultures of canine fundic mucosal cells. Am J Physiol 1984; 247:G567–73.

31. Soll AH, Amirian DA, Thomas LP, Park J, Beaven MA, Yamada T. Gastrin receptors on nonparietal cells isolated from canine fundic mucosa. Am J Physiol 1984; 247:G715–23.

32. Soll AH, Amirian D, Park J, Elashoff J, Yamada T. Cholecystokinin potently releases somatostatin from canine fundic mucosal cells in short term culture. Am J Physiol 1985; 248:G569–73.

33. Sugano K, Park J, Soll A, Yamada T. Phorbol esters stimulate somatostatin release from cultured cells. Am J Physiol 1986 (in press).

22

REGULATION OF SOMATOSTATIN RELEASE FROM
DISPERSED CANINE FUNDIC D-CELLS

Tsutomu Chiba, Jung Park, and Tadataka Yamada

Department of Internal Medicine
University of Michigan Medical School, Ann Arbor, MI

Somatostatin, initially isolated from the ovine hypothalamus (1), has potent inhibitory actions on gastric acid secretion (2,3) and gastrin release (4,5). In the stomach, somatostatin producing D-cells are found in both fundic and antral mucosa, where they have been described as possessing long cytoplasmic processes terminating on parietal cells and gastrin-producing G cells (6,7). The regulation of gastric somatostatin secretion has been studied extensively in vivo and in vitro organ perfusion experiments; however, such studies are complicated by a number of factors. Somatostatin is capable of functioning in many different roles: as a hormone, a paracrine transmitter, or a neurotransmitter. Moreover, the ubiquitous distribution of somatostatin in the body has made it difficult to identify the sources of released somatostatin without cannulating selected veins draining specific organs. Even within the stomach, there may be several distinct types of cells containing somatostatin-like immunoreactivity (SLI). Furthermore, the presence within or delivery to the stomach of endogenous mediators that influence somatostatin release may make the interpretation of results obtained with exogenously administered agents difficult. Studies using whole animals or intact organ and tissue preparations do not permit discrimination between direct and indirect effects of agents acting on gastric somatostatin cells. In order to examine the regulation of gastric SLI secretion more directly, we undertook studies using fundic somatostatin cells isolated by a technique developed by Soll and Yamada (8,9).

DISPERSION AND SEPARATION OF SOMATOSTATIN CELLS FROM CANINE FUNDIC MUCOSA AND CELL CULTURE (Table 1)

Stomachs were obtained from anesthetized dogs and divided into fundic and antral segments. The fundic mucosa was bluntly separated from the submucosa, and the mucosal fragments were incubated sequentially in crude collagenase (0.35 mg/ml) and EDTA (1 mM). The dispersed cells were further separated by counterflow elutriation in a Beckman elutriator rotor. This technique permits us to separate cells on the basis of sedimentation velocity, which is proportional to the square of the cell radius. The rotor was sterilized by flowing 70% ethanol through the chamber and tubing for 15 minutes. Fractions were collected according to the protocol described by Ayalon et al. (10). The elutriator fractions enriched in SLI-containing cells (8,9) were layered at a density of

Table 1. Method for isolation and enrichment
of canine fundic somatostatin cells.

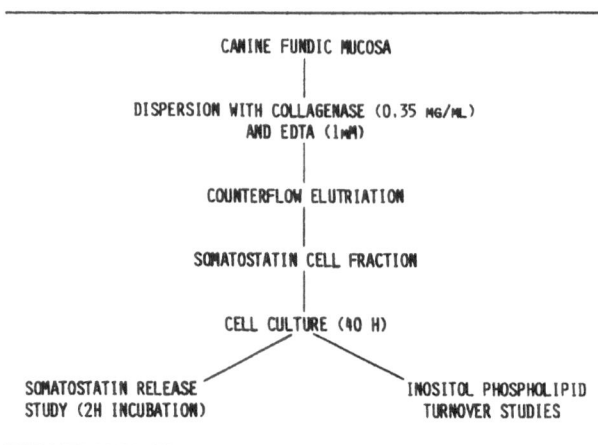

CANINE FUNDIC MUCOSA

DISPERSION WITH COLLAGENASE (0.35 MG/ML)
AND EDTA (1mM)

COUNTERFLOW ELUTRIATION

SOMATOSTATIN CELL FRACTION

CELL CULTURE (40 H)

SOMATOSTATIN RELEASE   INOSITOL PHOSPHOLIPID
STUDY (2H INCUBATION)   TURNOVER STUDIES

2.5–3.5 x 10^6 cells/ml on polymerized type I collagen in 1 ml medium
consisting of a mixture of Dulbecco's modified Eagle's and Ham's F-12
media (50:50) with 10% heat-inactivated dog serum added. Cultures were
maintained in a humidified environment of 95% air/5% CO_2. By using these
techniques SLI-containing cells selectively adhered to the collagen bed,
ultimately comprising 70% of the total cell population. After 40 hours of
incubation, the cultures were rinsed twice and covered with 1 ml of
Earle's balanced salt solution containing 0.1% gelatin and 15 mM HEPES
buffer. Agents to be tested were added and the cells were incubated at
37° for 2 hours. Aliquots (0.8 ml) of the medium were then removed and
centrifuged for 1 minute in a microfuge at 8,700 g to precipitate cells,
and the supernatant was frozen for subsequent SLI assay.

SOMATOSTATIN RELEASE VIA ADENYLATE CYCLASE–CYCLIC AMP–DEPENDENT MECHANISMS

Previous in vivo studies and in vitro perfusion experiments have
shown that in addition to the cyclic AMP analog dibutyryl cyclic AMP
(dbcAMP) by itself (11), agents which are known to increase intracellular
cyclic AMP production, such as epinephrine, peptides of the secretin
family, calcitonin and theophylline increase gastric somatostatin release.
These data clearly indicate the involvement of adenylate cyclase–cyclic
AMP-dependent mechanisms in mediating release of gastric somatostatin
(11–15). To explore the possibility that these effects result from direct
action on D-cells, we undertook studies with our isolated cell preparation.

As shown in Figure 1, epinephrine dose-dependently stimulated fundic
SLI release, and this increase was attenuated by propranolol. In contrast, phentolamine, an alpha-adrenergic antagonist, enhanced SLI secretion in response to epinephrine, which was reversed by the alpha-1 agonist
methoxamine but not by the alpha-2 agonist clonidine. Thus, it appears
that fundic D-cells possess stimulatory beta-adrenergic receptors, con-
firming data obtained from studies in perfused stomachs (12,13) although
the existence of an alpha adrenergic inhibitory receptor remains uncertain
(9). Of particular note was that SLI release induced by epinephrine was

potentiated by concomitant administration of gastrin. In contrast, dbcAMP enhanced epinephrine-induced SLI release only in an additive fashion (Fig. 2). These data indicate that gastrin and epinephrine may release SLI from D-cells via separate pathways.

The secretin-family peptides are inhibitors of acid secretion and some of its members have been proposed as candidate enterogastrones. Release of gastric somatostatin by these peptides has been demonstrated in previous studies and, indeed, the involvement of gastric somatostatin in mediating the inhibitory action of these peptides on gastrin release (15-16) as well as on gastric acid secretion (17,18) has been suggested. In dispersed fundic D-cells glucagon, secretin, VIP and GIP all stimulated SLI secretion (17). Moreover, the release of SLI induced by these peptides was potentiated by pentagastrin, but not by dbcAMP or isobutylmethylxanthine (IMX), a phosphodiesterase inhibitor, indicating the potential importance of adenylate cyclase-cyclic AMP mechanisms in mediating the action of SLI secretin family peptides.

SOMATOSTATIN RELEASE VIA PROTEIN KINASE C-DEPENDENT MECHANISMS

Recent studies in various tissues suggest the importance of a non-cAMP-dependent signal transduction mechanism for hormone release which appears to be initiated by breakdown of membrane inositol phospholipids (19,20). In the pancreas, for example, physiological secretagogues for

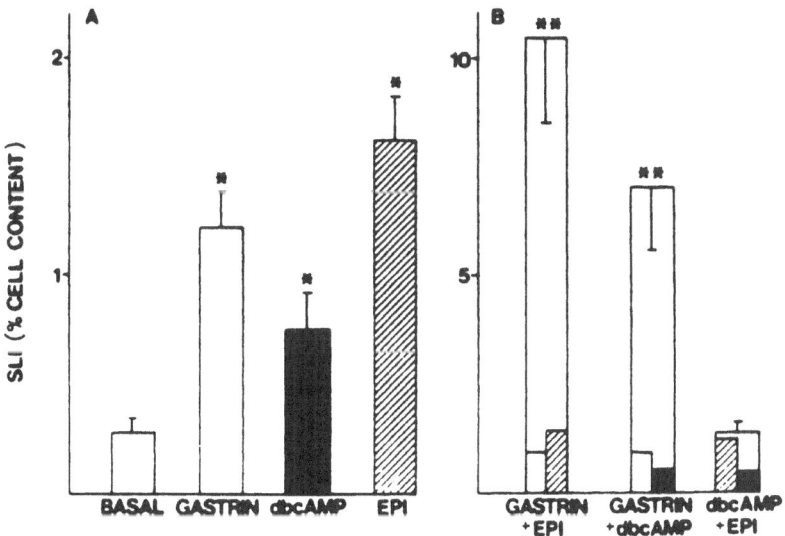

Fig. 1. Effects of alpha and beta-adrenergic blockade on epinephrine-stimulated release of somatostatin-like immunoreactivity (SLI). SLI response to epinephrine (E) was studied with (open circles) and without (closed circles) a background of 10 nM gastrin (G). Propranolol (0.1 and 1 μM) progressively shifted the dose response to epinephrine plus gastrin to right (open squares, triangles), whereas phentolamine (10 μM) increased the response (closed triangles). (Yamada et al., 9.)

amylase secretion such as acetylcholine and cholecystokinin appear to exert their effects by inducing the breakdown of phosphatidylinositol bisphosphate (PIP_2) through action of membrane phospholipase C (21-23). The resultant production of inositol trisphosphate (IP_3) and diacylglycerol induces an increase in cytosolic free calcium and activation of protein kinase C.

In order to elucidate whether such a mechanism is also involved in fundic somatostatin release, we first examine the effect of 12-0-tetradecanoyl phorbol-13-acetate (TPA), a direct activator of protein kinase C, on dispersed fundic D-cells. As depicted in Figure 3, TPA markedly stimulated SLI secretion from D-cells, and this effect was the most potent among all the agents thus far examined in our system (24). Another phorbol ester, phorbol-12, 13-dibutyrate (PDBu), which has only 50% of the tumor promoting activity of TPA, had a lesser effect on SLI secretion, and phorbol compounds with no tumor promoting activity did not affect fundic SLI release. The effects of the endogenous intracellular activators of protein kinase C, diacylglycerols, on D-cells, were also examined. We observed that 1-oleoyl-2-acetyl-sn-glycerol (OAG) had a significant stimulatory effect on SLI release when it was sonicated, but when it was not sonicated, it had a weaker action. On the other hand, diolein, a

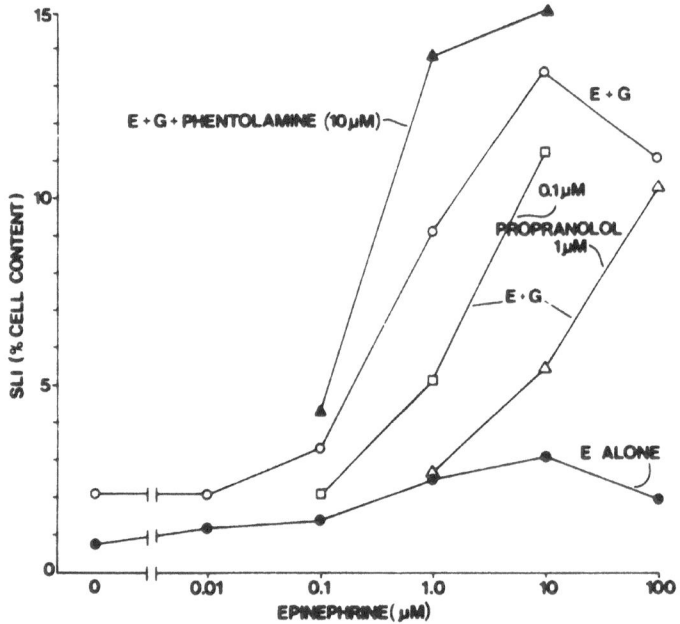

Fig. 2. Interactions of stimulants on somatostatin-like immunoreactivity (SLI) release. A. Cells were treated with 10 nM gastrin, 1 mM dibutyryl cAMP, and 1 μM epinephrine. Asterisks indicate significant increases over basal release (*P < 0.005). B. Total height of bars reflects mean of responses to combination of agents. Responses to individual agents are denoted by inset bars coded as in A. Double asterisk denotes that response to combination of agents is significantly greater than sum of individual responses (**P < 0.001). (Soll et al., 8.)

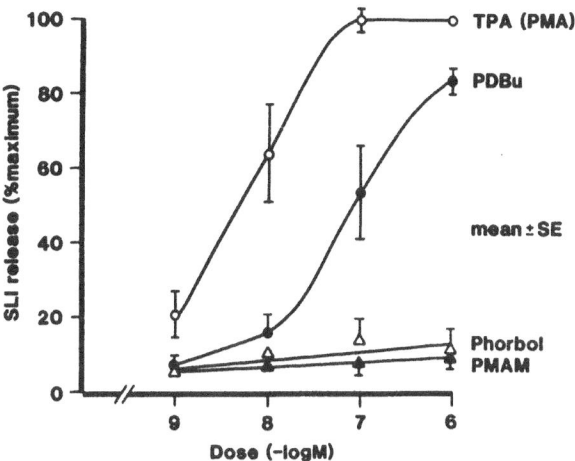

Fig. 3. Effects of phorbol esters on SLI release
from isolated fundic D-cells (Sugano et al., 24).

diacylglycerol with long chain fatty acids, had no effect on SLI secretion
even when sonicated. Thus, it is evident that diacylglycerol, once
setting into cells, stimulates SLI secretion. To determine the effect of
endogenously released diacylglycerols, we examined the effect of phospholipase C, the enzyme responsible for their generation from membrane
phospholipids and observed an increase in SLI release. SLI release
induced by TPA, OAG and phospholipase C was markedly potentiated by
dbcAMP, while only additive effects were observed with pentagastrin.
These data provide evidence for the involvement of protein kinase C-
dependent mechanisms in mediating the release of fundic SLI. The importance of intracellular free calcium ion in fundic SLI release remains
somewhat unclear. Although the calcium ionophore A23187 by itself did not
produce a significant stimulation of fundic SLI secretion, it potentiated
the effect of OAG. These results suggest a possible synergism between
intracellular Ca^{++} and protein kinase C.

INHIBITION OF SOMATOSTATIN RELEASE

Muscarinic cholinergic agents consistently inhibit SLI secretion in
vitro (25-27). This effect of cholinergic agonists was also demonstrated
in isolated fundic D-cells (Fig. 4). Of particular note was the observation that the cholinergic agonists appear to affect stimulatory mechanisms
that activate both adenylate cyclase-cyclic AMP and protein kinase C-
dependent pathways (Fig. 5) (9,17). Thus the site of muscarinic cholinergic action appears to be at a distal point in the intracellular signal
transduction cascade where stimulatory signals converge to cause SLI
release.

In addition to muscarinic agents, previous studies have suggested a
potential inhibitory role for somatostatin on its own secretion. To
determine whether this autoregulation is the result of a direct action of
somatostatin on D-cells, we examined the effect of a non-immunoreactive
but biologically active analogue of somatostatin, Leu[8]-D-Trp[22]-Tyr[25]-
somatostatin 28 on the release of SLI from our fundic cell cultures. The

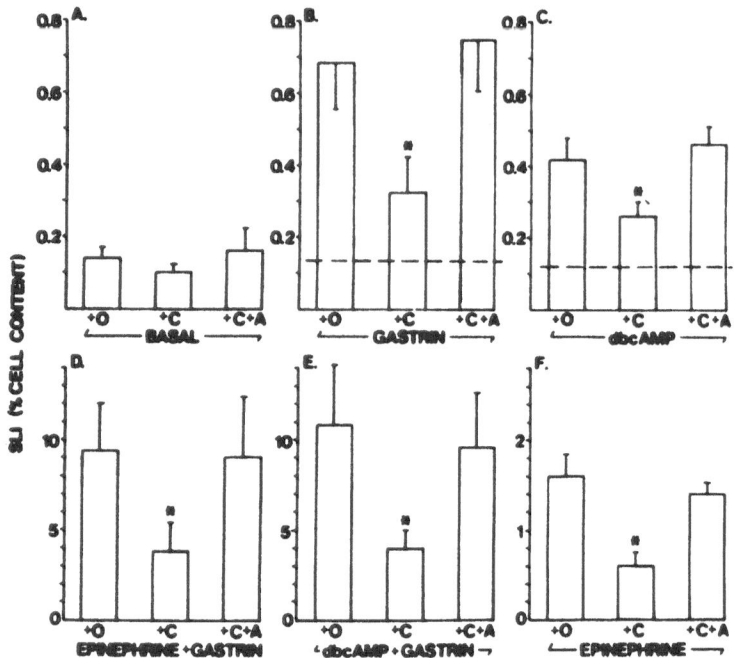

Fig. 4. Cholinergic inhibition of SLI release. SLI release was studied in untreated cells (A) and in cells treated with 10 nM gastrin (B), 1 mM dbcAMP (C), 1 μM epinephrine (D), 1 mM dbcAMP plus 10 nm gastrin (E), and 1 μM epinephrine plus 10 nM gastrin (F). Effects on these responses of 100 μM carbachol (+C) and of 100 μM carbachol plus 10 μM atropine (+C +A) are noted. *Significantly different (P < 0.05) from SLI responses to stimulants alone. (Yamada et al., 9.)

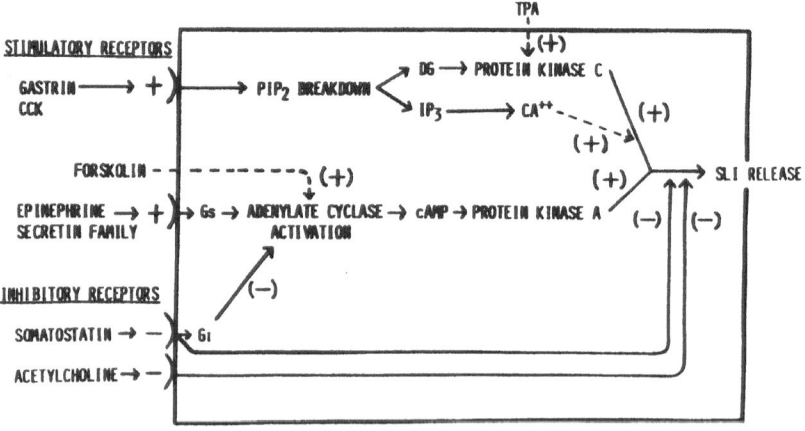

Fig. 5. Postulated intracellular mechanisms governing fundic somatostatin release.

234

somatostatin analogue inhibited SLI secretion in a dose-dependent manner and, like muscarinic agonists, the inhibitory effect was universal, again suggesting a distal site of action. Those agents which inhibited or stimulated SLI release from isolated fundic D-cells are summarized in Table 2.

CONCLUSION

Our experiments using isolated canine fundic D-cells, indicate that both adenylate cyclase-cyclic AMP- and protein kinase C-dependent mechanisms are involved in the release of gastric SLI. Moreover, D-cells appear to be under autoregulatory control by their secretory product, somatostatin. Both somatostatin and muscarinic agonists appear to inhibit somatostatin secretion at least in part at sites distal to the activation of intracellular signal transduction mechanisms.

Table 2. Agents which influence SLI release from isolated canine fundic D-cells.

STIMULATION
ADENYLATE CYCLASE-CYCLIC AMP DEPENDENT PATHWAY
SECRETIN
VIP
GLUCAGON
GIP
EPINEPHRINE
FORSKOLIN
IMX
DIBUTYRYL CYCLIC AMP
PHOSPHOLIPID-PROTEIN KINASE-C DEPENDENT PATHWAY
GASTRIN
CCK
TPA
1-OLEOYL-2-ACETYL-GLYCEROL (OAG)
PHOSPHOLIPASE C
INHIBITION
SOMATOSTATIN 28 (LEU^8-D-TRP^{22}-TYR^{25})
MUSCARINIC AGONISTS
NO EFFECT
HISTAMINE
BOMBESIN

REFERENCES

1. Brazeau P, Vale W, Burgus R, et al. Hypothalamic polypeptide that inhibits the secretion of immunoreactive pituitary growth hormone. Science 1973; 179:77.
2. Seal A, Yamada T, Debas H, et al. Somatostatin-14 and -28: clearance and potency on gastric function in dogs. Am J Physiol 1982; 243:G97.
3. Gomez-Pan A, Albinus M, Reed JD, et al. Direct inhibition of gastric acid and pepsin secretion by growth hormone release-inhibiting hormone in cats. Lancet 1975; 1:880.
4. Barros D'Sa AAJ, Bloom SR, Baron JH. Inhibition by somatostatin (growth hormone release inhibiting hormone, GH-RIH) of gastric acid and pepsin and G-cell release of gastrin. Gut 1978; 19:315.
5. Konturek SJ, Tasler J, Cieszkowski M, Coy DH, Schally V. Effect of growth hormone release inhibiting hormone on gastric secretion, mucosal blood flow and serum gastrin. Gastroenterology 1976; 70:737.
6. Kusumoto Y, Iwanaga T, Ito S, Fujita T. Juxtaposition of somatostatin cell and parietal cell in the dog stomach. Arch Histol Jpn 1979; 42:459.
7. Larsson LI, Goltermann N, Demagistris L, Rehfeld JF, Schwartz TW. Somatostatin cell processes as pathways for paracrine secretion. Science 1979; 205:1393.
8. Soll AH, Yamada T, Park J, Thomas LP. Release of somatostatin-like immunoreactivity from canine fundic mucosal cells in primary culture. Am J Physiol 1984; 247:G558.
9. Yamada T, Soll AH, Park J, Elashoff J. Autonomic regulation of somatostatin release: studies with primary cultures of canine fundic mucosal cells. Am J Physiol 1984; 247:G567.
10. Ayalon A, Sanders MJ, Thomas LP, Amirian DA, Soll AH. Electrical effects of histamine on monolayers formed in culture from enriched canine gastric chief cells. Proc Natl Acad Sci USA 1982; 79:7009.
11. Chiba T, Seino Y, Goto Y, et al. Somatostatin release from isolated perfused rat stomach. Biochem Biophys Res Commun 1978; 82:731.
12. Goto Y, Berelowitz M, Frohman L. Effect of catecholamines on somatostatin secretion by isolated perfused rat stomach. Am J Physiol 1981; 240:E274.
13. Koop H, Behrens I, Bothe E, et al. Adrenergic control of rat gastric somatostatin and gastrin release. Scand J Gastroenterol 1983; 18:65.
14. Chiba T, Taminato T, Kadowaki S, et al. Effects of (Asu 1, 7)-eel calcitonin on gastric somatostatin and gastrin release. Gut 1980; 21:94.
15. Chiba T, Taminato T, Kadowaki S, et al. Effects of glucagon, secretin, and vasoactive intestinal polypeptide on gastric somatostatin and gastrin release from isolated perfused rat stomach. Gastroenterology 1980; 79:67.
16. Wolfe MM, Reel GM, McGuigan JE. Inhibition of gastrin release by secretin is mediated by somatostatin in cultured rat antral mucosa. J Clin Invest 1983; 72:1586.
17. Chiba T, Park J, Yamada T. Glucagon and vasoactive intestinal polypeptide stimulate somatostatin secretion from isolated canine fundic mucosal cell cultures. Gastroenterology 1984; 88:1348.
18. Short GM, Doyle JW, Wolfe MM. Effect of antibodies to somatostatin on acid secretion and gastrin release by the isolated perfused rat stomach. Gastroenteroloy 1985; 88:984.
19. Nishizuka Y. Turnover of inositol phospholipids and signal transduction. Science 1984; 225:1365.
20. Berridge MJ, Irvine RF. Inositol trisphosphate, a novel second messenger in cellular signal transduction. Nature 1984; 312:315.
21. Farese RV, Larson RE, Sabir MA. Ca^{2+}-dependent and Ca^{2+}-independent effects of pancreatic secretagogues on phosphatidylinositol metab-

olism. Biochim Biophys Acta 1982; 710:391.

22. Orchard JL, Davis JS, Larson RE, Farese RV. Effects of carbachol and pancreozymin (cholecystokinin-octapeptide) on polyphosphoinositide metabolism in the rat pancreas in vitro. Biochem J 1984; 217:281.

23. Streb H, Heslop JP, Irvine RF, Schulz I, Berridge MJ. Relationship between secretagogue-induced Ca^{2+} release and inositol polyphosphate production in permeabilized pancreatic acinar cells. J Biol Chem 1984; 260:7309.

24. Sugano H, Park J, Soll AH, Yamada T. Phorbol esters stimulate somatostatin release from cultured cells. Am J Physiol (in press).

25. Martindale R, Kauffman GL, Levin S, Walsh JH, Yamada T. Differential regulation of gastrin and somatostatin secretion from isolated perfused rat stomachs. Gastroenterology 1982; 83:240.

26. Saffouri B, Weir GC, Bitar KN, Makhlouf GM. Gastrin and somatostatin secretion by perfused rat stomach: functional linkage of antral peptides. Am J Physiol 1980; 238:G495.

27. Chiba T, Kadowaki S, Taminato T, et al. Effects of acetylcholine and vagal stimulation on somatostatin and gastrin release from isolated perfused rat stomach. Regul Pept 1983; 52(suppl 2).

27. Chiba T, Kadowaki S, Taminato T, et al. Effects of acetylcholine and vagal stimulation on somatostatin and gastrin release from isolated perfused rat stomach. Regul Pept 1983; 52(suppl 2).

23

ANTRAL SOMATOSTATIN: A PARACRINE REGULATOR OF GASTRIN SECRETION

G. M. Makhlouf

Department of Medicine, Medical College of Virginia
Virginia Commonwealth University
Richmond, Virginia

PARACRINE ROLE OF ANTRAL SOMATOSTATIN

The first firm evidence for a paracrine role of somatostatin was obtained by Saffouri et al. (1) who showed that addition of somatostatin antiserum to the perfusate in the isolated vascularly perfused rat stomach produced a prompt, reversible increase in gastrin secretion (Fig. 1). The increase, two- to threefold above basal levels, was about 50% of the maximal gastrin response obtained with other stimulatory agents. This augmentatory effect of somatostatin antiserum has now been reproduced by other investigators using the vascularly perfused stomach preparation or segments of antral tissue (2,3). The finding implies that basal secretion of somatostatin exerts a continuous restraint on basal secretion of gastrin. The discovery of functional coupling between somatostatin and gastrin secretion coincided with the discovery of a close structural coupling between these two cell types, which in human and rat antral mucosa takes the form of cytoplasmic processes extending from somatostatin cells to gastrin cells (4).

Next, evidence was obtained that cholinergic stimulation of gastrin secretion was mediated in part by inhibition of basal somatostatin secretion (5). Muscarinic agonists increased gastrin and decreased somatostatin secretion in a dose-dependent manner (Fig. 2); however, the stoichiometry of increase in gastrin and decrease in somatostatin was such that virtual elimination of basal somatostatin secretion could account only for about 50% of the maximal gastrin response, consistent with the results obtained from the use of somatostatin antiserum. Inhibition of somatostatin secretion by muscarinic agonists has been repeatedly confirmed in a variety of in vitro preparations from different species (3,5-9). The residual response to maximal stimulation with muscarinic agonists represents either a direct effect of these agonists on the gastrin cell or an indirect effect via release of a neural stimulant of gastrin secretion.

BOMBESIN (GRP): A NEURAL STIMULANT OF GASTRIN WITHIN THE STOMACH

The most likely candidate for noncholinergic stimulant of gastrin secretion is bombesin (also known as gastrin releasing peptide or GRP because of its ability to stimulate gastrin secretion) which is found in intramural neurons that innervate fundic and antral mucosa (10). Bombesin

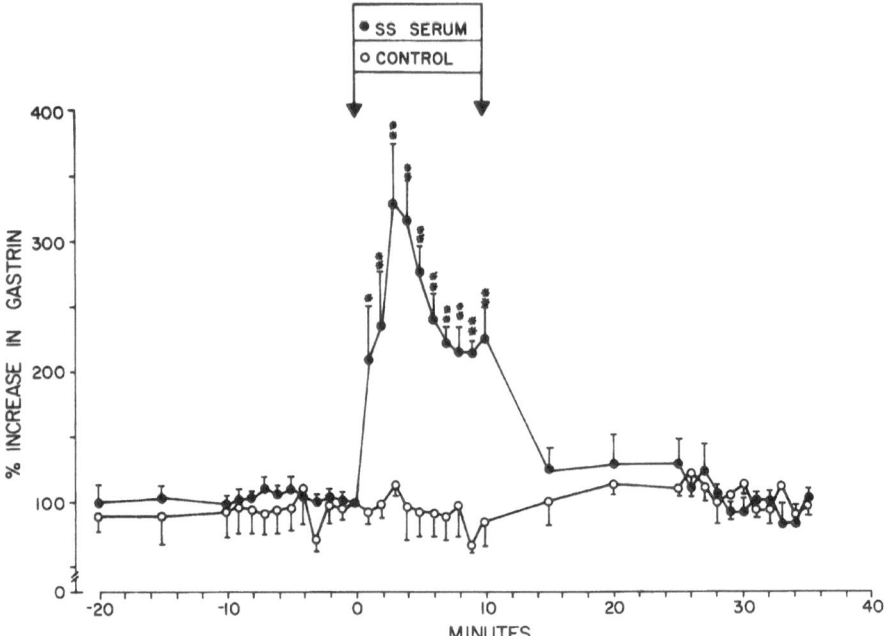

Fig. 1. Effect on gastrin secretion of addition of somatostatin
antiserum to vascular perfusate in isolated vascularly perfused
rat stomach. Final antiserum dilutions of 1:1 (Fig. 1) and 1:9
caused increments of 238% and 188%, respectively. From 1.

is the prototype of stimulants that cause stimulation of both gastrin and
somatostatin (11). Others include the ganglionic nicotinic agonist,
dimethyl phenylpiperazinium (DMPP) (12) and the beta-adrenergic agonist,
isoproterenol (6,13). These agents cause substantial, and in the case of
isoproterenol, predominant (up to 8-fold) increase in somatostatin secretion but only a moderate (2-fold) increase in gastrin secretion. Neutralization of ambient somatostatin, i.e., basal as well as incremental
somatostatin secretion, with somatostatin antiserum augments significantly
the gastrin response (11) (Fig. 3). In instances where this has been
examined, the gastrin response attains maximal levels. These results are
summarized in Table 1 and they clearly illustrate the fact that inhibition
of somatostatin determines the magnitude of gastrin secretion.

FUNCTIONAL LINKAGE BETWEEN GASTRIN AND SOMATOSTATIN SECRETION

The notion of functional linkage applies specifically to the influence of somatostatin on gastrin secretion. There is no evidence for
the converse, that is, for an effect of secreted gastrin on somatostatin
secretion. Although gastrin receptors are present on somatostatin cells
and gastrin itself added to cultures of somatostatin cells (14,15) or to
the vascular perfusate in the isolated stomach (2,5) causes an increase in
somatostatin secretion, there is no evidence that secreted gastrin has an
effect on somatostatin secretion. Addition of proglumide, a gastrin/CCK
receptor antagonist, to the vascular perfusate has no effect on the
magnitude of somatostatin secretion (M. L. Schubert and G. M. Makhlouf,
unpublished studies).

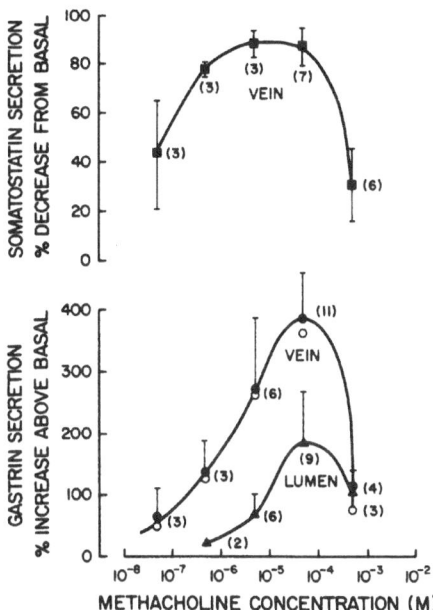

Fig. 2. Dose-response curves for the effect of methacholine on gastrin and somatostatin secretion. Secretion of peptides was predominantly (about 80%) into the vascular perfusate. Somatostatin secretion decreases invariably in response to muscarinic agonists. From 5.

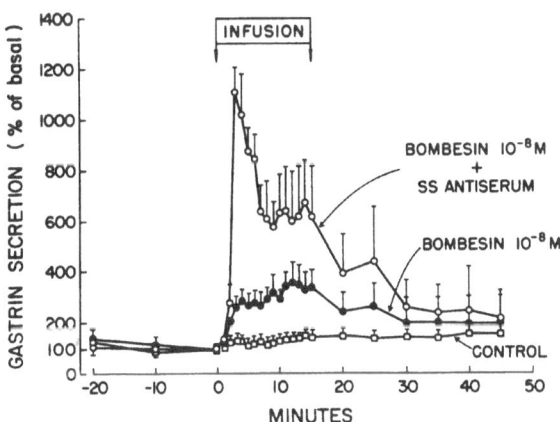

Fig. 3. Effect of somatostatin antiserum (final dilution 1:100) on gastrin response to bombesin in the isolated vascularly perfused rat stomach. From 11.

Table 1.

STIMULANT	SS RESPONSE	GASTRIN RESPONSE
METHACHOLINE ELECTRICAL STIMULUS	↓	⬆
ISOPROTERENOL BOMBESIN	↑	↑
ISOPROTERENOL + SS ANTISERUM BOMBESIN + SS ANTISERUM	⬇	⬆

Gastrin and somatostatin (SS) responses to various modes of stimulation in the isolated vascularly perfused rat stomach. Stimuli (e.g., methacholine and transmural, i.e., field, stimulation of the antrum) that cause a decrease in somatostatin secretion from basal levels elicit maximal gastrin responses, whereas stimuli (e.g., bombesin and beta-adrenergic agonists) that cause an increase in somatostatin secretion cause only a moderate increase in gastrin secretion. Neutralization of ambient somatostatin with somatostatin antiserum augments the gastrin response to bombesin or isoproterenol to maximal levels. Data from 5,11,13,22.

In addition to agents such as muscarinic agonists that cause inhibition of somatostatin and stimulation of gastrin secretion, and to agents such as bombesin that cause stimulation of both gastrin and somatostatin secretion, there are agents, for example, prostaglandins (5) and peptides of the secretin-glucagon family (3,16,17), that cause stimulation of somatostatin and inhibition of gastrin secretion. There is, however, no evidence that the increase in somatostatin secretion is functionally linked to the decrease in gastrin secretion. With some of these agents, addition of somatostatin antiserum restores and even augments gastrin secretion, but this could result from neutralization of basal somatostatin, thus eliminating its usual restraint on gastrin secretion. Furthermore, with secretin, inhibition of gastrin secretion persists despite the presence of somatostatin antiserum implying a direct inhibitory effect of secretin on the gastrin cell (17).

The notion of functional linkage between somatostatin and gastrin applies solely to the restraint exerted by basal somatostatin on gastrin secretion. Elimination of this restraint is responsible in part for the gastrin response and facilitates the effect of direct stimulants on gastrin secretion. There is no firm evidence that an increase in somatostatin secretion above basal levels has an additional inhibitory effect on gastrin secretion. There is also no evidence that either basal or stimulated gastrin has a reciprocal influence on somatostatin secretion.

MODEL FOR THE REGULATION OF GASTRIN AND SOMATOSTATIN SECRETION BY INTRAMURAL CHOLINERGIC AND NONCHOLINERGIC NEURONS

The pharmacological studies with muscarinic agonists and bombesin summarized above led to the formulation of a model according to which gastrin secretion is regulated by intramural cholinergic and noncholinergic neurons: stimulation of cholinergic neurons caused inhibitions of somatostatin secretion and thus, stimulation of gastrin secretion, whereas stimulation of noncholinergic neurons caused direct stimulation of gastrin secretion by releasing a peptide neurotransmitter, bombesin (11) (Fig. 4). Earlier in vivo studies in humans, dogs and cats had raised the possibility that both cholinergic and noncholinergic pathways were involved in the regulation of gastrin secretion. Activation of vagal pathways by sham-feeding (18) or by electrical stimulation of preganglionic fibers (19) induced atropine-resistant gastric secretion, whereas activation of intramural gastric pathways by instillation of a meal induced atropine-sensitive gastrin secretion (20). In vivo studies, however, did not disclose the nature of the noncholinergic transmitter or the interplay of cholinergic and noncholinergic pathways within the stomach. The isolated vascularly perfused whole stomach proved to be useful for this purpose: the preparation maintains the integrity of neural pathways and enables pharmacological, electrical and intraluminal stimulation of intramural neurons (21).

The participation of intramural neurons was examined pharmacologically with DMPP (12) and electrically by transmural (i.e., field) stimulation of the antral region (22). DMPP caused an increase in gastrin secretion that was abolished by hexamethonium but only partly (35%) inhibited by atropine. Transmural stimulation of the antral region using stimuli of increasing pulse duration (0.1 to 4 ms) caused increasing gastrin secretion that was progressively more resistant to atropine (Fig. 5). The maximal gastrin response elicited by 4 ms pulses was inhibited only 15% by atropine; the same dose of atropine (0.1 μM) inhibited the maximal gastrin response to muscarinic agonists by 70-90%.

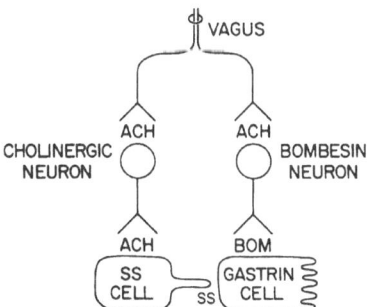

Fig. 4. Model illustrating the regulation of gastrin and somatostatin secretion in the antrum by intramural cholinergic and noncholinergic (bombesin) neurons. The somatostatin (SS) cell is shown to be structurally coupled to the gastrin cell by cytoplasmic processes. The cholinergic pathway is dominant in the regulation of somatostatin, causing inhibition of somatostatin secretion and thus, stimulation of gastrin secretion. The noncholinergic pathway is dominant in direct stimulation of gastrin secretion by causing the release of bombesin (GRP) in proximity of the gastrin cell (11).

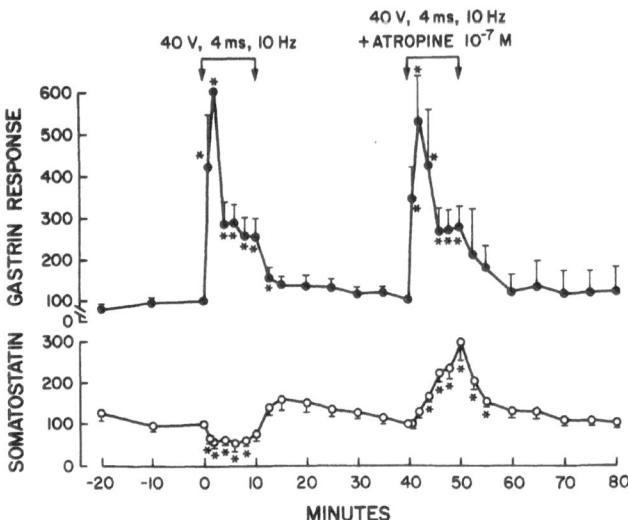

Fig. 5. Gastrin and somatostatin secretion in response to transmural (i.e., field) stimulation of the antral region at 40 V, 10 Hz, 4 ms, in the presence and absence of atropine. Atropine caused only minor (15%) inhibition of the gastrin response but converted the decrease in somatostatin secretion to increase above basal levels. Data expressed in percent of basal level (=100). Asterisks denote significance of difference from basal levels. From 22.

GASTRIC BOMBESIN (GRP): THE NEUROTRANSMITTER IN NONCHOLINERGIC PATHWAYS

The nature of the transmitter responsible for noncholinergic stimulation of gastrin secretion was tested with bombesin antiserum (23). Bombesin antiserum (final dilution 1:150) inhibited the maximal gastrin responses to either DMPP or field stimulation by 60% (Fig. 6). A combination of bombesin antiserum and atropine was additive, inhibiting the gastrin response by 75-95% (Fig. 7). The combined inhibitory effect of bombesin antiserum and atropine support the notion that endogenous acetylcholine and bombesin account for neural stimulation of gastrin secretion.

The results obtained in the rat have been confirmed recently in the isolated vascularly perfused pig antrum where electrical stimulation of preganglionic vagal fibers caused concomitant release of bombesin (GRP) and gastrin into the vascular perfusate (24). Addition of high doses of bombesin to the perfusate to desensitize the gastrin cell or addition of the substance P antagonist, (D-Arg^1, D-Pro^2, D-Trp^{7,9}, Leu^{11}) SP, which also acts as a bombesin antagonist, decreased the response to exogenous bombesin and abolished the effects of vagal stimulation.

The effects of DMPP and field stimulation on somatostatin secretion in the isolated rat stomach further demonstrate the involvement of cholinergic and noncholinergic (bombesin) neurons and the participation of somatostatin as a paracrine intermediate in the cholinergic pathway (23). Since bombesin and acetylcholine have opposite effects on somatostatin secretion, the net effect of a neural stimulus depends on whether the cholinergic or noncholinergic component is dominant. The net effect of

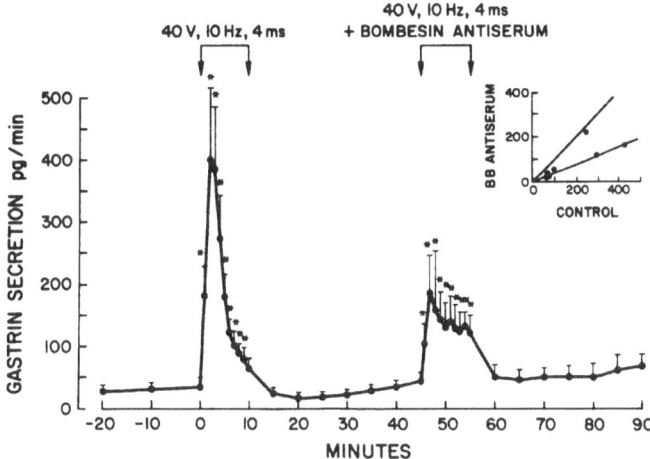

Fig. 6. Gastrin secretion (picogram/min) in response to transmural (i.e., field) stimulation of the antral region of the vascularly perfused rat stomach in the presence and absence of bombesin antiserum (final dilution 1:150). Inset: correlation between initial gastrin response in pg/min and response in the presence of bombesin (BB) antiserum. Points represent individual experiments (n = 7). Six out of seven lie on a slope of about 0.4 (inhibition = 60%). From 23.

DMPP is an increase in somatostatin secretion, reflecting a dominant noncholinergic influence (Fig. 8), whereas the net effect of field stimulation is a decrease in somatostatin secretion, reflecting a dominant cholinergic influence (Figs. 6 and 9). Addition of bombesin antiserum during stimulation with DMPP converts the increase in somatostatin to a decrease below basal levels: the results suggest that the initial increase was caused by bombesin and its conversion to a decrease was caused by the unmasking of a residual cholinergic (inhibitory) effect on somatostatin secretion (Fig. 8). In contrast, addition of bombesin antiserum during field stimulation does not alter the initial decrease in somatostatin secretion; addition of atropine, however, converts the decrease to an increase above basal levels (Fig. 9). The results suggest that the initial decrease was caused by a predominant cholinergic (inhibitory) effect on somatostatin secretion and that its blockade by atropine unmasked the residual noncholinergic (stimulatory) effect on somatostatin secretion.

SOURCE OF SECRETED GASTRIC SOMATOSTATIN

Although the somatostatin released into the vascular effluent of the isolated whole stomach is derived from both antrum and fundus, the patterns of secretion from both regions are similar; therefore, the pattern of secretion from whole stomach reflects the pattern of secretion from the antrum. The evidence for this notion is twofold: first, antral mucosa mounted in an Ussing chamber responds to cholinergic and noncholinergic stimulation in a similar fashion to the vascularly perfused whole stomach (25). Secondly, segments of antral and fundic mucosa perfused separately, release somatostatin identically in response to cholinergic and noncholinergic stimulation (26). It is worth emphasizing that the origin of

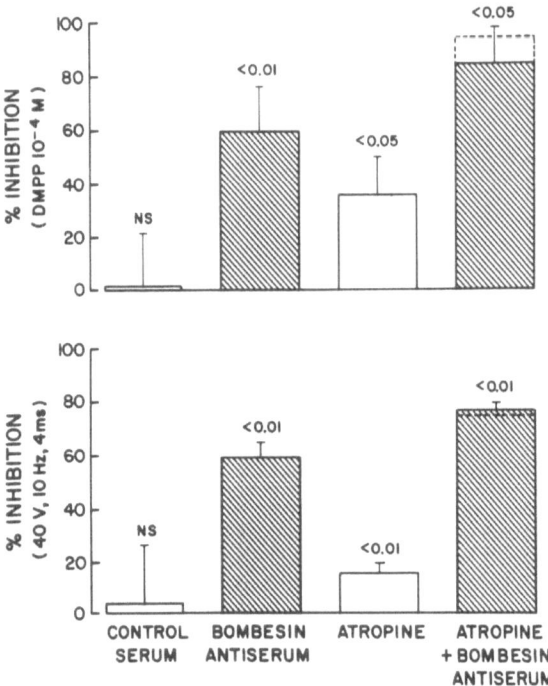

Fig. 7. Inhibition of the gastrin response to DMPP (upper panel) and field simulation (lower panel) by bombesin antiserum (final dilution 1:150), atropine 0.1 μM or a combination of both agents. Inhibition by bombesin antiserum (60%), by atropine (15-35%) and by both agents (75-95%). From 23.

somatostatin is not relevant when somatostatin antiserum is used as a probe of paracrine effects since the essential requisite is to determine the effect of immunoneutralization on gastrin secretion, the specific product of the antral region.

APPLICABILITY OF THE MODEL TO PHYSIOLOGICAL CONDITIONS

The model depicted in Fig. 4 holds also when physiological stimuli are applied via the lumen of the stomach such as during intraluminal perfusion with acidified or protein-containing solutions. Intraluminal perfusion of the isolated rat stomach with 0.5% peptone causes an increase in gastrin and decrease in somatostatin secretion (27) (Fig. 10). The effects appear to be mediated solely via intramural neurons, since addition of the axonal blocker, tetrodotoxin, to the vascular perfusate abolishes the gastrin and somatostatin responses. Addition of atropine, however, inhibits partly the gastrin response and converts the somatostatin response from decrease to increase above basal levels. The results mimic closely those obtained with field stimulation (23) (Fig. 5), demonstrating the involvement of intramural cholinergic and noncholinergic neurons in the regulation of gastrin, and the participation of somatostatin as a paracrine intermediate in the cholinergic pathway.

246

SUMMARY

Cholinergic neurons act predominantly to inhibit the paracrine secretion of somatostatin, eliminating the restraint exerted by basal somatostatin on gastrin secretion and enabling bombesin neurons to exert their potent stimulatory influence on gastrin secretion. The optimal physiological condition is thus realized by a combination of neural stimuli that cause cholinergic inhibition of somatostatin and stimulation of bombesin release. This combination of neural influences prevails when food, especially partially digested protein, is present in the lumen of the stomach.

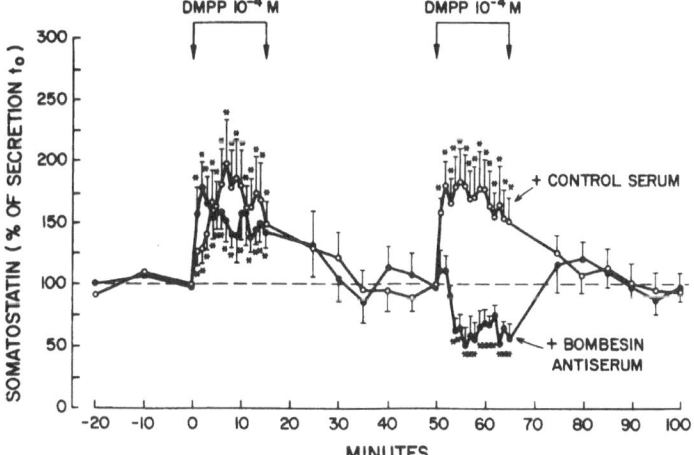

Fig. 8. Somatostatin secretion in response to DMPP in the presence of normal serum (open circles) and bombesin anti-serum (final dilution 1:150) (closed circles). The increase in somatostatin secretion caused by DMPP was converted to decrease below basal level by bombesin antiserum. Basal level (=100) denoted by dotted line. Data expressed in per-cent of basal response at time zero (t_0). Asterisks denote significance of difference from basal level. From 23.

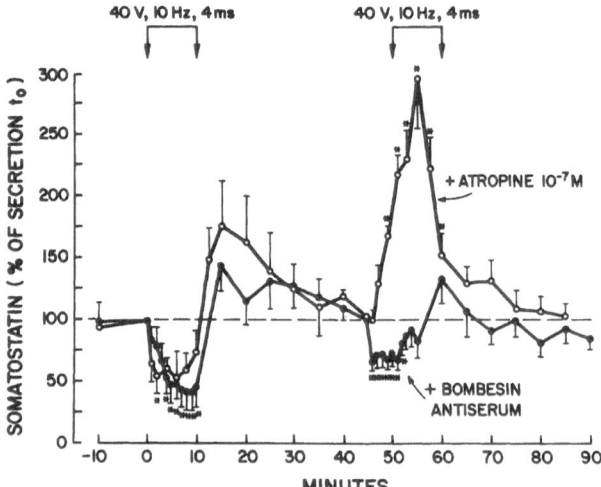

Fig. 9. Somatostatin secretion in response to transmural (i.e., field) stimulation of the antral region of the vascularly perfused rat stomach. The initial response (decrease from basal level during stimulation in the period 0–10 min) was not affected by addition of bombesin antiserum to the vascular perfusate (period 45–55 min) but was converted from decrease to significant increase above basal levels by 0.1 μM atropine. Open and closed circles represent two separate series of experiments each with its initial control response. Basal level (=100) denoted by dotted line. Data expressed in percent of basal response at time zero (t_0). Asterisks denote significance of difference from basal level. From 23.

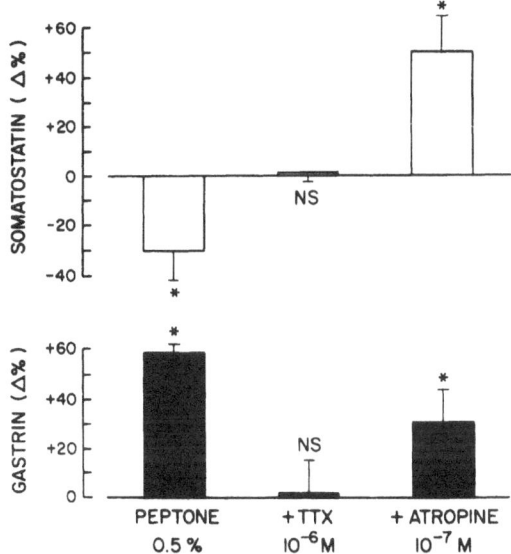

Fig. 10. Gastrin and somatostatin secretion in response to intraluminal perfusion with 0.5% peptone. In some experiments, tetrodo- toxin (TTX 1 μM) or atropine (0.1 μM) was added to the vascular perfusate of the isolated rat stomach. The axonal blocker TTX abolished all responses. Atropine partially inhibited the gastrin response and converted the decrease in somatostatin to increase above basal levels. Note similar- ity of responses to Figs. 5 and 9. Data expressed as percent increase or decrease from basal level. Asterisks denote signif- icance of difference from basal levels. NS = not significant. From 27.

ACKNOWLEDGMENTS

The studies reported in this review were done in the author's laboratory by Doctors B. Saffouri, J. W. DuVal, and M. L. Schubert. This research was supported by grant AM-15564 from the National Institutes of Health.

REFERENCES

1. Saffouri B, Weir GC, Bitar KN, Makhlouf CM. Stimulation of gastrin secretion from the vascularly perfused stomach by somatostatin antiserum. Life Sci 1979; 20:1749-54.
2. Chiba T, Kadowaki S, Taminato T, et al. Effect of antisomatostatin gammaglobulin on gastrin release in rats. Gastroenterology 1981; 81:321-6.
3. Wolfe MM, Reel GM, McGuigan JE. Inhibition of gastrin release by secretin is mediated by somatostatin in cultured rat antral mucosa. J Clin Invest 1983; 72:1586-93.

4. Larsson L-I, Goltermann N, De Magistri L, et al. Somatostatin cell processes as pathways for paracrine secretion. Science 1979; 205: 1393-5.

5. Saffouri B, Weir GC, Bitar KN, Makhlouf GM. Gastrin and somatostatin secretion by perfused rat stomach: functional linkage of antral peptides. Am J Physiol 1980; 238:G495-501.

6. Martindale R, Kauffman GL, Levin S, Walsh JH, Yamada T. Differential regulation of gastrin and somatostatin secretion from isolated perfused rat stomachs. Gastroenterology 1982; 83:240-4.

7. Koop H, Behrens I, Bothe E, et al. Adrenergic and cholinergic interactions in rat gastric somatostatin and gastrin release. Digestion 1982; 25:96-102.

8. McIntosh CHS, Pederson RA, Koop H, Brown JC. Gastric inhibitory polypeptide-stimulated secretion of somatostatin-like immunoreactivity from the stomach: inhibition by acetylcholine and vagal stimulation. Can J Physiol Pharmacol 1981; 59:468-72.

9. Richelsen B, Rehfeld JF, Larsson L-I. Antral gland cell column: a method for studying release of gastrin hormone. Am J Physiol 1983; 245(Gastrointest Liver Physiol 8):G463-9.

10. Dockray GJ, Vaillant C, Walsh JH. The neural origin of bombesin-like immunoreactivity in the rat gastrointestinal tract. Neuroscience 1970; 4:1561-8.

11. Duval JW, Saffouri B, Weir GC, et al. Stimulation of gastrin and somatostatin secretion from the isolated rat stomach by bombesin. Am J Physiol 1981; 241:G242-7.

12. Schubert ML, Makhlouf GM. Regulation of gastrin and somatostatin secretion by intramural neurons: effect of nicotinic receptor stimulation with dimethyl phenylpiperazinium. Gastroenterology 1982; 83:626-32.

13. Saffouri B, Duval JW, Makhlouf GM. Adrenergic regulation of gastrin and somatostatin secretion: evidence for functional linkage of the two peptides. Gastroenterology 1983; 84:1292.

14. Yamada T, Soll AH, Park J, Elashoff J. Autonomic regulation of somatostatin release: studies with primary cultures of canine fundic mucosal cells. Am J Physiol 1984; 247:G567-73.

15. Soll AH, Yamada T, Park J, Thomas LP. Release of somatostatin-like immunoreactivity from canine fundic mucosal cells in primary culture. Am J Physiol 1984; 247:G558-66.

16. Chiba T, Taminato T, Kadowaki S, et al. Effects of glucagon secretin and vasoactive intestinal polypeptide on gastric somatostatin and gastrin release from isolated perfused rat stomach. Gastroenterology 1980; 79:67-71.

17. Saffouri B, Duval JW, Arimura A, Makhlouf GM. Effects of vasoactive intestinal peptide and secretin on gastrin and somatostatin secretion in the perfused rat stomach. Gastroenterology 1984; 86:839-42.

18. Dockray GJ, Tracy HJ. Atropine does not abolish cephalic vagal stimulation of gastrin release in dogs. J Physiol 1980; 306:473-80.

19. Smith CL, Kewenter AM, Connell AM, et al. Control factors in the release of gastrin by direct electrical stimulation of the vagus. Am J Dig Dis 1975; 20:13-22.

20. Hirschowitz BI, Bigson R, Molina E. Atropine suppresses gastrin release by food in intact and vagotomized dogs. Gastroenterology 1981; 81:838-43.

21. Holst JJ, Jensen SL, Knuhtsen S, Nielsen OV, Rehfeld JF. Effect of vagus, gastric inhibitory polypeptide, and HCl on gastrin and somatostatin release from perfused pig antrum. Am J Physiol 1983; 244: G515-22.

22. Schubert ML, Bitar KN, Makhlouf GM. Regulation of gastrin and somatostatin secretion by cholinergic and noncholinergic intramural neurons. Am J Physiol 1982; 243:G442-7.

23. Schubert ML, Saffouri B, Walsh JH, Makhlouf GM. Inhibition of

neurally mediated gastrin secretion by bombesin antiserum. Am J Physiol 1985; 248:G456-62.

24. Holst JJ, Knuhtsen S, Orshov AC, Nielsen OV. GRP-producing nerves control the antral somatostatin (SS) secretion [Abstract]. International Conference on Somatostatin, Washington, DC, May 6-8,1986:54.

25. Schubert ML, Saffouri B, Makhlouf, GM. Neural regulation of gastrin and somatostatin secretion in isolated antral sheets. Gastroenterology 1984; 86:1238.

26. Schubert ML, Saffouri B, Makhlouf GM. Identical patterns of somatostatin secretion from the isolated antrum and fundus of rat stomach. Gastroenterology 1984; 86:1238

27. Schubert ML, Saffouri B, Makhlouf GM. Stimulation of gastrin secretion in vitro by intraluminal chemicals: regulation by intramural cholinergic and noncholinergic neurons. Gastroenterology 1984; 87:557-561.

24

SOMATOSTATIN INHIBITS INTESTINAL MOTILITY VIA MODULATION

OF CYCLIC AMP-DEPENDENT CHOLINERGIC TRANSMISSION

Chung Owyang and John Wiley

Department of Internal Medicine
University of Michigan Medical School
Ann Arbor, MI

Somatostatin (SRIF) is a tetradecapeptide that was initially isolated from ovine hypothalamus and described as an inhibitor of growth hormone release (1). In addition to its action as a modulator of the release of a wide variety of hormones and physiological secretions (2), SRIF is thought to function as a neurotransmitter, primarily because somatostatin-like immunoreactivity has been demonstrated in axons and nerve cell bodies of primary sensory neurons (3), sympathetic neurons (4), as well as in neurons in the central nervous system (5). In the gastrointestinal tract nerve cell bodies demonstrating somatostatin-like immunoreactivity have been found in both the myenteric and the submucous plexus (6). In the myenteric plexus they represent 4.7% of the total population of neurons. These somatostatin-containing neurons appear to project exclusively to other neurons in the myenteric plexus since no fibers are found in the muscle or in the tertiary plexus which is close to the muscle (6). Furthermore, somatostatin is not found in axons which project to the circular muscle or to the submucosa. Thus the somatostatin containing neurons appear to represent a population of interneurons in the myenteric plexus.

The presence of somatostatin containing neurons in the myenteric plexus points to a potential role for the peptide in regulating gastrointestinal motility. The overall effect of SRIF on gastrointestinal motility appears to be inhibitory (7). However, there may be some site-specific and species-specific stimulatory effects as well (8,9,10). The mechanism(s) by which SRIF acts to regulate gastrointestinal motility has not been clearly established. In isolated longitudinal muscle strips from guinea pig ileum SRIF has been shown to cause relaxation (11). Guillemin (12) demonstrated that SRIF inhibits ileal muscle contraction induced by electrical field stimulation which is atropine sensitive. In contrast, the contractile response of the ileal muscle strip to exogenous acetylcholine is not modified by large concentrations of SRIF. This suggests that SRIF is acting presynaptically to inhibit acetylcholine release. Similar observations have been made by Furness and Costa using isolated segments of ileum from the guinea pig (13). In addition these investigators observe that SRIF also causes the ileal muscle to relax under basal conditions. This relaxation is blocked by tetrodotoxin, but not by guanethidine. Thus under basal conditions SRIF may relax longitudinal muscle by inhibiting acetylcholine release resulting in a loss of cholinergic tone. In order to examine the modulation of cholinergic transmission by SRIF more directly, we investigated the ability of SRIF to alter acetylcholine release in ileal muscle strips and examined the second messenger pathways by which SRIF modulates acetylcholine release.

INHIBITION OF ACETYLCHOLINE RELEASE FROM THE MYENTERIC PLEXUS BY SOMATOSTATIN

To provide direct evidence that SRIF inhibits cholinergic transmission, the ability of SRIF to alter acetylcholine release in ileal muscle slices was examined using modifications of methods previously reported (14). Slices of guinea pig ileum without mucosa were incubated with tritiated choline and the release of synthesized tritiated acetylcholine was measured in the presence of physostigmine and hemicholinium. Sequential 10-min incubations and collections were performed for two hours. The effects of various agonists and antagonists were measured at 40 min and 90 min. Cation exchange chromatography was used to confirm that ^{3}H-ACh was the substance being released.

Mean ^{3}H-ACh release (expressed as percentage of tissue content) stimulated by 50 mM potassium was 3.2 ± 0.4%. This represents a 36 ± 7% increase over baseline. Similarly, depolarization by veratridine (10^{-4}M) increased ^{3}H-ACh release by 38 ± 6% over basal. Tetrodotoxin (10^{-6}M) abolished ^{3}H-ACh release evoked by veratridine but had no effect on potassium mediated release. This suggests that the major site of action for potassium is at the nerve terminal, whereas veratridine stimulates ACh release by axonal depolarization since this process is tetrodotoxin sensitive. SRIF (10^{-6}M) blocked ^{3}H-ACh release by veratridine but not that evoked by potassium. This indicates that SRIF acts on the cell body or the axon to modulate cholinergic transmission.

Electric field stimulation (1-20 Hz, 0.5 msec, 30 sec) evoked ^{3}H-ACh release in a dose-related manner. ^{3}H-ACh release induced by 5 Hz of electrical stimulation was completely abolished by tetrodotoxin (10^{-6}M) and partially inhibited by SRIF in a dose-related manner (10^{-9} to 10^{-6}M). SRIF (10^{-6}M) antagonized ^{3}H-ACh release by 57 ± 9%.

In separate studies we also demonstrated that octapeptide of cholecystokinin (CCK8) and substance P caused an increase in ^{3}H-ACh release in a dose-related manner. The ED50 for CCK8 and substance P were 2 x 10^{-8}M and 6 x 10^{-8}M respectively. Tetrodotoxin (10^{-6}M) abolished ^{3}H-ACh release evoked by CCK8 and substance P. In contrast SRIF (10^{-6}M) inhibited CCK8-induced release of ^{3}H-ACh by 58 ± 12% but had no effect on that evoked by substance P. This raises the possibility that CCK8 and substance P may stimulate cholinergic transmission by different intracellular messenger systems and SRIF may have differential effectiveness in inhibiting these systems. Thus we characterized the second messenger system(s) involved in cholinergic transmission and examined the effect of SRIF on these systems.

THE ROLE OF CYCLIC AMP IN CHOLINERGIC TRANSMISSION

Our initial studies were to identify the role of adenylate cyclase activation and cyclic AMP accumulation on the release of ^{3}H-ACh from myenteric plexus in ileal muscle slices. Forskolin, an activator of the adenylate cyclase system, stimulated the release of ^{3}H-ACh in a dose-related manner. The threshold dose was 10^{-7}M and a 28 ± 4% increase was observed with 10^{-6}M of forskolin. 8-bromo-cyclic AMP (10^{-4}M), a lipid soluble analogue of cyclic AMP, also caused a similar increase of ^{3}H-ACh. The release of ^{3}H-ACh evoked by forskolin and 8-bromo-cyclic AMP was abolished by tetrodotoxin (10^{-6}M). In contrast adenosine (10^{-4}M), an inhibitor of adenylate cyclase antagonized ^{3}H-ACh release evoked by forskolin but had no effect on that stimulated by 8-bromo-cyclic AMP. Adenosine is known to inhibit electrically-induced contractions in the guinea pig ileum via inhibition of acetylcholine release without having any effect on ACh generated contractions (15). Addition of theophylline (10^{-5}M) significantly enhanced forskolin (10^{-6}M) stimulated release of ^{3}H-ACh (52 ± 6% vs. 28 ± 4%). These data indicate that the cyclic AMP system participates in cholinergic transmission.

THE ROLE OF CALCIUM-PHOSPHATIDYLINOSITOL SYSTEM IN CHOLINERGIC TRANSMISSION

Increase in intracellular calcium concentration plays an important role in the release of neurotransmitter (16). Depolarization induced by electrical stimulation or appropriate agonists will lead to membrane phosphatidylinositide turnover (17), resulting in the liberation of inositol triphosphate (IP_3) and diacylglycerol (DAG). IP_3 subsequently mobilizes calcium from cellular stores (18). DAG, coupled with the rise in calcium, activates protein kinase C (19). In the following studies we evaluated the role of intracellular calcium and protein kinase C in cholinergic transmission using guinea pig ileum preloaded with ^{3}H-choline.

A23187, a calcium ionophore evoked ^{3}H-ACh release in a dose-related manner. At 10^{-6}M, A23187 increased ^{3}H-ACh by 15 ± 3% over basal. This stimulatory effect was abolished in calcium-free medium. Tumor-promoting phorbol esters such as 12-O-tetra-decanoyl phorbol 13-acetate (TPA) mimic the action of DAG to activate protein kinase C. In our ileal muscle strip system TPA up to 10^{-5}M did not have any obvious effect on ^{3}H-ACh release. However, a combination of TPA (10^{-7}M) and A23187 (10^{-6}M) caused a much larger release of ^{3}H-ACh compared to that released by A23187 alone (37 ± 9% vs. 15 ± 3%). The combination of A23187 and TPA-mediated release was similar to that observed with K$^+$ (50 mM) or electrical stimulation (36 ± 7% over basal). Addition of an inhibitor of protein kinase C, polymixin (10^{-7}M) abolished the potentiating effect of TPA resulting in a ^{3}H-ACh release (18 ± 5%) similar to that observed with A23187 alone. These data suggest that activation of protein kinase C can potentiate the action of intracellular calcium in modulating the release of acetylcholine. Thus both an increase in intracellular calcium and activation of protein kinase C are essential and act synergistically to induce cholinergic transmission.

MECHANISM OF INHIBITION OF CHOLINERGIC TRANSMISSION BY SOMATOSTATIN

To characterize the mechanism of action of SRIF on cholinergic transmission we compared the effect of SRIF on ^{3}H-ACh release evoked by the cyclic AMP and calcium-phosphoinositide second messenger systems.

Forskolin (10^{-6}M) and 8-bromo-cyclic AMP (10^{-4}M) stimulated ^{3}H-ACh release by 28 ± 4% and 30 ± 7% over basal respectively. SRIF (10^{-6}M) inhibited forskolin- and 8-bromo-cyclic AMP-evoked release of ^{3}H-ACh by 58 ± 15% and 16 ± 8% respectively. Thus SRIF acts mainly by inhibiting the adenylate cyclase and has little effect distal to cyclic AMP formation. In separate experiments we investigated the possibility that SRIF antagonizes forskolin-mediated release of ^{3}H-ACh via activation of the inhibitory (N_i) regulatory protein. Pertussis toxin has been shown to ribosylate N_i and, thereby, block its activation (20). Pretreatment with pertussis toxin (100 ng/ml) antagonized the inhibitory effect of SRIF on forskolin-stimulated release of ^{3}H-ACh but not that evoked by 8-bromo-cyclic AMP. This indicates the mechanism of inhibition probably involves activation of the N_1 subunit of adenylate cyclase.

In separate studies we evaluated the effect of SRIF on ^{3}H-ACh release stimulated by the calcium-phosphoinositide system. A21378 and a combination of A23178 plus TPA evoked ^{3}H-ACh release by 15 ± 3% and 37 ± 9% respectively. These were not antagonized by SRIF (10^{-6}M). Thus it appears that under the experimental conditions used SRIF exerts its action mainly via modulation of cyclic AMP-dependent cholinergic transmission in the myenteric plexus. Previous studies have demonstrated that calcium or calcium ionophore reversed SRIF's inhibition of insulin release from the pancreas (21,22). In pituitary tumor cell system SRIF may act through multiple mechanisms (20,23). Increasing the extracellular Ca^{++} concentration overcame SRIF's inhibition of ACTH release evoked by potassium but not that stimulated by forskolin or 8-bromo-cyclic AMP (24,25). Thus the effectiveness of SRIF to antagonize ^{3}H-ACh release evoked by A23178 plus TPA may be dependent on the intracellular calcium concentration. Further studies are needed to clarify this issue.

As indicated earlier we have demonstrated that both CCK8 and substance P stimulated ^{3}H-ACh release from the myenteric plexus. However, SRIF blocked ACh release evoked by CCK8 but not that evoked by substance P. Electrophysiological studies reveal that CCK8 and substance P generate slow excitatory postsynaptic potentials (EPSP's) in isolated myenteric plexus. Adenosine, an adenylate cyclase inhibitor antagonizes CCK8 mediated slow EPSP's but not those generated by substance P (26). These observations led us to hypothesize that in part CCK stimulates cholinergic transmission via a cyclic AMP pathway whereas substance P is acting via a cyclic AMP-independent mechanism. To test this hypothesis we examined whether or not CCK8- and substance P-evoked release of ^{3}H-ACh is inhibited by adenosine. Adenosine (10^{-4}M) partially antagonized CCK8-evoked release of ^{3}H-ACh by 45 ± 6% but had no effect on ^{3}H-ACh released by substance P. Furthermore, we also demonstrated that the inhibitory effect of SRIF on CCK8-evoked release of ^{3}H-ACh was reversed by pertussis toxin. These data indicate that CCK can stimulate acetylcholine release via the cyclic AMP pathway and SRIF antagonizes CCK-mediated release of acetylcholine via activation of the inhibitory (N_1) regulatory protein. Figure 1 presents a schematic representation of the proposed mechanism of regulation of adenylate cyclase by peptides.

CONCLUSION

Our studies using ileal muscle strips to investigate the release of ^{3}H-ACh-acetylcholine from myenteric plexus indicate that both the cyclic AMP and calcium-phosphatidylinositol second messenger systems participate in cholinergic transmission. SRIF exerts its inhibitory action mainly via modulation of cyclic AMP-dependent release of acetylcholine and its mechanism of action involves activation of N_1 subunit of adenylate cyclase. We have demonstrated that CCK can stimulate cholinergic transmission at least in part via the cyclic AMP pathway whereas substance P is acting via a cyclic AMP-independent mechanism. The differential effectiveness of SRIF on inhibiting the cyclic AMP and calcium-phosphatidylinositol second systems may explain the different action of SRIF on acetylcholine release evoked by CCK and substance P.

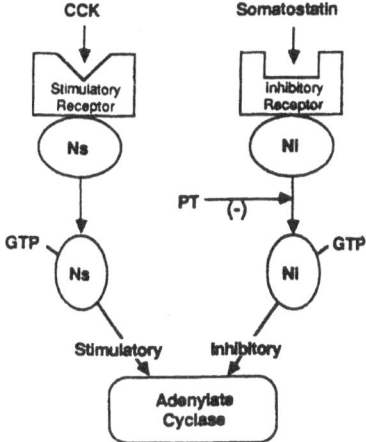

Fig. 1. Proposed regulation of adenylate cyclase by peptides. Somatostatin exerts its inhibitory action by activating the N_i subunit of the adenylate cyclase system which in turn inhibits adenylate cyclase. In contrast, stimulatory peptides such as cholecystokinin (CCK) stimulates the release of acetylcholine by activation of the adenylate cyclase system via the N_s subunit. Pertussis toxin (PT) ribosylates N_i subunit of the adenylate cyclase system to block its activation.

REFERENCES

1. Brazeau P, Vale W, Burgus R, et al. Hypothalamic polypeptide that inhibits the secretion of immunoreactive pituitary growth hormone. Science 1973; 179:77-9.
2. Vale W, Brazeau P, Rivier C, et al. Somatostatin. Recent Prog Horm Res 1975; 31:365-97.
3. Hokfelt T, Johansson O, Luft R, Arimura A. Immunohistochemical evidence for the presence of somatostatin, a powerful inhibitory peptide, in some primary sensory neurons. Neurosci Lett 1975; 1:231-5.
4. Hokfelt T, Elfvin LG, Elde R, Schultzberg M, Goldstein M, Luft R. Occurrence of somatostatin immunoreactivity in some peripheral sympathetic nonadrenergic neurons. Proc Natl Acad Sci USA 1977; 74:3587-91.
5. Hokfelt T, Efendic S, Johansson O, Luft R, Arimura A. Immunohistochemical localization of somatostatin (growth hormone release-inhibiting factor) in the guinea pig brain. Brain Res 1974; 80:165-9.
6. Costa M, Furness JB, Llewellyn-Smith IJ, Davies B, Oliver J. An immunohistochemical study of the projections of somatostatin-containing neurons in the guinea pig intestine. Neuroscience 1980; 5:841-52.
7. Johansson C, Efendic S, Wisen O, Uvnas-Wallensten K, Luft R. Effects of short-term somatostatin infusion on the gastric and intestinal propulsion in humans. Scand J Gastroenterol 1978; 13:481-3.

257

8. Lux G, Femppel J, Leaderer P. Somatostatin induces interdigestive intestinal motor and secretory complex-like activity in man. Gastroenterology 1980; 78:1212.

9. Peeters TL, Janssens J, Vantrappen GR. Somatostatin and the interdigestive migrating motor complex in man. Regul Pept 1983; 5:209-17.

10. Thor P, Krol R, Konturek SJ. Effect of somatostatin on myoelectrical activity of the small bowel. Am J Physiol 1978; 235:E249-54.

11. Cohen ML, Rosina E, Wiley KS, Slater IH. Somatostatin inhibits adrenergic and cholinergic neurotransmission in smooth muscle. Life Sci 1978; 23:1659-61.

12. Guillemin R. Somatostatin inhibits the release of acetylcholine induced electrically in the myenteric plexus. Endocrinology 1976; 99:1654.

13. Furness JB, Costa M. Actions of somatostatin on excitatory and inhibitory nerves in the intestine. Eur J Pharmacol 1979; 56:69-74.

14. Wu Z, Kisslinger SD, Gazinella TS. Functional evidence for the presence of cholinergic nerve endings in the colonic mucosa of the rat. J Pharmacol Exp Ther 1982; 221:664-9.

15. Gustafsson L, Hedquist P, Fredholm BB, Lundgren G. Inhibition of acetylcholine release in guinea pig ileum by adenosine. Acta Physiol Scand 1978; 104:469-78.

16. Katz B. Nerve, muscle, and synapse. New York: McGraw-Hill, 1966.

17. Berridge MJ. Inositol trisphosphate and diacylglycerol as second messengers. Biochem J 1984; 220:345-60.

18. Berridge MJ, Irvine RF. Inositol trisphosphate, a novel second messenger in cellular signal transduction. Nature 1984; 312:315-21.

19. Rasmussen H, Kojima I, Kojima K, et al. Calcium as intracellular messenger: sensitivity modulation, C-kinase pathway and sustained cellular response. Adv Cyclic Nucleotide Res 1984; 18:159-93.

20. Reisine TD. Somatostatin inhibition of cyclic AMP accumulation and adenocorticotropin release from mouse anterior pituitary tumor cells: mode of action and self-regulation. Adv Cyclic Nucleotide Res 1985; 19:169-77.

21. Reichlin S. Somatostatin. N Engl J Med 1983; 309:1495-501.

22. Curry D, Bennett L. Does somatostatin inhibition of insulin secretion involve two mechanisms of action? Proc Natl Acad Sci USA 1976; 73:248-51.

23. Koch BD, Donflinger LJ, Schonbrunn A. Pertussis toxin blocks both cyclic-AMP-mediated and cyclic AMP-independent actions of somatostatin. J Biol Chem 1985; 260:13138-45.

24. Richardson U, Schonbrunn A. Inhibition of adrenocorticotropin secretion by somatostatin in pituitary cells in culture. Endocrinology 1981; 108:281-90.

25. Reisine T. Multiple mechanisms of somatostatin inhibition of adrenocorticotropin release from mouse anterior pituitary tumor cells. Endocrinology 1985; 116:2259-66.

26. Palmer JM, Zafirov DH, Nemth PR, Wood JD. Peptidergic modulation of excitability in myenteric plexus neurons [Abstract]. Dig Dis Sci 1985; 30:786.

25

MULTIPLE MECHANISMS APPEAR TO UNDERLIE THE ANTISECRETORY

ACTION OF SOMATOSTATIN ON ACID SECRETION

Andrew H. Soll

Professor of Medicine, UCLA School of Medicine
Center for Ulcer Research and Education
Medical and Research Services
Wadsworth VA Hospital Center
Los Angeles, CA 90073

In recent years a reductionistic approach has been applied to study of the mechanisms regulating acid secretion. Although many of these regulatory events remain incompletely understood, a basis is beginning to emerge for understanding the mechanisms by which antisecretory agents inhibit acid secretion. One reason that the picture is far from complete is the complexity of the mechanisms regulating acid secretion. Three pathways deliver chemical messengers that regulate acid secretion: neural (transmitters released from postganglionic nerves in the stomach wall); endocrine (hormones, such as gastrin, delivered by blood), and paracrine (transmitters released from local storage sites move across the intercellular space to their local target cell). The latter point is important, because the fundic mucosa is composed of a heterogenous cell population and several of these cells have potential as endocrine/paracrine modulators of the secretory response. These cells include ones containing histamine, somatostatin, glucagon, dopamine, and serotonin. Therefore, in vivo the parietal cell is potentially exposed to many chemical transmitters that may modulate its function. Therefore, it has been difficult in vivo to sort out the direct and indirect regulators of secretion.

An additional factor complicating the physiology of acid secretion is an interdependency that exists between the pathways regulating acid secretion. This interdependency is most evident by the apparent nonspecificity of H_2 and muscarinic receptor blockers. These drugs not only inhibit the response to histamine and cholinergic stimulation respectively, but they also block the gastric acid response to gastrin, food, and vagal stimulation. From in vivo studies it is unclear whether the receptors mediating the three pathways regulating acid secretion reside on the parietal cell itself, or, alternatively, whether acetylcholine and gastrin act indirectly by inducing the release of histamine from its fundic mucosal stores.

To study this regulation we have dispersed cells and gastric glands from fundic mucosa using enzymes, and have developed techniques for studying function. Because of the cellular heterogeneity of the stomach mucosa, cell separation is necessary; both size (velocity) and density separation have been useful. Since isolated parietal cells lose their polar orientation in the mucosa, acid secretion cannot be used as an index of cell function; acid secreted at the apical surface is neutralized by bicarbonate secreted from the basal surface. Therefore, partial cell function is monitored indirectly using techniques such as the intracellular accumulation of the weak base aminopyrine or the consumption of oxygen or glucose. Resting parietal cells contain tubulovesicles in their cytoplasm; with stimulation these structures coalesce into secretory channels that, in the intact mucosa, drain secreted acid into the gland lumen. In the isolated parietal cell these channels also coalesce into large acidic compartments. Aminopyrine accumulates into these acidic spaces by pH partition; since it is a weak base, it picks up a hydrogen ion at low pH and, becoming ionized, is locked in by the surrounding plasma membranes.

PARIETAL CELL RESPONSES AND RECEPTORS

Regardless of the index monitored, canine parietal cells respond to histamine, acetylcholine, and gastrin (1). Specific antagonists for the histamine H_2, gastrin and muscarinic receptor have allowed characterization of the receptors involved. One interesting aspect of inhibitor action is an apparent nonspecificity displayed by all inhibitors in vivo. Although H_2 blockers and antimuscarinic agents display an apparent nonspecificity in vivo, these drugs are specific respectively against histamine (2,3) and cholinergic (2,4) stimulation of the isolated parietal cell. Studying canine parietal cells, gastrin caused a small stimulation of function that was not inhibited by muscarinic or H_2 receptor antagonists, suggesting that gastrin was acting at a separate receptor site. Specific receptor blockers are also available for the gastrin receptor. Proglumide, a glutaramic acid derivative, preferentially blocks the canine parietal cell response to gastrin (5). The existence of specific receptors for gastrin has been confirmed using a gastrin analogue labeled with radioactive iodine, ^{125}I-[Leu^{15}]-gastrin. Receptors for this biologically active tracer were localized to parietal cells in studies that produced highly enriched parietal cells using sequential velocity and density cell separation techniques. Gastrin inhibition of tracer binding and stimulation of parietal cell function were correlated over the gastrin dose response curve and both gastrin binding and action were proportionately inhibited by proglumide. Therefore, current data indicate that the parietal cell has specific receptors for histamine, acetylcholine and gastrin.

POTENTIATING INTERACTIONS AMPLIFY PARIETAL CELL RESPONSES

Potentiating interactions between stimulants are evident in studies of parietal cell function. Such amplification is evident by a response to a combination of stimulants that was greater than the sum of the individual responses and greater than the maximal response to either agent alone. Such potentiating interactions were found between histamine and gastrin and histamine and acetylcholine in their effects on parietal cell function. The studies of glucose oxidation illustrate such potentiation. As noted above when parietal cells were treated with single agents, H_2, muscarinic and gastrin receptor antagonists displayed specificity. However, when parietal cells were treated with combinations of agents, cimetidine and atropine displayed an apparent lack of specificity, reminiscent of that found in vivo and probably reflecting blockade of the histamine and cholinergic components of the amplification process (6). Although potentiating interactions at the parietal cell are likely to be a component of the interactions that occur between the pathways regulating acid secretion, other mechanisms of interaction exist, as considered subsequently.

PARIETAL CELL ACTIVATION BY CYCLIC AMP

Parietal cells are similar to many cell types in that their activation mechanisms fall into two categories, those related to the generation of cyclic adenosine monophosphate (AMP) from ATP and those related to increases in calcium concentration in the cell. Stimulation of parietal cell function by histamine, but not by cholinergics or gastrin, is closely linked to enhanced formation of cyclic AMP (3,7). Prostaglandins potently inhibit acid secretion in vivo and also directly inhibit the function of isolated parietal cell (8). This inhibition, studied most extensively for prostaglandin E_2 (PGE_2), is selective against histamine-stimulated parietal cell function; the responses to gastrin and acetylcholine are not blocked. PGE_2 also reduces the cellular accumulation of cyclic AMP in response to histamine, indicating effects at an early point in the histamine response (8,9). Current evidence indicates that prostaglandin inhibition is related to the inhibitory GTP binding protein of adenylate cyclase. Several inhibitory receptors, including the somatostatin receptor on several cell types, decrease the generation of cAMP via a link to G_i; cyclic AMP generation is reduced in proportion to the reduction in cell function. One important tool for dissecting these mechanisms is provided by the toxin produced by Bordetella pertussis. Pertussis toxin inactivates G_i and therefore blocks inhibition mediated by this inhibitory side of the adenylate cyclase complex. Pertussis toxin treatment of parietal cells has been found to remove PGE_2 inhibition or parietal cell function while not impairing stimulatory responses, suggesting that prostanoids act via G_i to turn off the parietal cell (10).

PARIETAL CELL ACTIVATION BY CALCIUM-DEPENDENT MECHANISMS

In contrast to histamine, cholinergic agents and gastrin act via calcium dependent mechanisms. There is good evidence that cholinergic agents enhance calcium uptake into the cell from the extracellular space (11). Cell stimulation by cholinergic agents and gastrin—but not histamine—is blocked by removal of extracellular calcium or by adding lanthanum, a trivalent cation that blocks calcium fluxes across the plasma membrane. This calcium uptake is probably via selective receptor-activated calcium channels in the cell membrane, but these channels are probably different from the channels present in muscle, nerve and other tissues that are blocked by the calcium channel antagonists such as verapamil or nifedipine.

NONPARIETAL GASTRIN AND ACETYLCHOLINE RECEPTORS

The picture painted regarding the receptors on the parietal cell is unfortunately an oversimplification. It has become clear from recent studies that gastrin and acetylcholine receptors are also present on other cells, such as the histamine cell. In our studies of gastrin receptors, specific gastrin binding was found to a small cell(s), in addition to the parietal cell (5,12). These small cell elutriator fractions are a heterogenous cell population that includes histamine cells and endocrine cells containing somatostatin or glucagon. We separated this small cell fraction by density and found that gastrin receptors were closely associated with the presence of somatostatin cells. Since the presence of specific receptors means little without testing functional responses, techniques were sought for determining if gastrin altered release of somatostatin from canine fundic endocrine cells (13). For these studies, the small cell elutriator fraction was placed in short term culture. Gastrin was found to stimulate the release of somatostatin from these cultured cells. Epinephrine also stimulated SLI release and marked potentiation was found between gastrin and epinephrine. The beta adrenergic antagonist propranolol, but not alpha adrenergic receptor antagonists, competitively inhibited this epinephrine response. Of interest, muscarinic receptors also regulated somatostatin cell function, but cholinergic agents inhibited—rather than stimulated—somatostatin release. This cholinergic effect was blocked by atropine acting at a typical muscarinic receptor (14).

HISTAMINE CEELS IN THE CANINE FUNDIC MUCOSA

Despite the central role for histamine in the regulation of gastric acid secretion, knowledge remains quite incomplete regarding the identity of the cells that store histamine within the gastric mucosa and the regulation of histamine formation and release. In the dog, morphologically typical mast cells appear to fully account for the histamine content present in the dispersed cells population (15). To determine the factors regulating histamine release, this small cell elutriator fraction was placed in overnight suspension culture and factors regulating histamine release then studied. These mast cells released histamine in response to a calcium ionophore that increases cytosolic calcium. Cross-linking of IgE receptors also induces histamine release. However, neither acetylcholine nor gastrin caused histamine release in this system. The absence of gastric and muscarinic receptors on canine fundic mast cells contrasted with their presence on fundic mucosal somatostatin cells, as discussed above. Of interest, mast cells also have two receptors that inhibit histamine release. Prostaglandin E_2 inhibited histamine release; concentrations above $10^{-7}M$ are necessary for this effect, but these levels may be achieved locally under certain circumstances. Additionally, adrenergic agents inhibit histamine release, acting at a $beta_2$ receptor site.

SOMATOSTATIN INHIBITION OF ACID SECRETION

In light of the above, the effects of somatostatin on acid secretion will be considered. Despite the potent antisecretory action of somatostatin (SRIF) the cellular mechanisms accounting for its effects remain uncertain. From present data, the antisecretory action of somatostatin probably reflects several components, the first of which is due to inhibition of gastrin release. Recent studies with isolated antral gastrin cells placed in short-term culture indicate a direct inhibitory effect of somatostatin on bombesin-stimulated gastrin release (16). However, the inhibitory effects of somatostatin also must reflect a direct action on the fundic mucosa, because in vivo SRIF also inhibits the acid secretory response to pentagastrin and cholinergic stimuli.

Several studies indicate that SRIF directly inhibits parietal cell function. Somatostatin inhibits histamine-stimulated aminopyrine accumulation by parietal cells isolated from rabbit, rat, and guinea pig (17,18,19) and by rabbit gastric glands (18,20). Somatostatin inhibits histamine-activation of adenylate cyclase; histamine-stimulated increases in cAMP are decreased over the same dose range in which inhibition of parietal cell function is found (17,19,21,22). The mechanism for this inhibition of adenylate cyclase by somatostatin has not been established, but it is likely to reflect interaction with the inhibitory GTP-binding protein of adenylate cyclase. It is of interest that in studies with canine parietal cells, somatostatin had either a very weak inhibitory effect against histamine (10% inhibition) (23), or no statistically significant effect (24; Soll, unpublished observations). In our studies, the weak inhibitory effect of somatostatin on histamine stimulation was found in cells which prostaglandins had marked inhibitory effects mediated via N_1 (10). The data indicating inhibition of histamine stimulation in these reductionistic in vitro systems are somewhat difficult to reconcile with data from in vivo studies; in the rat, dog, and cat somatostatin is a poor inhibitor of the response to exogenous histamine.

Somatostatin also inhibits the response of rabbit gastric glands to gastrin plus IBMX (18,20), but did not block the small response of isolated rabbit parietal cells to gastrin or to carbachol (18). These findings reflect an additional component of somatostatin action on rabbit gastric glands; somatostatin blocks pentagastrin and cholinergic stimulation of histamine release from cellular stores within the gastric gland (20). The sulfhydryl reducing agent dithiothreitol was found to enhance somatostatin action (18), although its presence was not essential for the somatostatin effect (20). In the rat (25) and presumably the rabbit, histamine in the fundic mucosa is stored in endocrine-like cells; it is these cells that presumably account for the somatostatin effects on histamine release. In our studies we found that mast cells accounted for the identified histamine stores in the fundic mucosa. However, although we found inhibitory prostaglandin and adrenergic receptors, as noted above, we failed to find inhibition of histamine release by somatostatin over a concentration range from 10 pM to 1 μM. These data contrast to the report that somatostatin inhibits histamine release from basophils (26).

A point that remains controversial is whether SRIF also directly inhibits the parietal cell response to gastrin and/or acetylcholine. SRIF inhibited the response to gastrin plus the phosphodiesterase inhibitor IBMX, but the inhibition was modest and required a higher dose range than one might expect from the in vivo potency of somatostatin (23). Others had previously not found somatostatin effects on canine parietal cells (24). In our studies with canine parietal cells, we also have not found reproducible somatostatin inhibition of carbachol- or gastrin-stimulated parietal cell function (A. H. Soll, D. Amirian, unpublished observation); this failure to find somatostatin inhibition did not reflect a failure of somatostatin to inhibit isolated canine cells; somatostatin markedly inhibited neurotensin and enteroglucagon release from ileal endocrine cells in short-term culture (27) and gastrin release from cultured antral G cells (16). Either the parietal cell response to somatostatin is impaired by the trauma of cell separation and culture, or another fundic somatostatin receptor remains to be identified.

Several other mechanisms have been proposed for mediating somatostatin action on acid secretion. One hypothesis was that somatostatin induced the production of prostaglandins (28). However, other studies failed to support the hypothesis that somatostatin acts via enhanced prostanoid production; indomethacin did not block somatostatin inhibition of rabbit gastric gland function (20) nor did indomethacin block somatostatin inhibition of acid secretion in vivo (29,30,31).

It is also quite possible that somatostatin has a neuromodulatory effect on acid secretion, inhibiting the release of a stimulatory neurotransmitter, such as acetylcholine. However, this possibility remains to be directly tested in the fundic mucosa.

OVERVIEW

The regulation of acid secretion is indeed complex, with several pathways and cell types involved. To further complicate the picture, receptors for several of these transmitters are present on more than one cell type. Examples of this point are the presence in canine fundic mucosa of gastrin and acetylcholine receptors on parietal cells, as well as on somatostatin and possibly other cells. Gastrin thus activates both stimulatory and inhibitory pathways regulating acid secretion via receptors on parietal cells and somatostatin cells respectively. In contrast, muscarinic receptors on the somatostatin cell attenuate release of this acid-inhibitory peptide while stimulating parietal cell function. Cholinergic input may therefore be an important balancing element in regulation of the secretory response. Anticholinergic agents may inhibit acid secretion by both enhancing somatostatin release and inhibiting the parietal cell. Receptors for somatostatin also are present on several cell types. Somatostatin inhibits release of gastrin via an antral G cell receptor. Somatostatin also appears to directly inhibit parietal cell function in response to histamine and possibly gastrin and acetylcholine. Somatostatin also blocks histamine release from rabbit gastric glands, presumably as a result of a direct effect on endocrine-like cells storing histamine. There are probably other somatostatin receptors that also contribute to its antisecretory action that remain to be identified.

REFERENCES

1. Soll AH, Berglindh T. Physiology of isolated gastric glands and cells: receptors and effectors regulating secretion. In: Johnson LR, ed. Physiology of gastrointestinal tract. New York: Raven Press, 1986 (in press).
2. Soll AH. Secretagogue stimulation of ^{14}C-aminopyrine accumulation by isolated canine parietal cells. Am J Physiol 1980; 238:G366-75.
3. Chew CS, Hersey SJ, Sachs G, Berglindh T. Histamine responsiveness of isolated gastric glands. Am J Physiol 1980; 238:G312-20.
4. Ecknauer R, Dial E, Thompson WJ, Johnson LR, Rosenfeld GC. Isolated rat gastric parietal cells: cholinergic response and pharmacology. Life Sci 1981; 28:609-21.
5. Soll AH, Amirian DA, Thomas LP, Reedy TJ, Elashoff JD. Gastrin receptors on isolated canine parietal cells. J Clin Invest 1984; 73:1434-47.
6. Soll AH. Potentiating interactions of gastric stimulants on ^{14}C-aminopyrine accumulation by isolated canine parietal cells. Gastroenterology 1982; 83:216-23.
7. Soll AH, Wollin A. Histamine and cyclic AMP in isolated canine parietal cells. Am J Physiol 1979; 237:E444-50
8. Soll AH. Specific inhibition by prostaglandins E_2 and I_2 of histamine-stimulated [^{14}C]aminopyrine accumulation and cyclic adenosine monophosphate generation by isolated canine parietal cells. J Clin Invest 1978; 65:1222-9.
9. Major JS, Scholes P. The localization of a histamine H_2-receptor adenylate cyclase system in canine parietal cells and its inhibition by prostaglandins. Agents Actions 1978; 8:324-31.
10. Soll AH, Chen M, Amirian DA, Toomey M, Sanders MJ. Enprostil and PGE_2 inhibition of canine parietal cells: mediation by the inhibitory GTP binding protein of adenylate cyclase [Abstract]. Gastroenterology 1986; 90(5):1642.
11. Soll AH. Extracellular calcium and cholinergic stimulation of isolated canine parietal cells. J Clin Invest 1981; 68:270-8.
12. Soll AH, Amirian DA, Thomas LP, Park J, Beaven MA, Yamada T. Gastrin receptors on nonparietal cells isolated from canine fundic mucosa. Am J Physiol 1984; 247(Gastrointest Liver Physiol 10):G715-23.
13. Soll AH, Yamada T, Park J, Thomas LP. Release of somatostatin-like immunoreactivity from canine fundic mucosal cells in primary culture. Am J Physiol 1984; 247(Gastrointest Liver Physiol 10):G567-73.
14. Yamada T, Soll AH, Park J, Elashoff J. Autonomic regulation of somatostatin release: studies with primary cultures of canine fundic

mucosal cells. Am J Physiol 1984; 247(Gastrointest Liver Physiol 10):G567-73.

15. Soll AH, Lewin K, Beaven MA. Isolation of histamine containing cells from canine fundic mucosa. Gastroenterology 1979; 77:1283-90.

16. Giraud AS, Walsh JH, Soll AH. Prostanoids of the PGE_2 series differentially affect gastrin (G) release from canine G-cells in short term culture [Abstract]. Gastroenterology 1986; 90(5):1428.

17. Batzri S. Direct action of somatostatin on dispersed mucosal cells from guinea pig stomach. Biochem Biophys Acta 1981; 677:521-4.

18. Chew CS. Inhibitory action of somatostatin on isolated gastric glands and parietal cells. Am J Physiol 1983; 245 (Gastrointest Liver Physiol 8):G221-9.

19. Schepp W, Heim H-K, Ruoff H-J. Comparison of the effect of PGE_2 and somatostatin on histamine stimulated ^{14}C-aminopyrine uptake and cyclic AMP formation in isolated rat gastric mucosal cells. Agents Actions 1983; 13(2/3):200-6.

20. Nylander O, Bergqvist E, Obrink KJ. Dual inhibitory actions of somatostatin on isolated gastric glands. Acta Physiol Scand 1985; 125:111-9.

21. Gespach C, Bouhours D, Bouhours JF, Rosselin G. Histamine interaction on surface recognition sites of H_2-type in parietal and non-parietal cells isolated from the guinea pig stomach. FEBS Lett 1982; 149:85-90.

22. Becker M, Ruoff H-J. Inhibition by prostaglandin E_2, somatostatin and secretin of histamine-sensitive adenylate cyclase in human gastric mucosa. Digestion 1982; 23:194-200.

23. Chiba T, Park J, Yamada T. Glucagon and vasoactive intestinal polypeptide stimulate somatostatin secretion from isolated canine fundic mucosal cell cultures. Gastroenterology 1985; 88(5):1348.

24. Perez-Reyes E, Payne NA, Gerber JG. Effect of somatostatin, secretin, and glucagon on secretagogue stimulated aminiopyrine uptake in isolated canine parietal cells. Agents Actions 1983; 13(4):265-8.

25. Soll AH, Lewin KJ, Beaven MA. Isolation of histamine-containing cells from rat gastric mucosa: biochemical and morphologic differences from mast cells. Gastroenterology 1981; 80:717-27.

26. Goetzl EJ, Payan DG. Inhibition by somatostatin of the release of mediators from human basophils and rat leukemic basophils. J Immunol 1984; 133:3255-9.

27. Barber DJ, Buchan AMJ, Walsh JH, Soll AH. Regulation of neurotensin release from canine enteric primary cell cultures. Am J Physiol 1986; 250:G385-90.

28. Ligumsky M, Goto Y, Debas H, Yamada T. Prostaglandins mediate inhibition of gastric acid secretion by somatostatin in the rat. Science 1983; 219:301-3.

29. Mogard MH, Maxwell V, Kovacs T, et al. Somatostatin inhibits gastric acid secretion after gastric mucosal prostaglandin synthesis inhibition by indomethacin in man. Gut 1985; 26:1189-91.

30. Mogard MH, Kauffman GL Jr, Pehlevanian M, Golanska E, Elashoff JD, Walsh JH. Prostaglandins may not mediate inhibition of gastric acid secretion by somatostatin in the rat. Regul Pept 1985; 10:231-6.

31. Feldman M, Colturi TJ. Effect of indomethacin on gastric acid and bicarbonate secretion in humans. Gastroenterology 1984; 87:1339-43.

26

SOMATOSTATIN IN GASTROINTESTINAL FUNCTION:

INTESTINAL ABSORPTION AND SECRETION

Kiertisin Dharmsathaphorn

Department of Medicine, University of California
San Diego Medical Center, San Diego, California 92103

INTRODUCTION

Somatostatin, a 14-amino acid peptide with a growth hormone release inhibition property, was initially isolated from sheep hypothalami (1). Later, the peptide was isolated or detected in many organ systems of all mammalians as well as lower animals. Different molecular forms of somatostatin have been recognized. In the intestine, somatostatin-containing cells, the D cells, are widely distributed in the gastrointestinal mucosa, with the highest number found in the upper intestine. These cells are located in the region of the crypt of Lieberkuhn and are in contact with the gut lumen (2-4). Beneath the epithelial cells of the intestine, in the lamina propria, somatostatin is widely distributed in the neural elements, e.g., the submucosal plexus, myenteric plexus, and vagus nerve (3-6).

Somatostatin undoubtedly has a wide spectrum of functions in the gut. It inhibits the release and/or function of a large variety of regulatory peptides in the intestine. Examples include gastrin, secretin, cholecystokinin, vasoactive intestinal polypeptide, gastric inhibitory polypeptide, motilin, pancreatic polypeptide, and enteroglucagon (7-12). Somatostatin-containing cells are in close proximity to other endocrine cells and may directly affect their secretion (13). Alternatively, somatostatin may inhibit the action of the hormones released by these endocrine cells. Besides its possible paracrine or neurocrine functions, somatostatin may also have a classical endocrine function. This is suggested by the detection of somatostatin-like immunoreactivity in portal blood in response to stimuli (14-16). Although many pharmacological actions of somatostatin have been observed, the physiological roles of somatostatin are yet to be defined. This chapter discusses only the effect of somatostatin on intestinal water and electrolyte absorption without taking into consideration the effect of somatostatin on gut motility or other factors. In the future, when the relation between these other factors and intestinal transport mechanisms is better understood, a discussion will have to take these factors into account.

INTESTINAL WATER AND ELECTROLYTE TRANSPORT

The following discussion will emphasize the intestinal antisecretory function of somatostatin in the intestine. This property of somatostatin

has been observed in the small and large intestine of a variety of animals, including man. In the rat, somatostatin inhibits PGE_1- and the-
ophylline-induced water and electrolyte secretion, while having little or
no effect on unstimulated intestine (17-19) (Fig. 1). Similar antisecretory effects have been observed in the rabbit and dog intestine (20-22).
In man, somatostatin inhibits water secretion, particularly that caused by
over-production of endogenous peptides or other regulatory substances.
Similar to the rat, somatostatin has little or no significant effect at
the basal state in man (23-26). Since somatostatin appears to inhibit
hypersecretory states, while having little or no effect in normal subjects, we believe that it inhibits or interferes with the secretory
process after secretion has been initiated. Alternatively, somatostatin
may restore the absorptive function which is impaired by the disease
process. Unfortunately, little is known about the effect of somatostatin
on intestinal absorptive functions. Our recent study, utilizing a crypt
cell-like human colonic cell line which exhibits only secretory properties, provides support for an antisecretory effect of somatostatin (27).
In this study, somatostatin partially reversed VIP-, PGE_1-, or A23187-
induced short circuit current, which reflects chloride and water secretion
(28-30). The mechanisms by which somatostatin reverses or inhibits
chloride secretion in the intestine are not yet determined. The fact that
somatostatin affects both cAMP- and Ca^{++}-mediated secretion without
altering the cAMP or free cytosolic calcium levels suggest that somatostatin inhibits an intermediate step in the secretory process common to
both cAMP- and Ca^{++}-mediated secretion. This may occur at the very distal
step in the chloride secretory process, i.e., at the electrolyte transport
pathways. A number of transport pathways, including the Na^+ K^+, Cl^-
cotransport, K^+ channels and Cl^- channels have been shown to be intimately

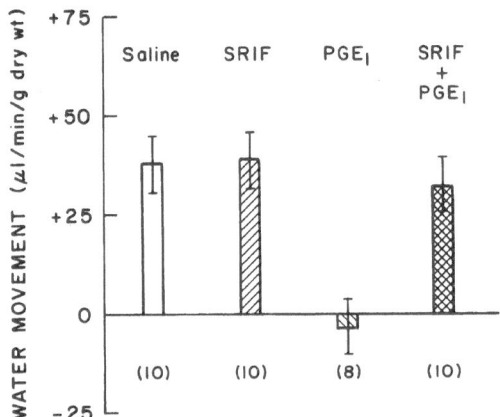

Fig. 1. The effect of somatostatin (SRIF) on water
secretion induced by prostaglandin E_1 (PGE_1) in the
rat jejunum. Water absorption was determined over
45-min intervals, utilizing jejunal perfusion techniques. Basal absorption (saline) was determined
before SRIF (10 µg/ kg/min) or PGE_1 (5 µg/kg/minute)
infusions. PGE_1 abolished net water absorption and
caused a small net secretion. Pretreatment with
somatostatin (SRIF + PGE_1) inhibited the response to
PGE_1. (Adapted from Gastroenterology 1980; 78:1554.)

involved in the chloride secretory process. Somatostatin may interfere with the function of any one of these pathways. It is also possible that regulation by somatostatin occurs at the protein kinase or other secondary messenger level. The homogeneity of cultured cells allows better elucidation of the mechanism of action of somatostatin once the secretory mechanism itself is well understood.

CLINICAL APPLICATION OF SOMATOSTATIN IN DIGESTIVE DISEASE

The effectiveness of somatostatin has been demonstrated in patients suffering from severe watery diarrhea due to carcinoid syndrome (23,24) (Fig. 2), VIPoma (25), colonic pseudoobstruction (31), and short bowel syndrome (32). The fact that somatostatin is quite effective in controlling diarrhea in a wide variety of illnesses suggests its potential as an antidiarrheal agent. However, the use of somatostatin in clinical medicine is limited by two drawbacks. One is the lack of an orally active form, and thus the need for intravenous or intramuscular injection. Another is the concern regarding the side effects of somatostatin on other organ systems. Fortunately, the side effects usually are minor. Only elevation of blood sugar levels is potentially troublesome (23,28).

Synthesis of somatostatin analogs, which are smaller and more resistant to digestion by intestinal peptides, may allow the drug to be administered orally. The intestine can absorb a small amount of peptide hormones intact, although little is known about the mechanism of absorption and the structural requirements. Clinical trials of other orally-active peptides, e.g., enkephalin analog, may provide useful information

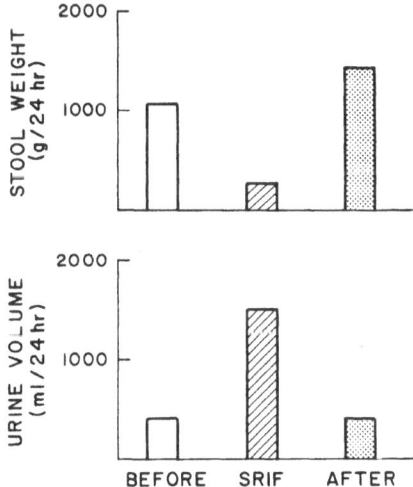

Fig. 2. The effect of somatostatin (SRIF) infusion (4 µg/min) on fecal and urinary excretion in patient with the carcinoid syndrome and diarrhea. Stool weight decreased significantly on the day that somatostatin was infused and diarrhea recurred with discontinuation of somatostatin infusion. The reverse was observed with the urine volume. (Adapted from Ann Int Med 1980; 92:68.)

269

applicable to somatostatin. As a matter of fact, cyclic hexapeptide analogs of somatostatin have been administered orally in animals with encouraging results (33).

Regarding the systemic side effects, it may be possible to eliminate many side effects provided that: (1) receptors for somatostatin in the intestine are different from receptors in other organs and (2) gut specific somatostatin analog can be developed. Different structural requirements for somatostatin's action in different organ systems suggest the feasibility of developing a gut selective analog (34-39). In collaboration with Dr. Jean Rivier, Dr. Wylie Vale, and Dr. Marvin Brown, we have tested a series of somatostatin analogs for intestinal action (40). In this study, each amino acid in the somatostatin molecule was systematically substituted, deleted, or altered. The potency of each analog for ion transport was determined in the rabbit ileum and rat colon using the modified Ussing chamber technique. Results were then compared to the non-enteric effect of somatostatin, including inhibition of the stimulated release of growth hormone from cultured rat anterior pituitary cells and inhibition of arginine stimulated insulin and glucagon release in the rat in vivo (see Table 1). We found that substitution with L-alanine, or deletion of amino acids at Phe^6, Phe^7, Trp^8, and Lys^9 in the somatostatin molecule, or deletion of Thr^{10}, reduced the ion transport property as well as the inhibition of growth hormone, insulin, and glucagon releases to near zero. This indicates that Phe^6, Phe^7, Trp^8, and Lys^9 are necessary for somatostatin receptor binding, while Thr^{10} may serve as an essential spacer. More importantly, we have observed that substitution or deletion of Phe^{11} and substitution with alanine or the D-isomer at Lys^4 resulted in compounds with selective intestinal ion transport properties. These analogs demonstrated little or no inhibition of insulin or glucagon release. Therefore, Phe^{11} and Lys^4 do not appear to be critical for the electrolyte transport property in the rabbit ileum and rat colon, as they

Table 1. Relative potency of somatostatin analogs.

| Analog | Release inhibition of | | | Ion transport | |
	Growth hormone	Insulin	Glucagon	Rat colon	Rabbit ileum
Somatostatin (S-14)	100	100	100	100	100
$[D-Lys^4]$-S-14	22	1	1	100	139
$[Ala^4]$-S-14	60	12	12	Not tested	94
$[Ala^{11}]$-S-14	3	<10	<10	27	52
des-Phe^{11}-S-14	2	< 1	< 1	9	34

Ion transport potencies were obtained from the rat colon and rabbit ileum in vitro utilizing the Ussing chamber technique. Inhibition of the stimulated release of growth hormone was obtained from cultured rat anterior pituitary cells in vitro and inhibition of arginine-stimulated insulin and glucagon release from the rat in vivo. (Adapted from J Clin Invest 1983; 71: 840.)

are for some other endocrine effects. Alteration of either one of these amino acids results in gut-specific analogs in the rat and rabbit. Whether these results also apply to man still remains to be tested. These results suggest that somatostatin receptor subtypes in the gut may be different from those in other organs and that it may be possible to design a gut-specific analog. Hopefully, further development of somatostatin analogs will make clinical use of somatostatin in diarrheal diseases more realistic.

ACKNOWLEDGMENT

This study was supported by grant AM 28305 from the National Institutes of Health. Dr. K. Dharmsathaphorn is the recipient of an NIH Research Career Development Award AM 1146 and an American Gastroenterological Association/Glaxo Research Scholar Award. We would like to thank Mr. Gary L. Deming who typed the manuscript.

REFERENCES

1. Brazeau P, Vale W, Burgus R, et al. Hypothalamic polypeptide that inhibits the secretion of immunoreactive pituitary growth hormone. Science 1973; 179:77.
2. Polak JM, Pearse AGE, Grimelius L, Bloom SR, Arimura A. Growth hormone release-inhibiting hormone in gastrointestinal and pancreatic D cells. Lancet 1977; 1:1220.
3. Ferri G-L, Adrian TE, Ghatei MA, et al. Tissue localization and relative distribution of regulatory peptides in separated layers from the human bowel. Gastroenterology 1983; 84:777.
4. Penman E, Wass JAH, Butler MG, et al. Distribution and characterization of immunoreactive somatostatin in human gastrointestinal tract. Regul Pept 1983; 7:53.
5. Hokfelt T, Schultzberg M, Johansson O, et al. Central and peripheral peptide producing neurons. In: Bloom SR, ed. Gut hormones. Edinburgh: Churchill Livingstone, 1978:423.
6. Uvnas-Wallenstein K, Efendic S, Luft R. The occurrence of somatostatin-like immunoreactivity in the vagal nerves. Acta Physiol Scand 1978; 102:248.
7. Konturek SJ, Tasler J, Cieszkowski M, Coy DH, Schally AV. Effect of growth hormone release-inhibiting hormone on gastric secretion, mucosal blood flow and serum gastrin. Gastroenterology 1976; 70:737.
8. Boden G, Sivitz MC, Owen EO, Essa-Koumar N, Landor JH. Somatostatin suppresses secretin and pancreatic exocrine secretion. Science 1975; 190:163.
9. Konturek SJ, Tasler J, Obtulowicz W, Coy DH, Schally AV. Effect of growth hormone-release inhibiting hormone on hormones stimulating exocrine pancreatic secretion. J Clin Invest 1976; 58:1.
10. Mitznegg P, Bloom SR, Domschke W, Domschke S, Wunsch E, Demling L. Pharmacokinetics of motilin in man. Gastroenterology 1977; 72:413.
11. Kayasseh L, Haecki WH, Gyr K, et al. The endogenous release of pancreatic polypeptide by acid and meal in dogs. Scand J Gastroenterol 1978; 13:385.
12. Gerich JE, Patton GS. Somatostatin. Physiology and clinical applications. Med Clin North Am 1978; 62:375.
13. Larsson LI, Goltermann N, DeMagistris L, Rehfeld JF, Schwartz TW. Somatostatin cell process as pathways for paracrine secretion. Science 1979; 205:1393.
14. Schusdziarra V, Harris V, Conlon JM, Arimura A, Unger R. Pancreatic and gastric somatostatin release in response to intragastric and

intraduodenal nutrients and HCl in the dog. J Clin Invest 1978; 62:509.

15. Penman E, Wass JAH, Medbak S, et al. Response of circulating immuno-reactive somatostatin to nutritional stimuli in normal subjects. Gastroenterology 1981; 81:692.

16. Rouiller D, Schusdziarra V, Conlon JM, Harris V, Unger RH. Release of somatostatin-like immunoreactivity from the lower gut. Gastro-enterology 1979; 77:700.

17. Dharmsathaphorn K, Sherwin RS, Dobbins JW. Somatostatin inhibits fluid secretion in the rat jejunum. Gastroenterology 1980; 78:1554.

18. Carter RF, Bitar KN, Zfass AM, Makhlouf GM. Inhibition of VIP-stimulated intestinal secretion and cyclic AMP production by somato-statin in the rat. Gastroenterology 1978; 74:726.

19. Dharmsathaphorn K, Racusen L, Dobbins JW. Effect of somatostatin on ion transport in the rat colon. J Clin Invest 1980; 66:813.

20. Dharmsathaphorn K, Binder HJ, Dobbins JW, Leo L. Somatostatin stimulates sodium and chloride absorption in the rabbit ileum. Gastroenterology 1980; 78:1559.

21. Guandalini S, Kachur JF, Smith PL, Miller RJ, Field M. In vitro effects of somatostatin on ion transport in rabbit intestine. Am J Physiol 1980; 238:G67.

22. Barbezat GO, Reasbeck PG. Somatostatin inhibition of glucagon-stimulated jejunal secretion in the dog. Gastroenterology 1981; 81:471.

23. Dharmsathaphorn K, Sherwin RS, Cataland S, Jaffe B, Dobbins J. Somatostatin inhibits diarrhea in the carcinoid syndrome. Ann Intern Med 1980; 92:68.

24. Davis GR, Camp RC, Raskin P, Krejs GJ. Effect of somatostatin infusion on jejunal water and electrolyte transport in a patient with secretory diarrhea due to malignant carcinoid syndrome. Gastro-enterology 1980; 78:346.

25. Ruskone A, Rene E, Chayvialle JA, et al. Effect of somatostatin on diarrhea and on small intestinal water and electrolyte transport in a patient with pancreatic cholera. Dig Dis Sci 1982; 27:459.

26. Krejs GJ, Browne R, Raskin P. Effect of intravenous somatostatin on jejunal absorption of glucose, amino acids, water, and electrolytes. Gastroenterology 1980; 78:26.

27. Dharmsathaphorn K, McRoberts JA, Mandel KG, Tisdale LD, Masui H. A human colonic tumor cell line that maintains vectorial electrolyte transport. Am J Physiol 1984; 246:G204.

28. Dharmsathaphorn K, McRoberts JA, Masui H, Mandel KG. VIP-induced chloride secretion by a colonic epithelial cell line: direct partic-ipation of a basolaterally localized Na^+,K^+,Cl^- cotransport system. J Clin Invest 1985; 75:462.

29. Mandel KG, McRoberts JA, Beuerlein G, Foster ES, Dharmsathaphorn K. Ba^{++} inhibition of VIP and A23187 stimulated Cl^- secretion by T_{84} cell monolayers. Am J Physiol 1986; 259:C486.

30. Weymer A, Huott P, McRoberts JA, Dharmsathaphorn K. Chloride secre-tory mechanism induced by prostaglandin E_1 in a colonic epithelial cell line. J Clin Invest 1985; 76:1828.

31. Mulvihill S, Passaro E Jr, Debas H, Yamada T. Severe diarrhea after colonic pseudo-obstruction: treatment with somatostatin. N Engl J Med 1984; 310:467.

32. Dharmsathaphorn K, Gorelick FS, Sherwin RS, Cataland S, Dobbins JW. Somatostatin decreases diarrhea in patients with the short-bowel syndrome. J Clin Gastroenterol 1982; 4:521.

33. Veber DF, Freidinger RM, Schwenk Perlow D, et al. A potent cyclic hexapeptide analogue of somatostatin. Nature 1981; 292:58.

34. Murphy WA, Meyers CA, Coy DH. Potent, highly selective inhibition of growth hormone secretion by position 4 somatostatin analogs. Endo-crinology 1981; 109:491.

35. Meyers CA, Coy DH, Murphy W, Redding TW, Arimura A, Schally AV. [Phe[4]] Somatostatin: a potent, selective inhibitor of growth hormone release. Proc Natl Acad Sci USA 1980; 77:577.
36. Sarantakis D, McKinley WA, Jaunakais I, Clark D, Grant NH. Structure activity studies on somatostatin. Clin Endocrinol 1976; 5:275.
37. Brown M, Rivier J, Vale W. Somatostatin: analogs with selected biological activities. Science 1977; 196:1467.
38. Vale W, Rivier J, Brown M. Biologic and immunologic activities and applications of somatostatin analogs. Metabolism 1978; 27:1391.
39. Brown M, Rivier J, Vale W. Somatostatin: central nervous system action on glucoregulation. Endocrinology 1979; 104:1709.
40. Rosenthal LE, Yamashiro DJ, Rivier J, Vale W, Brown M, Dharmsathaphorn K. Structure-activity relationships of somatostatin analogs in the rabbit ileum and the rat colon. J Clin Invest 1983; 71:840.

27

EFFECT OF SOMATOSTATIN ON EXOCRINE PANCREAS

Travis E. Solomon

Departments of Medicine and Physiology,
University of Missouri Medical School, and
Research Service, Truman VA Hospital, Columbia, MO

The exocrine pancreas serves an important function in digestion and absorption of nutrients by secreting digestive enzymes into the lumen of the small intestine. Pancreatic secretion of fluid and bicarbonate aids the digestive function of these enzymes by providing an appropriate intraluminal pH for their action, as well as protecting intestinal mucosa from damage by neutralizing gastric acid. Although most attention has been focused on stimulatory factors which regulate exocrine pancreatic secretion, there is also evidence which supports an inhibitory component in overall regulation of pancreatic enzyme and bicarbonate production. Somatostatin is one candidate for mediation of physiologic inhibition of the exocrine pancreas because of its known effects on secretory responses to endogenous and exogenous stimulants. Somatostatin may also affect growth of the exocrine pancreas. Therefore, characterization of the role of somatostatin as a regulator of the exocrine pancreas has important implications for understanding both normal and abnormal pancreatic function.

Evidence for inhibitory factors which mediate pancreatic responses to a meal and intraluminal nutrients has recently been reviewed in detail (1). Most of the relevant studies on this topic have been performed using dogs or humans as experimental subjects. In both species, the maximal pancreatic enzyme response to exogenous cholecystokinin (CCK) is a reproducible measure of maximal secretory capacity since there is no evidence for additive or potentiated effects of other stimulants and CCK (2,3). The maximal bicarbonate secretory response to exogenous secretin is also a useful and reproducible measurement in these two species, but it underestimates the maximal capacity of the pancreas to secrete bicarbonate because there are potentiating interactions among secretin, CCK, and cholinergic mechanisms (2,3). Enzyme and bicarbonate responses to a meal are distinctly submaximal when compared to CCK- and secretin-induced maximal responses in the same subjects (4,5). Submaximal pancreatic enzyme secretion is also observed during sham feeding (6), distention of a gastric pouch with food (7), and intestinal perfusion with amino acids (8,9). One of several possible explanations for these observations is that each type of pancreatic stimulation also releases an inhibitory hormone or local pancreatic or intestinal inhibitory peptide which counteracts the stimulatory actions of CCK, cholinergic reflexes, secretin, and other factors thought to mediate pancreatic secretion in response to food. Other observations which suggest the existence of a circulating or intrapancreatic factor which inhibits the exocrine pancreas include: (1) suppression of CCK- and secretin-induced secretion by intestinal perfusion with hypertonic solutions (10), and (2) similar suppression of stimulated enzyme and bicarbonate secretion by intraileal administration of fatty acids (11). (3) Finally, intravenous administration of glucose (12) or amino acids (13,14) to simulate the postabsorptive phase of a meal has been shown to inhibit exocrine pancreatic secretion.

While these observations suggest the existence of an inhibitory component of the regulatory mechanisms for exocrine pancreatic secretion, the factors which mediate this inhibition and the details of their method of action on the pancreas are poorly characterized. Evidence for and against somatostatin being one such inhibitory factor will be presented here.

ACTION OF SOMATOSTATIN ON EXOCRINE PANCREATIC SECRETION

Administration of somatostatin has been shown in many studies to inhibit exocrine pancreatic responses to many different stimulants in several species. It is important in such studies to distinguish between the effects of somatostatin on pancreatic response to exogenous stimulants such as intravenous CCK and secretin and endogenous stimulation by meals and intraluminal substances, since in the latter case somatostatin may act to inhibit the release of hormones and other factors from the intestine as well as the action of these mediators on the pancreas. Useful information could also be gained from comparing the sensitivity of the pancreas and other target organs to exogenous somatostatin under identical conditions in the same subjects and comparing the sensitivity of intestinal hormone release versus hormone action to somatostatin. Very little information of this type is available. There are also only a few studies which have examined multiple doses of exogenous somatostatin and endogenous and exogenous pancreatic stimulants. In some cases this has led to erroneous conclusions about the ability of somatostatin to inhibit exocrine pancreatic secretion.

Exogenous Stimulants

In vivo administration of somatostatin inhibits pancreatic bicarbonate secretion in response to exogenous secretin in humans (15,16), dogs (17,18), and cats (19). In rats, somatostatin has been reported to have little (20) or no (21,22) effect on bicarbonate responses to large doses of secretin. The inhibitory effect of somatostatin is most pronounced when low doses of secretin are studied in humans (16) and dogs (17,18), probably accounting for the apparent lack of somatostatin-induced inhibition in the rat experiments and in other studies in humans (23) and dogs (24) which used only very large doses of secretin.

Exogenous somatostatin also strongly decreases the pancreatic enzyme response to exogenous CCK in humans (23), dogs (18), rats (22), and rabbits (25), and inhibition is most pronounced at low doses of CCK (18). Somatostatin has also been reported to inhibit the enzyme response to exogenous acetylcholine (22), electrical stimulation of the vagus nerves (22), and exogenous bombesin (26).

From available data, it seems clear that exogenous somatostatin produces strong inhibition of the primary mediators of pancreatic bicarbonate secretion (secretin) and enzyme secretion (CCK, acetylcholine). The question of whether somatostatin has more marked effects on bicarbonate versus enzyme secretion is unanswered because no comparable detailed dose response studies which include very low doses of stimulants have been done. The effects of somatostatin on other possible mediators of pancreatic secretion in vivo (such as VIP, motilin, and neurotensin) have not been reported.

Endogenous Stimulants

Basal pancreatic secretion in vivo is strongly inhibited by exogenous somatostatin (18,21), an effect which must be taken into account when assessing inhibition of responses to exogenous stimulants. Particularly for enzyme secretion, basal outputs may be a significant portion of stimulated outputs; somatostatin could appear to inhibit the response to a stimulant when in fact it has only removed the basal component of secretion. In a single report, giving a very large bolus dose of somatostatin increased basal pancreatic enzyme secretion in rats (27); this is not likely to be a physiologically important effect.

Exogenous somatostatin has been found to inhibit both bicarbonate and enzyme secretion in response to a normally ingested solid meal (17,28). This inhibitory effect is probably due to many actions of somatostatin, both directly on the pancreas and indirectly on gastric secretion, gastro-intestinal motility, release of hormones, and initiation of reflexes. An example of the difficulty in interpreting such results is a report that a somatostatin analog decreased plasma secretin and pancreatic bicarbonate responses to a meal in dogs (29). In addition to a direct effect on secretin release, somatostatin may have inhibited gastric acid secretion and gastric emptying, both of which could lead to decreased release of secretin.

The effect of somatostatin on components of the pancreatic secretory response to food—the cephalic, gastric, and intestinal phases—are more amenable to interpretation. However, there has been limited investigation of this area. An analog of somatostatin has been reported to cause marked inhibition of sham feeding-induced pancreatic enzyme secretion (29). Sham feeding is thought to stimulate pancreatic secretion mainly by activating efferent vagal cholinergic fibers in the pancreas (1), indicating that the inhibitory effect of somatostatin is due to inhibition of ganglionic transmission or release of acetylcholine by postganglionic fibers or the action of acetylcholine on acinar cells. There have been no studies on the effect of somatostatin on the gastric phase of pancreatic secretion. The major activators of the intestinal phase of pancreatic secretion in most species are intraluminal acid, amino acids and peptides, and fatty acids and monoglycerides (1). Exogenous somatostatin has been shown to inhibit pancreatic bicarbonate secretion in response to intestinal perfusion with HCl (17) and enzyme secretion in response to amino acids (17) and sodium oleate (17). The bicarbonate response to intestinal acid is thought to be due to release of secretin into the circulation, with potentiation of secretin's effects by cholinergic intrapancreatic neurons (1). In addition to the above described inhibition of the pancreatic response to secretin by somatostatin, it has also been reported that somatostatin inhibits acid-induced release of secretin (30). There have been no detailed comparisons of the sensitivity to somatostatin of secretin release versus secretin-induced bicarbonate secretion. There is also no information on whether somatostatin interferes with the cholinergic component of acid-induced bicarbonate secretion.

The pancreatic enzyme response to intestinal amino acids and fatty acids is thought to be due to activation of a vago-vagal, cholinergic reflex from intestine to pancreas and by the release of CCK into the circulation (1). There is no published information to indicate whether somatostatin inhibits some aspect of reflex stimulation of enzyme secretion other than by inhibiting the action of acetylcholine on acinar cells

277

as described above. There is also no reliable information on the effect of somatostatin on CCK release; only recently have sensitive, specific assays for plasma CCK become available, and they have not been applied to this question. The notion that somatostatin inhibits CCK release because the pancreatic response to intestinal amino acids or fatty acid is inhibited (17) cannot be accepted until actual measurements of plasma CCK levels are made.

Two other hormones which may regulate exocrine pancreatic enzyme secretion are motilin (31) and neurotensin (32). Surges of motilin secretion in the basal state are correlated with cyclic increases in enzyme secretion in dogs, and exogenous motilin initiates an "early" peak of enzyme secretion (31). Somatostatin has been demonstrated to block the cyclic pattern of plasma motilin levels (33), perhaps accounting for some of the inhibition of basal pancreatic secretion noted above. Whether somatostatin also blocks the secretory response to exogenous motilin has not been determined. Plasma levels of neurotensin increase in response to intestinal perfusion with fatty acid (32), and exogenous neurotensin stimulates both enzyme and bicarbonate secretion (32). Somatostatin blocks fatty acid-induced neurotensin release (34), but the effect of somatostatin on the pancreatic response to neurotensin has not been examined.

HORMONAL VERSUS LOCAL EFFECTS OF SOMATOSTATIN

Somatostatin could act as both an endocrine (circulating) and paracrine (local) inhibitor of (1) the release of intestinal factors which stimulate exocrine pancreatic secretion, and (2) of the action of these factors on the pancreas. Most information available to date concerns the role of somatostatin as a circulating inhibitor of exocrine pancreatic secretion, reflecting the simpler nature of examining this mechanism.

Hormonal Effects of Somatostatin

If somatostatin acts as a circulating inhibitor of the release of pancreatic stimulants or their effects on pancreatic secretion, it should be possible to fulfill several criteria regarding such an action. (1) Plasma levels of somatostatin should increase in situations where inhibition is known to occur. (2) Copying these plasma levels of somatostatin by exogenous infusion of the same molecular form of endogenous somatostatin should reproduce the inhibition. (3) Specific blockade of somatostatin release should remove the inhibition. (4) Removal of circulating somatostatin (such as by immunoneutralization) or blocking its action by a specific receptor antagonist should remove the inhibition. (5) A target cell population with receptors of the correct affinity and efficacy for several analogs of somatostatin should be demonstrable. Only the first two of these criteria have been satisfied to any degree at present.

Is somatostatin released into the circulation in situations where inhibition of exocrine pancreatic secretion may occur? The answers are yes for systemic plasma somatostatin levels after a normal solid meal in dogs (35,36) and humans (37) and sham feeding in dogs (38), no for intestinal perfusion with L-phenylalanine (36), and not studied for other situations. Are the plasma levels of somatostatin sufficient to account for inhibition of pancreatic secretion? In dogs, infusion of exogenous somatostatin-14 at rates of 200 to 400 pmol/kg/hour or somatostatin-28 at about 40 pmol/kg/hour reproduces postprandial plasma somatostatin levels (35,39). Intravenous infusion of doses of somatostatin in these ranges clearly inhibits pancreatic bicarbonate and enzyme secretion in response to exogenous secretin and CCK (24,35). The inhibitory effects of somato-

278

statin-14 and -28 appeared to be similar at equivalent plasma levels (35). There have been no studies in humans or other species with infusion of somatostatin doses shown to reproduce postprandial levels of plasma somatostatin. There have also been no studies in any species to indicate whether physiologic doses of somatostatin-14 or -28 inhibit pancreatic secretion elicited by endogenous factors during the cephalic, gastric, or intestinal phases.

Local Effects of Somatostatin

Somatostatin is present in both endocrine cells and neurons of the enteric nervous system in the small intestine (40,41). While it is possible that both these pools of intestinal somatostatin might act locally to inhibit the release of secretin and CCK or to inhibit some aspect of the enteropancreatic reflex, there is no evidence at present which confirms or denies this possibility.

Several observations suggest that somatostatin present in D-cells in the endocrine pancreas may act locally on the exocrine pancreas. Pancreatic D-cells have cellular projections which end on islet capillaries (42), implying that selective release of somatostatin could occur into these islet capillaries. It has been demonstrated that islet capillaries are the first arborization in an intrapancreatic, insular-exocrine portal system (43) and that most or all of islet capillary blood flows into venules which arborize again to supply exocrine duct and acinar cells (44). Finally, the pancreas has been shown to selectively extract a much larger proportion of arterial somatostatin compared to insulin or glucagon (45,46). Thus, the much higher concentrations of somatostatin which probably occur in capillary plasma in some areas of the exocrine pancreas could act locally to suppress neurotransmitter release from cholinergic and peptidergic neurons or to directly inhibit duct and acinar cell secretion. Again, no other evidence exists to confirm or deny this possibility.

MECHANISM OF SOMATOSTATIN-INDUCED INHIBITION

The site and mechanism of action of somatostatin-induced inhibition of pancreatic responses to endogenous and exogenous stimulants is unknown. So little is known about a possible effect of somatostatin on release of intestinal endocrine and neural mediators that further discussion is unwarranted.

Two classes of receptors for somatostatin have been demonstrated using isolated pancreatic acini from guinea pigs in vitro (47,48). One receptor possesses almost equal affinity for somatostatin-14 and -28, has an EC_{50} of about 0.5 nM for somatostatin-14, and is sensitive to extracellular calcium (47). The second class of receptors actually appears to be a CCK receptor to which somatostatin-28 binds with low affinity (48); somatostatin-14 does not bind to this receptor (48). In spite of the existence of two different binding sites for somatostatin on acinar cells, neither somatostatin-14 or -28 inhibits the enzyme secretory response to cerulein, secretin, or VIP in guinea pig pancreatic acini in vitro (48). In fact, very high concentrations of somatostatin-28 actually stimulated enzyme secretion (48), probably due to crossreactivity with the CCK receptor. It has also been reported that somatostatin-14 did not inhibit bicarbonate or enzyme secretion in response to secretin and carbachol in an isolated, arterially perfused preparation of cat pancreas (49). Two other reports indicate that somatostatin-14 does not inhibit enzyme secretory response to a large concentration of CCK in rat pancreas fragments in vitro (50), but that somatostatin-14 and -28 did inhibit basal amylase secretion, the amylase response to a low concentration of secretin, and the potentiated amylase response to secretin plus insulin in rat pancreatic acini in vitro (51). Somatostatin has also been shown to inhibit the increase in cellular cyclic AMP levels induced by secretin and VIP in rat pancreatic duct cells in vitro (52) and guinea pig acini in vitro (48). Although cyclic AMP is thought to mediate acinar cell enzyme response to secretin and VIP, the lack of inhibition of enzyme secretion by somatostatin in guinea pig acini in the face of inhibition of cyclic AMP levels makes this observation difficult to interpret. Overall, it would appear that somatostatin does not act directly on pancreatic acinar duct cells to inhibit their secretory responses to stimulants. It should be kept in mind, however, that the direct in vitro effects of somatostatin on pancreatic secretion have been examined only in species in which there is little or no information about the in vivo actions of somatostatin, not all agonists for enzyme secretion have been studied in detail for sensitivity to inhibition by somatostatin, and the effects of somatostatin on acinar cell response to combinations of stimulants have not been characterized. Nevertheless, the difficulty in demonstrating a direct effect of somatostatin on pancreatic exocrine secretory cells, compared to the relative ease with which this can be shown in other primary targets of somatostatin, strongly suggests that inhibition of pancreatic response to stimulants by somatostatin must occur through an indirect mechanism.

Of several hypothetical mechanisms for an indirect effect of somatostatin on the exocrine pancreas—release of a second inhibitory peptide or neurotransmitter, release of a local inhibitor such as a prostaglandin in in vivo but not in vitro preparations, suppression of circulating factors which augment the pancreatic response to a given stimulant, or suppression of intrapancreatic release of neurotransmitters or islet hormones which augment the response to primary stimulants—the last possibility at least has some experimental support. In pigs, electrical stimulation of the vagus nerves releases both acetylcholine and VIP (53). Exogenous somatostatin has been shown to block the release of VIP in this case, but not to block the secretory effect of exogenous VIP on bicarbonate secretion (53). In rats, pancreatic polypeptide (PP) is another inhibitory peptide which is effective in vivo but not in vitro (54). Recently, PP has been shown to inhibit the release of acetylcholine from intrapancreatic, postganglionic neurons in the rat (55), suggesting that PP exerts its inhibitory effect on pancreatic secretion by removing the additive and potentiating effects of acetylcholine on enzyme and bicarbonate secretion. Because somatostatin has been shown to suppress acetylcholine release in other organs (56), this may also occur in the pancreas and account for some of the inhibitory action of somatostatin.

REFERENCES

1. Solomon TE. Control of exocrine pancreatic secretion. In: Johnson LR, ed. Physiology of the gastrointestinal tract. New York: Raven Press (in press).
2. Beglinger C, Grossman MI, Solomon TE. Interaction between stimulants of exocrine pancreatic secretion in dogs. Am J Physiol 1984; 246: G173-9.
3. You CH, Rominger JM, Chey WY. Potentiation effect of cholecystokinin-octapeptide on pancreatic bicarbonate secretion stimulated by a physiologic dose of secretin in humans. Gastroenterology 1983; 85:40-5.
4. Henriksen FW, Worning H. External pancreatic response to food and its relation to the maximal secretory capacity in dogs. Gut 1969; 10:209-14.

5. Beglinger C, Fried M, Whitehouse I, Jansen JB, Lamers CB, Gyr K. Pancreatic enzyme responses to a liquid meal and to hormonal stimulation. Correlation with plasma secretin and cholecystokinin levels. J Clin Invest 1985; 75:1471-6.

6. Defillipi C, Solomon TE, Valenzuela JE. Pancreatic secretory response to sham feeding in humans. Digestion 1982; 23:217-23.

7. Debas HT, Yamagishi T. Evidence for pyloropancreatic reflex for pancreatic exocrine secretion. Am J Physiol 1978; 234:E468-71.

8. Debas HT, Grossman MI. Pure cholecystokinin: pancreatic protein and bicarbonate response. Digestion 1973; 9:469-81.

9. Malegelada JR, Go VLW, Dimagno EP, Summerskill WHJ. Interactions between luminal bile acids and digestive products on pancreatic and gallbladder function. J Clin Invest 1973; 52:2160-5.

10. Dyck WP. Influence of intrajejunal glucose on pancreatic exocrine function in man. Gastroenterology 1971; 60:864-9.

11. Harper AA, Hood AJC, Mushens J, Smy JR. Inhibition of external pancreatic secretion by intracolonic and intraileal infusions in the cat. J Physiol (Lond) 1979; 292:445-54.

12. MacGregor IL, Deveney C, Way LW, Meyer JH. The effect of acute hyperglycemia on meal-stimulated gastric, biliary, and pancreatic secretion, and serum gastrin. Gastroenterology 1976; 70:197-202.

13. DiMagno EP, Go VLW, Summerskill WHJ. Intraluminal and postabsorptive effects of amino acids on pancreatic enzyme secretion. J Lab Clin Med 1973; 82:241-8.

14. Stubbs RS, Stabile BE. Inhibition of the stimulated exocrine pancreas by absorbed amino acids. J Surg Res 1984; 36:395-400.

15. Domschke S, Domschke W, Rosch W, et al. Inhibition by somatostatin of secretin-stimulated pancreatic secretion in man: a study with pure pancreatic juice. Scand J Gastroenterol 1977; 12:59-63.

16. Vatn MH, Schrumpf E, Hanssen KF, Myren J. A small dose of somatostatin inhibits the secretin stimulated secretion of bicarbonate, amylase, and chymotrypsin in man. J Endocrinol Invest 1980; 3:279-82.

17. Konturek SJ, Tasler J, Obtulowicz W, Coy DH, Schally AV. Effect of growth hormone-release inhibiting hormone on hormones stimulating exocrine pancreatic secretion. J Clin Invest 1976; 58:1-6.

18. Susini C, Esteve JP, Bommelaer G, Vaysse N, Ribet A. Inhibition of pancreatic secretion by somatostatin in dogs. Digestion 1978; 18:384-93.

19. Konturek SJ, Radecki T, Pucher A, Coy DH, Schally AV. Effect of somatostatin on gastrointestinal secretions and peptic ulcer production in cats. Scand J Gastroenterol 1977; 12:379-83.

20. Moriga M, Kojima K, Aono M, Uchino H, Yajima H. Effect of intravenous infusion of somatostatin on gastric, pancreatic and biliary secretion in the rat. Gastroenterol Jpn 1978; 13:190-6.

21. Folsch UR, Lankisch PC, Creutzfeldt W. Effect of somatostatin on basal and stimulated pancreatic secretion in the rat. Digestion 1978; 17:194-203.

22. Chariot J, Roze C, Vaille C, Debray C. Effects of somatostatin on the external secretion of the pancreas of the rat. Gastroenterology 1978; 75:832-7.

23. Dollinger HC, Raptis S, Pfeiffer EF. Effects of somatostatin on exocrine and endocrine pancreatic function stimulated by intestinal hormones in man. Horm Metab Res 1976; 8:74-8.

24. Lin TM, Evans DC, Shaar CJ, Root MA. Action of somatostatin on stomach, pancreas, gastric mucosal blood flow, and hormones. Am J Physiol 1983; 244:G40-5.

25. Miller TA, Tepperman FS, Fang WF, Jacobson ED. Effect of somatostatin on pancreatic protein secretion induced by cholecystokinin. J Surg Res 1979; 26:488-93.

26. Konturek SJ, Krol R, Tasler J. Effect of bombesin and related

peptides on the release and action of intestinal hormones on pancreatic secretion. J Physiol (Lond) 1976; 257;663–72.

27. Robberecht P, Deschodt-Lanckman M, De Neff P, Christophe J. Effects of somatostatin on pancreatic exocrine function. Interaction with secretin. Biochem Biophys Res Commun 1975; 67;315–23.

28. Wilson RM, Bodan G, Shore LS, Essa-Koumar N. Effect of somatostatin on meal-stimulated pancreatic exocrine secretions in dogs. Diabetes 1977; 26:7–10.

29. Konturek SJ, Cieszkowski M, Bilski J, Konturek J, Bielanski W, Schally AV. Effects of cyclic hexapeptide analog of somatostatin on pancreatic secretion in dogs. Proc Soc Exp Biol Med 1985; 178:68–72.

30. Hanssen LE, Hanssen KF, Myren J. Inhibition of secretin release and pancreatic bicarbonate secretion by somatostatin infusion in man. Scand J Gastroenterol 1977; 12:391–4.

31. Magee DF, Naruse S. The role of motilin in periodic interdigestive pancreatic secretion in dogs. J Physiol (Lond) 1984; 355:441–7.

32. Konturek SJ, Jaworek J, Cieszkowski M, Pawlik W, Kania J, Bloom SR. Comparison of effects of neurotensin and fat on pancreatic stimulation in dogs. Am J Physiol 1983; 244:G590–8.

33. Poitras P, Steinbach JH, Van Deventer G, Code DF, Walsh JH. Motilin-independent ectopic fronts of the interdigestive myoelectric complex in dogs. Am J Physiol 1980; 239:G215–20.

34. Ferris CF, Parker MC, Armstrong MJ, Leeman SE. Inhibition of neurotensin release by a cyclic hexapeptide analog of somatostatin. Peptides 1985; 6:945–8.

35. Vaysse N, Chayvialle JA, Pradayrol L, et al. Somatostatin 28: comparison with somatostatin 14 for plasma kinetics and low dose effects on the exocrine pancreas in dogs. Gastroenterology 1981; 81:700–6.

36. Beglinger C, Ribes G, Whitehouse I, Loubatieres-Mariani MM, Grotzinger U, Gyr K. Effect of exocrine pancreatic secretagogues on circulating somatostatin in dogs. Am J Physiol 1986; 250:G15–20.

37. Colturi TJ, Unger RH, Feldman M. Role of circulating somatostatin in regulation of gastric acid secretion, gastrin release, and islet cell function. Studies in healthy subjects and duodenal ulcer patients. J Clin Invest 1984; 74:417–23.

38. DeGraef J, Woussen-Colle MC. Effects of sham feeding, bethanechol, and bombesin on somatostatin release in dogs. Am J Physiol 1985; 248:G1–7.

39. Seal A, Yamada T, Debas H, et al. Somatostatin-24 and -28: clearance and potency on gastric function in dogs. Am J Physiol 1982; 243:G97–102.

40. Alumets J, Sundler F, Hakanson R. Distribution, ontogeny and ultrastructure of somatostatin immunoreactive cells in the pancreas and gut. Cell Tissue Res 1977; 185:465–79.

41. Keast JR, Furness JB, Costa M. Somatostatin in human enteric nerves. Distribution and characterization. Cell Tissue Res 1984; 237:299–308.

42. Aponte G, Gross D, Yamada T. Capillary orientation of rat pancreatic D-cell processes: evidence for endocrine release of somatostatin. Am J Physiol 1985; 249:G599–606.

43. Henderson JR, Daniel PM. A comparative study of the portal vessels connecting the endocrine and exocrine pancreas, with a discussion of some functional implications. Q J Exp Physiol 1979; 64:267–75.

44. Lifson N, Kramlinger KG, Mayrand RR, Lender EJ. Blood flow to the rabbit pancreas with special reference to the islets of Langerhans. Gastroenterology 1980; 79:466–73.

45. Kawai K, Orci L, Unger RH. High somatostatin uptake by the isolated perfused dog pancreas consistent with an "insulo-acinar" axis. Endocrinology 1982; 110:660–2.

46. Taborsky GJ, Ensinck JW. Extraction of somatostatin by the pancreas.

Endocrinology 1983; 112:303-7.

47. Esteve JP, Susini C, Vaysse N, et al. Binding of somatostatin to pancreatic acinar cells. Am J Physiol 1984; 247:G62-9.

48. Esteve JP, Vaysse N, Susini C, et al. Bimodal regulation of pancreatic exocrine function in vitro by somatostatin-28. Am J Physiol 1983; 245:G208-16.

49. Albinus M, Blair EL, Case RM, et al. Comparison of the effect of somatostatin on gastrointestinal function in the conscious and anesthetized cat and on the isolated cat pancreas. J Physiol (Lond) 1977; 269:77-91.

50. Imamura K, Miyazawa T, Abe Y, Nakamura T, Takebe K. Effect of several polypeptide hormones and 5-HT on exocrine pancreatic function. Biomed Res 1980; 1(suppl):171-4.

51. Susini C, Vaysse N, Esteve JP, Pradayrol L, Slassi C, Ribet A. Action of somatostatin 28 and somatostatin 14 on amylase release and cyclic AMP content in rat pancreatic acini. In: Ribet A, Pradayrol L, Susini C, eds. Biology of normal and cancerous exocrine pancreatic cells. Amsterdam: Elsevier North Holland Biomedical Press, 1980.

52. Vaysse N, Susini C, Esteve JP, Pradayrol L, Balas D, Ribet A. Action of somatostatin, big somatostatin and secretin on rat pancreatic duct cells. In: Rosselin G, Fromageot P, Bonfils S, eds. Hormone receptors in digestion and nutrition. Amsterdam: Elsevier North Holland Biomedical Press, 1979.

53. Fahrenkrug J, Schaffalitzky de Muckadell OB, Holst JJ, Lindkaer JS. Vasoactive intestinal polypeptide in vagally mediated pancreatic secretion of fluid and HCO_3. Am J Physiol 1979; 237:E535-40.

54. Louis DS, Williams JA, Owyang C. Action of pancreatic polypeptide on rat pancreatic secretion: in vivo and in vitro. Am J Physiol 1985; 249:G489-95.

55. Jung G, Louie D, Owyang C. Pancreatic polypeptide inhibits pancreatic enzyme secretion by presynaptic modulation of acetylcholine release [Abstract]. Gastroenterology 1986; 90:1794.

56. Guillemin R. Somatostatin inhibits the release of acetylcholine induced electrically in the myenteric plexus. Endocrinology 1976; 99:1653-4.

28

SOMATOSTATIN, CLEARANCE AND INHIBITION OF

GASTRIC ACID SECRETION IN DUODENAL ULCER PATIENTS

Mats Mogard, Vern Maxwell, Terry Reedy, Gary Van Deventer,
Janet Elashoff and John Walsh

Center for Ulcer Research and Education, V. A. Wadsworth
Medical Center and UCLA, Los Angeles, California, USA

INTRODUCTION

Somatostatin is one of several gastrointestinal peptides of potential physiological significance in the inhibitory regulation of gastric acid secretion. It is produced and released in the gastric mucosa and exogenous administration of this peptide strongly inhibits acid secretion stimulated by a variety of secretagogues in man (1). Gastric acid hypersecretion may be of major significance in the pathogenesis of duodenal ulcer disease. The etiology of this excessive acid secretion is not fully understood and may differ for individual ulcer patients. Increased stimulation, hypersensitivity to normal stimuli or defective inhibitory mechanisms have been suggested to be involved. It has been suggested that duodenal ulcer patients may have a reduced sensitivity to somatostatin, resulting in acid hypersecretion due to lack of inhibition (2). The present study reevaluates the role of somatostatin as inhibitor of acid secretion in duodenal ulcer patients.

METHODS

Studies were performed on 8 healthy male volunteers and 8 male duodenal ulcer patients. The patients had a history of peptic ulcer disease verified by x-ray examination and/or endoscopy. All were asymptomatic at the time of study and all medications were withheld during the present study. Age and weight for the normal subjects and ulcer patients were 35 ± 6 years, 75 ± 3 kg and 58 ± 3 years, 78 ± 2 kg, respectively. The study was approved by the V. A. Wadsworth Human Studies Committee and informed consent was obtained from each subject. Synthetic somatostatin, S-14, was administered under IND 20799 of the Food and Drug Administration.

Meal stimulated gastric acid secretion was quantified by intragastric titration (3). Following an overnight fast a double lumen tube was introduced into the stomach, through which test meals were administered. An isotonic glucose solution was administered for 30 min and followed by 4 consecutive 8% peptone (Difco Laboratories, Inc.) meals, 45 + 3 x 30 min. The pH of the gastric contents was maintained constant at 5.5 by automatic titration (Autoburette, Copenhagen) with 0.5 M NaOH. Acid output was calculated from the amount of titrant added. All subjects were studied on two separate days. On one day, somatostatin dissolved in saline containing 0.25% human serum albumin was infused intravenously during the last 3 peptone meals at sequentially increasing doses: 200, 400 and 800 pmol kg^{-1} h^{-1}. A control day was identical but no somatostatin was infused. Venous blood samples were collected every 15 min into chilled tubes containing 500 KIU aprotinin (Trasylol, FBA) and 0.13 mg EDTA per ml whole blood and centrifuged at 4°C for 10 min. The plasma was stored at -20°C until subsequent radioimmunoassay of somatostatin-like immunoreactivity (SLI) and gastrin as previously described using antisera 1001 (4) and 1611 (5), respectively. After the acid secretory test on the control day was completed, somatostatin was infused intravenously at a dose of 1600 pmol kg^{-1} h^{-1} for 15 min for a pharmacokinetic study. Venous blood samples were drawn at -15, -5, -2, 0, 0.5, 1.0, 1.5, 2.0, 2.5, 3.5, 5.0, 7.5, 10.0, 12.5, 15, 20 and 30 min.

Plasma SLI data were fitted by computer to the following exponential up-and-down one-compartment mathematical model.

During the infusion period; $\qquad s = b + p\ (1 - e^{-rt_i})$

During the decay period; $\qquad s = b + p\ (e^{rt_d} - e^{-rt_i})$

Let,

s = the plasma somatostatin level, (pM)
b = the basal plasma somatostatin level, (pM)
p = the plateau plasma somatostatin level, (pM)
t_i = the time since the infusion started, (min)
t_d = the time since the infusion stopped and decay started, (min)
$t_{\frac{1}{2}}$ = the plasma half-life, (min)
r = disappearance rate constant = $\log 2\ t_{\frac{1}{2}}^{-1}$, (min^{-1})

The clearance rates were calculated from the equation: $\quad C = dp^{-1}$
where,

C = the clearance rate, (1 kg^{-1} h^{-1})
d = the somatostatin dose administered IV, (pmol kg^{-1} h^{-1})

Statistics

The results are presented as mean and standard error of the means. Repeated measures analysis of variance was used to evaluate significances of differences between experimental groups, $P < 0.05$ was considered as significant.

RESULTS

Acid secretion (Figs. 1 and 2)

In the control experiments, peptone stimulated acid output reached plateau levels within 45 min of 11 and 16 mmol per 30 min for normals and ulcer patients respectively, Figure 1. Intravenous administration of somatostatin significantly and equally inhibited the stimulated acid output in ulcer patients and normals, Figure 2. In the ulcer patient group, the 30 min acid output was reduced from 16.5 ± 3.8, 15.4 ± 3.0 and 16.8 ± 3.7 mmol to 8.3 ± 2.1, 3.3 ± 1.0 and 1.4 ± 0.7 mmol by the 200, 400 and 800 pmol kg^{-1} h^{-1} doses respectively. Corresponding reduction in the normal group was from 11.0 ± 0.9, 11.2 ± 0.8 and 10.8 ± 0.8 mmol to 6.8 ± 1.3, 3.3 ± 1.3 and 1.4 ± 0.8 mmol. Although the mean peptone-stimulated acid output was noticeably higher in ulcer patients than in the normals, the difference is not significant due to the large variation of acid output in the ulcer patient group. The intravenous infusion of somatostatin resulted in increased plasma somatostatin-like immunoreactivity (SLI), Figure 3. The subsequent inhibition of acid secretion was associated with suppression of gastrin release, Figure 4.

Pharmacokinetics

Somatostatin was cleared from the blood circulation similarly in ulcer patients and normals. Basal plasma somatostatin levels were 96 ± 5 and 88 ± 5 pM; plateau plasma somatostatin levels 581 ± 21 and 527 ± 13 pM; disappearance rate constants -0.13 ± 0.01 and -0.16 ± 0.03 min^{-1}, the clearance rates 3.02 ± 0.41 and 3.12 ± 0.17 $1\ kg^{-1}\ h^{-1}$, and the half-lives were 2.5 ± 0.1 and 2.4 ± 0.1 min in normal volunteers and duodenal ulcer patients, respectively.

DISCUSSION

Somatostatin administration inhibited acid output in ulcer patients and normals to a similar extent. Gastric acid hypersecretion in duodenal ulcer patients therefore cannot be explained by a reduced sensitivity to somatostatin. This present observation is in agreement with a recent report (6), but in contrast to the findings of others (2). The somatostatin induced inhibition of acid output was associated with a suppression

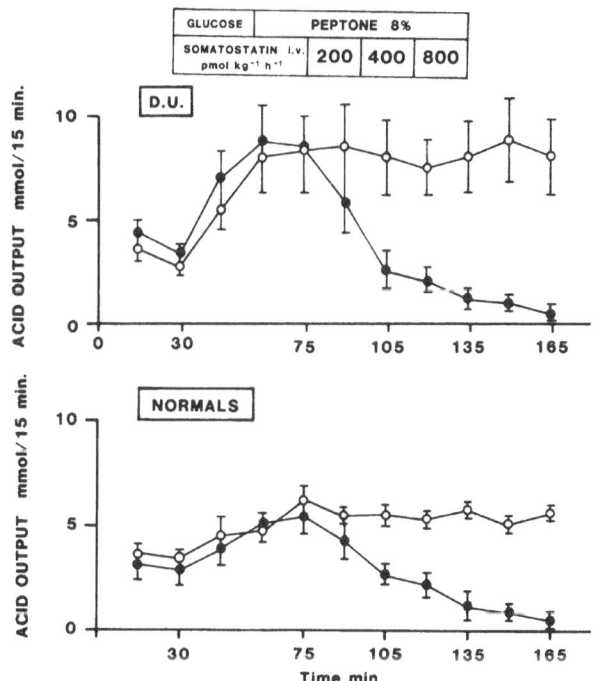

Fig. 1. Glucose and peptone stimulated gastric acid secretion in duodenal ulcer patients (D.U.) and normal subjects (NORMALS). Somatostatin infusion (●) significantly inhibited the stimulated acid output as compared to control (o), P < 0.05. x̄ ± SEM, n = 8.

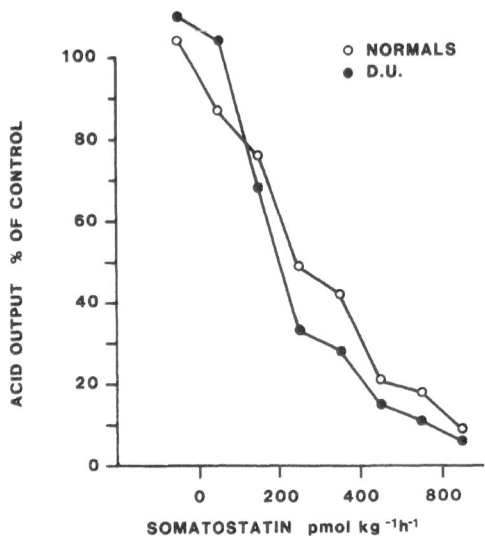

Fig. 2. Acid output in duodenal ulcer patients (●) and normal
subjects (o), during increasing doses of somatostatin. The acid
output in the somatostatin infusion experiment is expressed in per
cent of the acid output in the control experiment. Duodenal ulcer
patients and normals are equally sensitive to somatostatin.

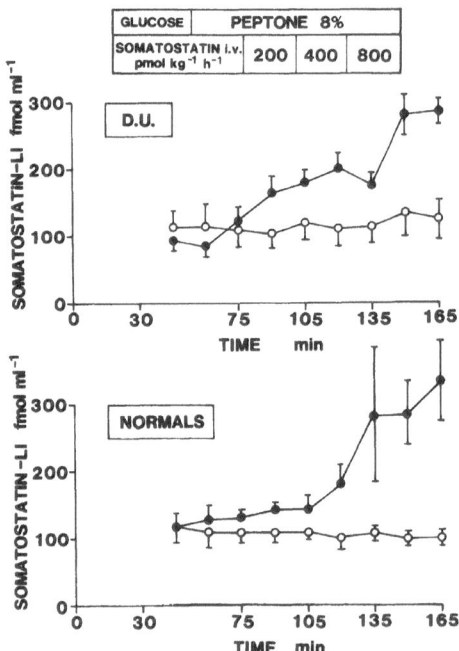

Fig. 3. Glucose and peptone stimulated plasma somatostatin-like immunoreactivity in duodenal ulcer patients (D.U.) and normal subjects (NORMALS).
(o) control, (●) somatostatin infusion. $\bar{x} \pm$ SEM, n = 8.

288

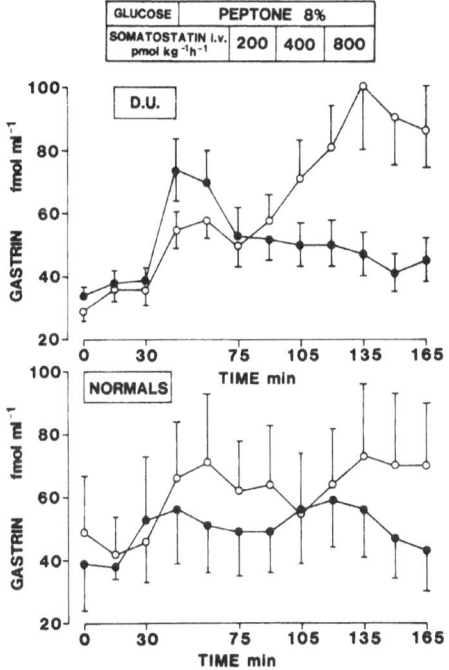

Fig. 4. Glucose and peptone stimulated plasma gastrin release in duodenal ulcer patients (D.U.) and normal subjects (NORMALS). $\bar{x} \pm$ SEM, n = 8.

of gastrin release, but suppression of acid occurred at lower doses. Other human studies showed both effects (1), and the higher sensitivity of parietal cells than gastrin cells to somatostatin has been shown previously (4). Thus, the inhibition of acid secretion by somatostatin cannot be accounted for by decreased serum gastrin.

The half-lives of somatostatin in plasma determined in this study, 2.4 and 2.5 min for duodenal ulcer patients and normals respectively, are in agreement with previous studies in healthy volunteers (7), and indicate that acid hypersecretion in ulcer patients cannot be explained by an abnormal clearance of somatostatin.

ACKNOWLEDGMENTS

This study was supported by grants from the National Institute of Health, AM 17328 and AM 35445. Mats Mogard was, in part, supported by Soderbergs Stiftelse and Karolinska Institutet, Stockholm, Sweden. Somatostatin, Stilamin®, was generously supplied by Serono Laboratories, Inc., MA, USA. We thank Anita Starlight for typing the manuscript.

REFERENCES

1. Creutzfeldt W, Arnold R. Somatostatin and the stomach: exocrine and endocrine aspects. Metabolism 1978; 27:1309-15.
2. Konturek SJ, Swierczek J, Kwiecieu N, et al. Effect of somatostatin on meal-induced gastric secretion in duodenal ulcer patients. Dig Dis Sci 1977; 11:981-8.
3. Fordtran JS, Walsh JH. Gastric acid secretion rate and buffer content of the stomach after eating. Results in normal subjects and patients with duodenal ulcer. J Clin Invest 1973; 52:645-57.
4. Seal A, Yamada T, Debas H, et al. Somatostatin 14 and 28: clearance and potency on gastric function in dogs. Am J Physiol 1982; 243:G97-102.
5. Walsh JH. Radioimmunoassay of gastrin. In: Rothfield B, ed. Nuclear medicine in vitro. Philadelphia: Lippincott, 1974:231-48.
6. Colturi JT, Unger RH, Feldman M. Role of circulating somatostatin in regulation of gastric acid secretion, gastrin release and islet function. J Clin Invest 1984; 74:417-23.
7. Sheppard M, Shapiro B, Pimstone B, et al. Metabolic clearance and plasma half-disappearance time of exogenous somatostatin in man. J Clin Endocrinol Metab 1979; 48:50-3.

V. CLINICAL APPLICATIONS

29

EFFECT OF A LONG-ACTING SOMATOSTATIN ANALOG (SMS 201-995) ON GLUCOSE HOMEOSTASIS IN TYPE I DIABETES AND IN ACROMEGALY

E. del Pozo,* S. W. J. Lamberts,[2] C. Sieber,*
A. Gomez-Pan[3]

Clinical Research* Sandoz Ltd., Basle, Switzerland
Erasmus University,[2] Rotterdam, The Netherlands
Faculty of Medicine,[3] Madrid, Spain

INTRODUCTION

Recently, Bauer et al. (1) have reported the synthesis of an octapeptide SMS 201-995 (DPhe-Cys-Phe-DTrp-Lys-Thr-Cys-Thr-ol), found in animal experiments to be about 45 times more potent than native somatostatin (SRIF). Studies in normal volunteers have shown SMS 201-995 to exhibit a 20-fold higher potency than SRIF in the suppression of growth hormone (GH) secretion and a shorter lasting effect on insulin (2,3). Otherwise, SMS 201-995 possesses endocrine properties similar to the natural peptide. Thus, it blocks insulin and glucagon secretion (3) and also retards intestinal absorption of sugar (2). Its high potency and prolonged plasma half-life (3) following subcutaneous administration of 50 and 100 μg prompted the investigation of its clinical usefulness. Acute and chronic administration of SMS 201-995 to acromegalic subjects has produced a rapid and sustained reduction in circulating GH (4,5,6,7). This was accompanied by improvement of clinical features typical of the disease.

More recently, a beneficial action of this peptide on insulin hypersensitivity has been reported in brittle diabetes (8,9). Because of its clinical potential, the results of acute and repeated administration of SMS 201-995 to insulin-dependent diabetics and to acromegalic patients will be analyzed in the following sections.

SOMATOSTATIN AND GLUCOSE HOMEOSTASIS: A RATIONALE FOR CLINICAL USE IN DIABETES

Abnormal glucose homeostasis in insulin-dependent diabetes mellitus (IDDM) seems to be a multifactorial phenomenon. Excessive sensitivity to exogenous insulin, marked blood glucose oscillations and undue counter-regulation by diabetogenic hormones are factors contributing to the perpetuation of a situation of maladjustment (10). Thus, augmented insulin sensitivity is compensated by a series of hormonal mechanisms preventing supraphysiological hypoglycemia. Among these, GH exerts a diabetogenic effect probably by enhancing peripheral insulin resistance. Elevated circulating GH may be found in insulin-dependent diabetes (11,12) and its possible role in the derangement of glucose control has been evaluated. Thus, juvenile diabetics may exhibit not only elevated basal

GH levels, but also exaggerated nocturnal surges (13) and enhanced response to exercise and other stimulation tests (14,15). Moreover, recent studies indicate that the dawn phenomenon may be mediated by GH elevated during sleep (16) and that it can be ameliorated by administration of somatostatin (17). Also, the effect of nocturnal insulin deprivation can be improved by the same procedure (18).

Increased circulating glucagon is a common finding in IDDM (19), although the causative mechanism of this phenomenon remains unclear. Mobilization of liver glycogen by glucagon may also play an important role in insulin counterregulation. Indeed, glucagonomas are almost invariably associated with elevated blood sugar concentrations (20) and glucagonemia in poorly controlled diabetics can be readily suppressed by adequate insulin therapy (21). In turn, endogenous hyperglucagonemia may stimulate function and growth of pancreatic D-cells to hypersecrete somatostatin (22) establishing a link between the A- and D-cellular systems. Thus, pancreatic islets contain an increased number of somatostatin cells in juvenile type of diabetes (23). This intercellular connection is further supported by the fact that somatostatin directly inhibits insulin and glucagon release by the pancreas (24), composing a kind of regulatory short-loop.

As already mentioned in the introduction, intravenous or subcutaneous administration of the somatostatin derivative SMS 201-995 to humans has delineated an action profile similar to that described for the native peptide. Thus, SMS 201-995 inhibits the secretion of growth hormone, insulin and glucagon in normal volunteers, and retards glucose absorption from the gastrointestinal tract (2,3). It has also been found to diminish the output of practically all gastrointestinal hormones tested (25).

The effect of somatostatin on glucose regulation deserves a more detailed analysis. Once its negative effect on insulin secretion has been obviated through exogenous replacement, the spectrum of activity of somatostatin may be of assistance in the readjustment of glucose homeostasis in unstable diabetes. Thus, inhibition of GH secretion may represent a kind of "medical" partial hypophysectomy, whereas by suppressing glucagon release somatostatin may facilitate blood glucose control. This effect would further be supported by attenuation of entry of glucose into the circulation in order to prevent exaggerated counterregulation. Moreover, in the long run, potentiation of insulin sensitivity (26) may contribute to the prevention of vascular complications by lowering the insulin requirements in IDDM, possibly in conjunction with a substantial reduction in circulating GH and glucagon (27,28,29).

EFFECT OF ACUTE AND REPEATED ADMINISTRATION OF SMS 201-995 ON INSULIN-DEPENDENT DIABETES MELLITUS

A first study with SMS 201-995 in this condition was conducted by Spinas et al. (30). They reported considerable dampening of postprandial blood glucose excursions following a single subcutaneous injection of 50 or 100 μg SMS 201-995 (Fig. 1). This effect was accompanied by a marked decrease in plasma GH and glucagon. Free plasma insulin following injection of identical doses was not modified by SMS 201-995 in comparison with placebo. At the same time, Gomez-Pan et al. (31) obtained similar results in a brittle diabetic. Administering 50 μg SMS 201-995 twice in the same day, the authors were able to reduce postprandial blood glucose oscillations observing a tendency toward lower levels after supper despite reduction of the evening insulin and SMS 201-995 doses. Prolongation of therapy for 7 days in another patient revealed persistence of this effect. Figure 2 presents the course of treatment: administration of 50 μg SMS

201-995 twice daily allowed stabilization of glucose profiles at lower level in comparison with a control day on insulin alone. Accordingly, daily insulin doses could be reduced by approximately 40%.

More recently, Serrano-Rios et al. (8) conducted another study in 6 type I diabetics after glucose stabilization by means of a Biostator™. Three standardized mixed meals were ingested after injection of 50 μg SMS 201-995 or placebo. Postprandial hyperglycemia was significantly diminished (Fig. 3) and insulin requirements, both total and 2 hours postprandially, also decreased in a significant way with a parallel reduction

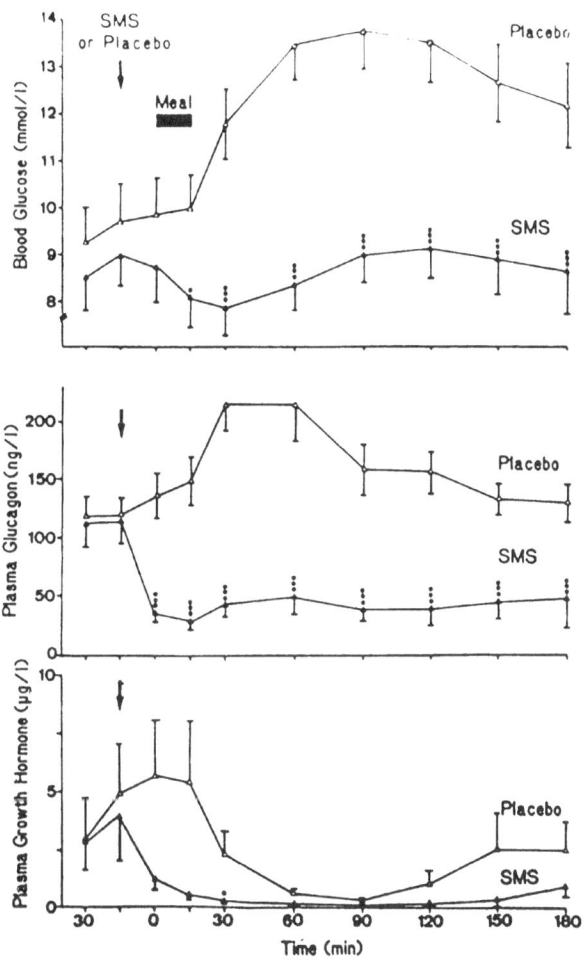

Fig. 1. Blood glucose, glucagon and GH levels after subcutaneous injection of 100 μg SMS 201-995 simultaneously with the morning insulin prior to a standard breakfast in type I diabetes mellitus. Glucagon and GH secretion are inhibited and the blood glucose profile is blunted, adopting a typical sinusoidal pattern. Reproduced from Spinas et al. (30) with permission.

in free insulin levels (Fig. 4). Postprandial glucagon levels were also significantly decreased.

The effect of SMS 201-995 on hormonal mechanisms controlling glucose metabolism was tested by Plewe et al. (9) in 8 type I diabetics over a 3-day period. In addition to dietary measures and conventional insulin therapy, the patients received a subcutaneous dose of 50 μg SMS 201-995 three times daily.

Basal GH and plasma somatomedin-C had decreased significantly by the third day. In all cases, the insulin requirements could be reduced (mean 28%) without deterioration of metabolic control. Moreover, blood glucose profiles showed a tendency to lower morning postprandial peaks after SMS 201-995 treatment. The authors concluded that dampening of glucose oscillations and counterregulatory mechanisms by SMS 201-995 may enable a better control of unstable diabetes.

Data recorded in this section are not surprising since a similar effect on glucose counterregulatory mechanisms was already reported for natural somatostatin in the mid-seventies (for review see 32). Indeed, the native peptide has been found to decrease postprandial hyperglycemia and prevent ketoacidosis in diabetic subjects probably through a dual mechanism: dampening of blood glucose surges transforming the supply of

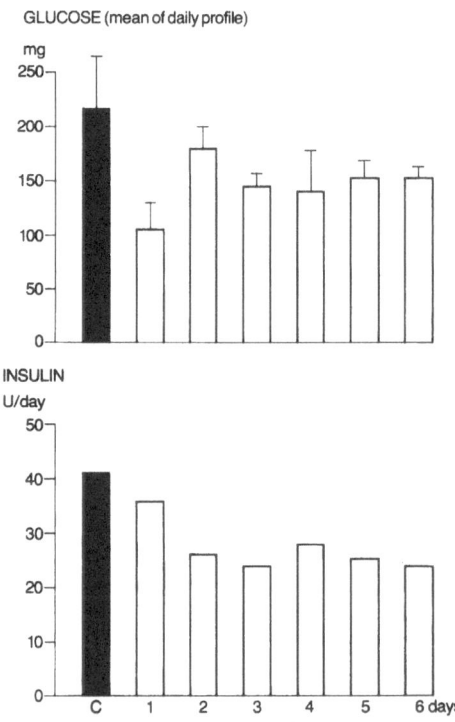

Fig. 2. Decrease in mean daily blood glucose values (upper panel) and 40% daily insulin reduction (lower panel) in a type I diabetic female, receiving 50 μg SMS 201-995 twice daily for 7 days.

sugar to peripheral tissues into a more physiological way and reducing ketone formation through inhibition of glucagon secretion (33). This effect has been demonstrated under standardized clinical conditions (34) and after glucose stabilization with an artificial pancreas (35). The former is probably favored by the delay in sugar uptake from the gut as already mentioned earlier in this paper (36,37). It is interesting to note that the typical biphasic blood glucose pattern induced by somatostatin is clearly reproducible in diabetic subjects accentuating the

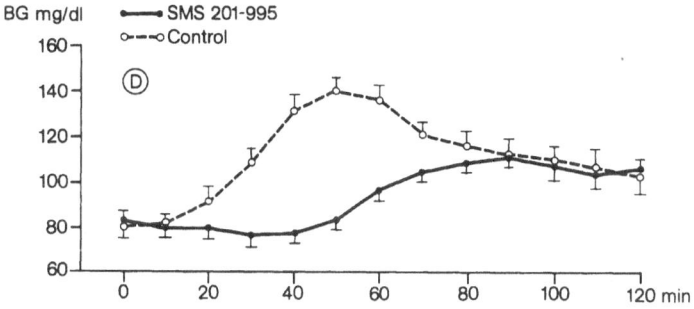

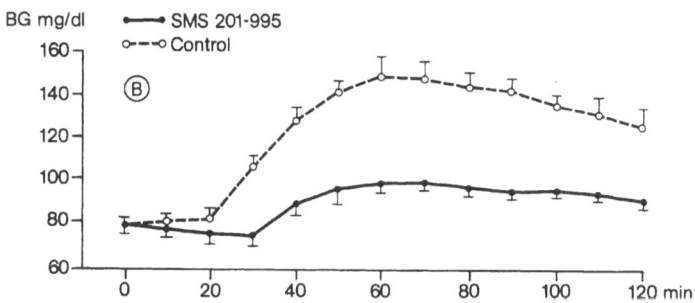

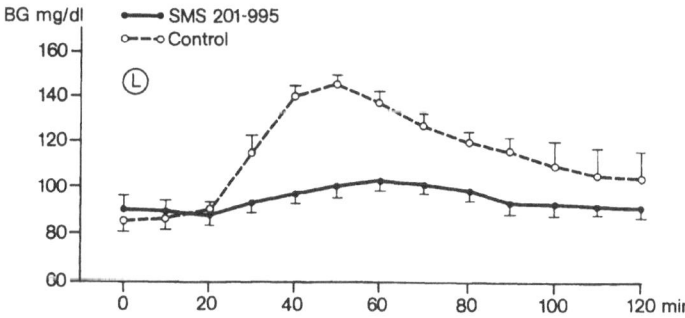

Fig. 3. Six subjects with type I diabetes mellitus received 50 μg SMS 201-995 subcutaneously before dinner, breakfast and lunch after blood glucose stabilization by means of a Biostator™. Glucose oscillations are considerably diminished in comparison with the placebo control. Reproduced from Serrano-Rios et al. (8) with permission.

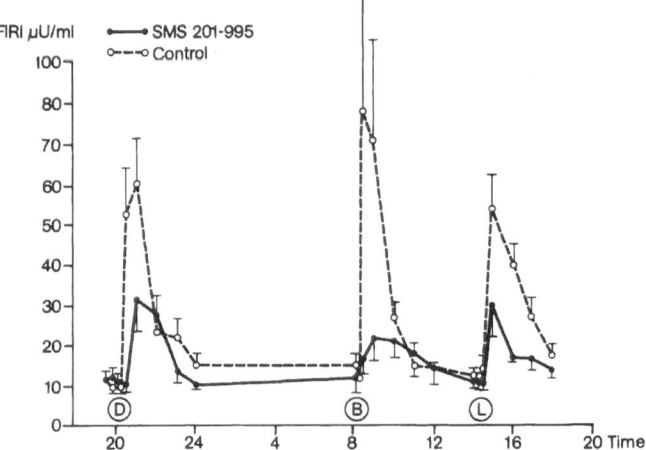

Fig. 4. Plasma free insulin values in stabilized (Biostator™) diabetes type I. Subcutaneous administration of 50 μg SMS 201-995 is followed by a marked insulin saving effect. Reproduced from Serrano-Rios et al. (8) with permission.

importance of hypoglucagonemia in this particular condition once hyperglycemia has been obviated by exogenous insulin. This effect may also explain the attenuation by somatostatin of the ketogenic reaction following discontinuation of exogenous insulin in diabetic patients (38). Indeed, diminution of ketone body formation can be antagonized by glucagon administration (33).

Generally speaking, the spectrum of actions recorded following the administration of somatostatin to humans faithfully reproduces some of the biochemical substrate of the somatostatinoma syndrome as originally defined by Unger (39). Thus, insulin sensitive, non-ketotic diabetes is a distinctive feature of this syndrome described in cases of pancreatic localization (for review see 20). The rare occurrence of hypoglycemia associated with a somatostatinoma may be due to the co-existence of an insulin-producing cell line within the tumor or to a double secretory mechanism, again stressing the importance of the interplay between insulin, growth hormone and glucagon in the maintenance of glucose homeostasis (40,41).

CHRONIC TREATMENT OF ACROMEGALY WITH SMS 201-995:   EFFECT ON GLUCOSE HOMEOSTASIS

A salient feature of acromegaly is moderate insulin resistance. Similar to type II diabetes, this peripheral disturbance is compensated in many instances by enhanced insulin secretion. Chronic treatment of acromegaly with the long-acting somatostatin derivative SMS 201-995 has been made available only recently. In agreement with previous reports (42,43), clinical diabetes was detected in 12 out of 46 (12%) acromegalics entering long-term therapy with this analog (44). An abnormal glucose tolerance test was found in another 10 subjects without evidence of the disease, bringing the total number of overt or latent diabetics to 22 (48%). As expected, hyperinsulinemia was a common finding. Out of this collective, 6 cases without evidence of disturbance of sugar metabolism were selected for special testing.

Figure 5 depicts the effect of acute and chronic treatment with SMS 201-995 on the glucose and insulin response to a standard mixed meal in the 6 subjects. First administration of the peptide was followed by a dramatic fall in plasma GH and insulin concentrations. B-cell blockade precluded the insulin discharge required to meet the glucose challenge and produced a diabetogenic postprandial blood sugar profile. This effect was still present after long-term therapy with SMS 201-995. However, there were some differences in comparison with the acute trial: despite a similar degree of insulin inhibition, the glucose curve in the chronic trial was somewhat dampened. It was therefore assumed that the peripheral blocking effect of GH on insulin receptors was not removed in the acute experiment, so that a dual situation originated through transient insulinopenia in addition to the disturbance at receptor level. In the chronic trial, normalization of GH secretion led to an improvement in the abnormal glucose tolerance after elimination of the latter factor.

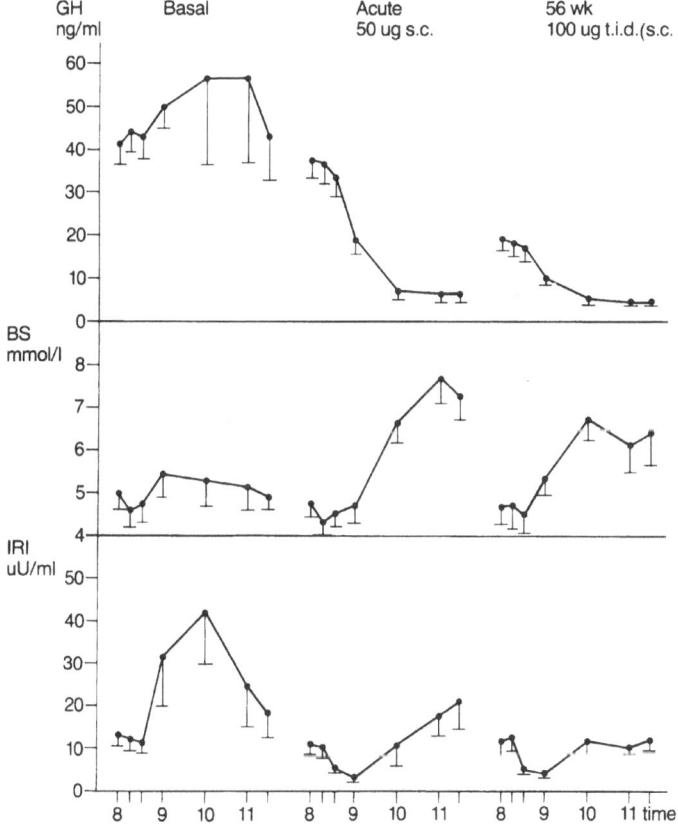

Fig. 5. Blood GH, glucose and insulin profiles in 6 acromegalic subjects following a standard breakfast under basal conditions, after single subcutaneous administration of 50 μg SMS 201995, and at the end of a 56-week treatment period with 100 μg t.i.d. (explanation in text).

In theory, treatment with somatostatin may have reversed the original picture of insulin receptor hyposensitization by increased circulating GH, close to type II diabetes, into a juvenile insulinopenic type I in the absence of peripheral blockade. Results of acute experiments supporting this view have been published previously (45). However, limited experience to date has shown no deterioration of the glucose metabolic substrate of acromegalics on long-term therapy with SMS 201-995. Nevertheless, larger collectives should be investigated under strict metabolic surveillance before a definitive prognostic statement can be made.

REFERENCES

1. Bauer W, Briner U, Doepfner W, et al. SMS 201-995: a very potent and selective octapeptide analogue of somatostatin with prolonged action. Life Sci 1982; 31:1133.
2. del Pozo E, Kutz K. Pharmacological properties and effect on glucose homeostasis of a somatostatin derivative (SMS 201-995): studies in humans. In: Ludecke D, Tolis G, eds. Growth factors and acromegaly. New York: Raven Press (in press).
3. del Pozo E, Neufeld M, Schluter K, et al. Endocrine profile of a long-acting somatostatin derivate SMS 201-995. Study in normal volunteers following subcutaneous administration. Acta Endocrinol 1986; 11:433.
4. Plewe G, Beyer J, Krause U, Neufeld M, del Pozo E. Long-acting and selective suppression of growth hormone secretion by somatostatin analogue SMS 201-995 in acromegaly. Lancet 1984; 2:782.
5. Lamberts SWJ, Oosterom R, Neufeld M, del Pozo E. The somatostatin analog SMS 201-995 induces long-acting inhibition of growth hormone secretion without rebound hypersecretion in acromegalic patients. J Clin Endocrinol Metab 1985; 60:1161.
6. Ching LJC, Sandler LM, Kraenzlin ME, Burrin JM, Joplin GF, Bloom SR. Long-term treatment of acromegaly with a long-acting analogue of somatostatin. Br Med J 1985; 290:284.
7. Lamberts SWJ, Uitterlinden P, Verschoor L, van Dongen KJ, del Pozo E. Long-term treatment of acromegaly with the somatostatin analogue SMS 201-995. N Engl J Med 1985; 313:1576.
8. Serrano-Rios M, Navascues J, Saban J, Ordonez A, Sevilla F, del Pozo E. Effect of a somatostatin analog (SMS 201-995) on insulin needs in IDDM by means of an artificial pancreas. J Clin Endocrinol Metab (in press).
9. Plewe G, Noelken G, Krause U, Beyer J, del Pozo E. Suppression of growth hormone and somatomedin C by the long-acting somatostatin analog SMS 201-995 in type I diabetes mellitus. Horm Res (in press).
10. Schade DS, Eaton RP. The controversy concerning counterregulatory hormone secretion. A hypothesis for the prevention of diabetic ketoacidosis? Diabetes 1977; 26:596.
11. Hansen AP, Johansen K. Diurnal patterns of blood glucose, serum free fatty acids, insulin, glucagon and growth hormone in normals and juvenile diabetics. Diabetologia 1970; 6:27.
12. Molnar GD, Taylor WF, Longworthy A, Fatourechi V. Diurnal growth hormone and glucagon abnormalities in unstable diabetics: studies in ambulatory-fed subjects during continuous blood glucose analysis. J Clin Endocrinol 1972; 34:837.
13. Press M, Tamborlane WV, Sherwin RS. Importance of raised growth hormone levels in mediating the metabolic derangements of diabetes. N Engl J Med 1984; 310:810.
14. Hansen AP. Abnormal serum growth hormone response to exercise in juvenile diabetics. J Clin Invest 1970; 49:1467.
15. Meek JC, Reitz RP, Bolinger RE. Plasma growth hormone response to

glucocorticoids in diabetics. Proc Soc Exp Biol Med 1970; 135(1):
123-6.

16. Campbell PJ, Bolli GB, Cryer Ph.E, Gerich JE. Parthenogenesis of the
dawn phenomenon in patients with insulin-dependent diabetes mellitus.
N Engl J Med 1985; 312:1473.

17. Campbell PJ, Bolli GB, Gerich JE. Nasal somatostatin analogue: a
practical and effective approach to treatment of the dawn phenomenon.
Diabetes Research and Clinical Practice 1985; 1(suppl):84.

18. Scheen AJ, Krzentowski G, Castillo M, Lefebvre PJ, Luyckx AS. A
6-hour nocturnal interruption of a continuous subcutaneous insulin
infusion: 2. Marked attenuation of the metabolic deterioration by
somatostatin. Diabetologia 1983; 24:319.

19. Unger RH, Aguilar-Parada E, Muller W, Eisentraut A. Studies of
pancreatic alpha cell function in normal and diabetic subjects. J
Clin Invest 1970; 49:837.

20. Berelowitz M. Somatostatin-producing tumors: clinical aspects.
Neuroendocrine Perspectives 1985; 4:59.

21. Muller W, Faloona G, Unger RH. Hyperglucagonemia in diabetic ketoacidosis: its prevalence and significance. Am J Med 1973; 54:52.

22. Patton GS, Ipp E, Dobbs RE, Orci L, Vale W, Unger RH. Pancreatic
immunoreactive somatostatin release. Proc Natl Acad Sci USA 1977;
74:2140.

23. Orci L, Baetens D, Rufener C. Hypertrophy and hyperplasia of somatostatin-containing D-cells in diabetes. Proc Natl Acad Sci USA 1976;
73:1338.

24. Guillemin R, Gerich JE. Somatostatin: physiology and clinical
significance. Annu Rev Med 1976; 27:379.

25. Kraenzlin ME, Wood SM, Neufeld M, Adrian TE, Bloom SR. Effect of
long-acting somatostatin-analogue SMS 201-995 on gut hormone secretion in normal subjects. Experientia 1985; 41:738.

26. Gerich JE, Haymond M, Rizza R, Verdonk C, Miles G. Hormonal and
substrate determinants of hepatic glucose production in man. In:
Veneziale CM, ed. The regulation of carbohydrate formation and
utilization in mammals. Baltimore: University Park Press, 1981.

27. Pyoeraelae K. Relationship of glucose tolerance and plasma insulin
to the incidence of coronary heart disease: results from two population studies in Finland. Diabetes Care 1979; 2:131.

28. Welborn TA, Wearne K. Coronary heart disease incident and mortality
in Busselton with reference to glucose and insulin levels. Diabetes
Care 1979; 2:154.

29. Hillson RM, Hochaday TDR, Mann JI, Newton DJ. Hyperinsulinemia is
associated with development of electrocardiographic abnormalities in
diabetics. Diabetes Research 1984; 1:143.

30. Spinas GA, Bock A, Keller U. Reduced postprandial hyperglycemia
after subcutaneous injection of a somatostatin analogue (SMS 201-995)
in insulin-dependent diabetes mellitus. Diabetes Care 1985; 8:429.

31. Gomez-Pan A, Rodriguez-Arnao MD, del Pozo E. Advances in somatostatin research. In: del Pozo E, Fluckiger E, eds. Dopamine and
neuroendocrine active substances. London: Academic Press, Inc.,
1985.

32. Gottesman JS, Mandarino LJ, Gerich JE. Somatostatin: its role in
health and disease. Spec Top Endocrinol Metab 1982; 4:177.

33. Greco A, Ghirlanda G, Altomonte A, Manna R, Rebuzzi A, Bertoli A.
Somatostatin and insulin infusion in the management of diabetes
ketoacidosis. Horm Metab Res 1981; 13:310.

34. Gerich JE, Schultz T, Tsalikian E, Lorenzi M, Lewis S, Karam J.
Clinical evaluation of somatostatin as a potential adjunct to insulin
in the management of diabetes mellitus. Diabetologia 1977; 13:537.

35. Meissner C, Thurn C, Beischer W, Winkler G, Schroder K, Pfeiffer E.
Antidiabetic action of somatostatin—assessed by the artificial
pancreas. Diabetes 1975; 24:988.

36. Felig P, Wahren J. Somatostatin and diabetes: suppression of glucose absorption rather than stimulation of glucose disposal. Metabolism 1976; 25:1509.
37. Wahren J, Efendic S, Luft R, Hagenfeldt L, Bjorkman O, Felig P. Influence of somatostatin on splanchnic glucose metabolism in post absorptive and 60 hours fasted humans. J Clin Invest 1977; 59:299.
38. Gerich JE, Lorenzi M, Bier D, et al. Prevention of human diabetic ketoacidosis by somatostatin: evidence for an essential role of glucagon. N Engl J Med 1975; 292:985.
39. Unger RH. Somatostatinoma. N Engl J Med 1977; 296:998.
40. Wright J, Abolfathi A, Penman E, Marks U. Pancreatic somatostatinoma presenting with hypoglycaemia. Clin Endocrinol 1980; 12:603.
41. Pipeleers D, Couturier E, Gepts W, Reynders J, Somers G. Five cases of somatostatinoma: clinical heterogeneity and diagnostic usefulness of basal and tolbutamide-induced hypersomatostatinemia. J Clin Endocrinol Metab 1983; 56:1236.
42. Gordon DA, Mill FM, Ezrin C. Acromegaly: a review of 100 cases. Can Med Assoc J 1962; 87:1106.
43. Emmer M, Gordon P, Roth J. Diabetes in association with other endocrine disorders. Med Clin North Am 1971; 55:1057.
44. del Pozo E, Chiodini PG, Lamberts SWJ, et al. Long-term treatment of acromegaly with the somatostatin analog SMS 201-995: report of 46 cases (submitted).
45. Lamberts SWJ, del Pozo E. The acute and long-term effects of SMS 201-995 in acromegaly. Scand J Gastroenterol (in press).

30

TREATMENT OF DIABETES WITH L363,586

J. Gerich, I. Gottesman, G. Bolli, P. Campbell, F. Kennedy

Endocrine Research Unit
Mayo Clinic
Rochester, Minnesota

L363,586 (now referred to as MK-678) is a cyclic hexapeptide analog of somatostatin. This compound, whose amino acid sequence is shown in Figure 1, was developed by chemists at Merck, Sharp and Dohme Research laboratories on the basis of modeling of the active site of the somatostatin molecule in a project which involved the synthesis of more than 150 analogs (1).

Based on its prolonged duration of action and potency of more than 50 times that of somatostatin in animal and in vitro studies (1), L363,586 was chosen to undergo evaluation in patients with insulin-dependent diabetes mellitus (IDDM).

Initial studies (2) were therefore undertaken to assess its metabolic clearance rate and half-life during 5-hour intravenous infusions, as well as its concomitant effect on postprandial plasma glucose, glucagon, growth hormone and triglyceride levels.

Three doses (2.5, 10 and 40 µg/hour) of L363,586 were compared with placebo and a 200 µg/hour somatostatin infusion. Xylose (5 gm) was incorporated into the standard test meal given six patients with IDDM to assess the effect of the analog on carbohydrate absorption. The subjects had been withdrawn from their intermediate-acting (lente or NPH) insulin at least 24 hours prior to entering the Clinical Study Unit. During this period they were managed on multiple subcutaneous injections of regular insulin (Iletin II®, Eli Lilly, Indianapolis, Indiana).

After receiving a standard supper, the subjects were connected to a closed-loop insulin infusion device (Biostator™, GCIIS, Life Science Instruments, Elkhart, Indiana) and were maintained euglycemic with it overnight. The following morning, subjects received a standard injection of regular insulin (Iletin II®, 0.15 U/kg) 30 minutes prior to beginning breakfast which was consumed over 15 minutes. Infusions of L363,586, somatostatin or placebo were begun at the time of meal ingestion.

Cyclo(N-Me-Ala-Tye-D-Trp-Lys-Val-Phe)

Fig. 1. Amino acid sequence of L363,586.

Figure 2 shows the plasma L363,586 levels found during the three infusions. Levels during the 2.5 μg/hour infusion were too low to reliably calculate a half-life, but from values obtained during the other two infusions, the metabolic clearance rate was approximately 300 ml/min and the half-life was 45 minutes.

Plasma glucagon (Fig. 3) and growth hormone (Fig. 4) were suppressed to a comparable extent with all three doses of L363,586 and somatostatin, but after termination of the intravenous somatostatin infusion, a rebound increase in plasma concentrations of the hormones was observed, whereas none occurred during the infusion of L363,586.

Postprandial plasma glucose levels in the diabetic subjects (Fig. 5) were significantly reduced with all three doses of L363,586 and with somatostatin. L363,586 infused at 10 μg/hour was as effective as somatostatin infused at a rate of 200 μg/hour, producing approximately a 70% reduction in the area under the postprandial plasma glucose curve (67 ± 23 vs. 224 ± 22 mM/1/5 hour with placebo, P < 0.01).

The diminution of postprandial hyperglycemia by L363,586 does not appear to be wholly explicable on the basis of a delaying of carbohydrate absorption since there was a dissociation between reduction in postprandial plasma xylose responses (Fig. 6) and the reduction in postprandial hyperglycemia. Thus, the 10 μg/hour infusion of L363,586 that had produced a maximal (~70%) reduction in postprandial hyperglycemia produced only a 25% reduction in postprandial plasma xylose responses (9.5 ± 0.7 vs. 12.9 ± 0.5 mM/1/5 hour with placebo, P < 0.05).

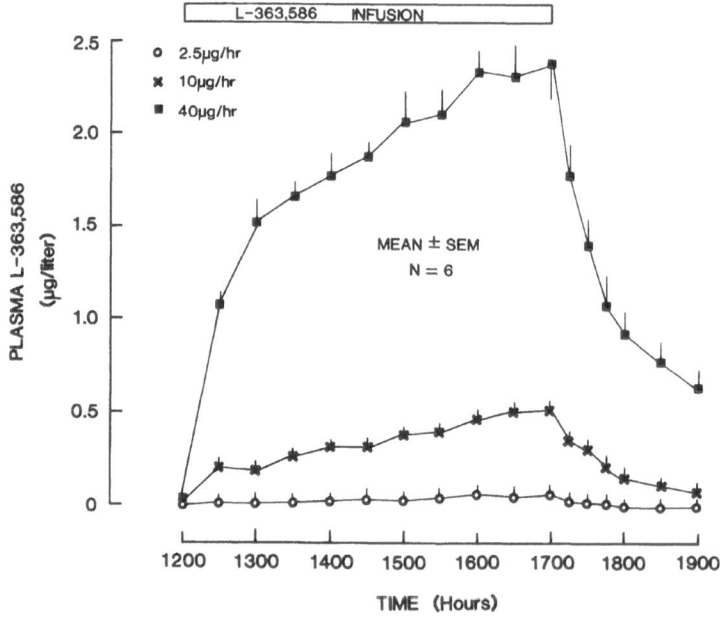

Fig. 2. Plasma L363,586 levels during intravenous infusion of L363,586 at 3 concentrations in 6 subjects with IDDM.

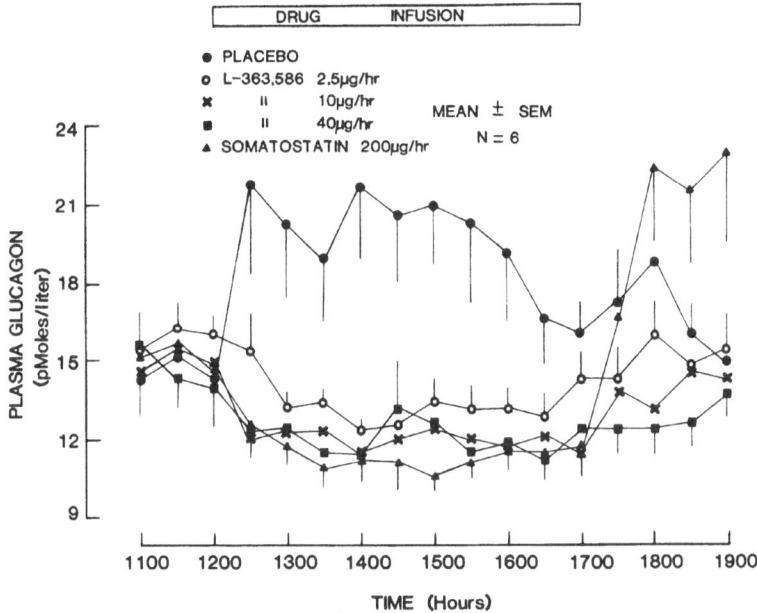

Fig. 3. Effects of L363,586 infusions at 3 concentrations and somatostatin (200 µg/hour) on postprandial plasma glucagon levels in 6 IDDM patients compared to placebo.

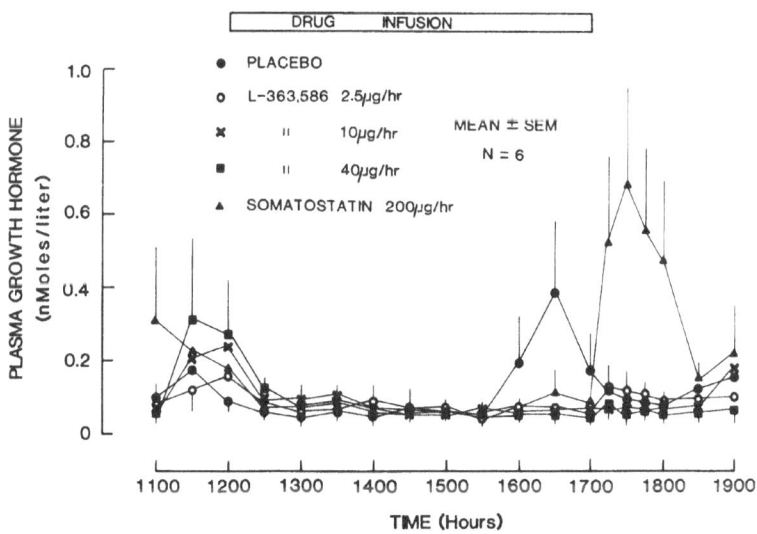

Fig. 4. Effects of L363,586 infusions at 3 concentrations and somatostatin (200 µg/hour) on postprandial plasma growth hormone levels in 6 IDDM patients compared to placebo.

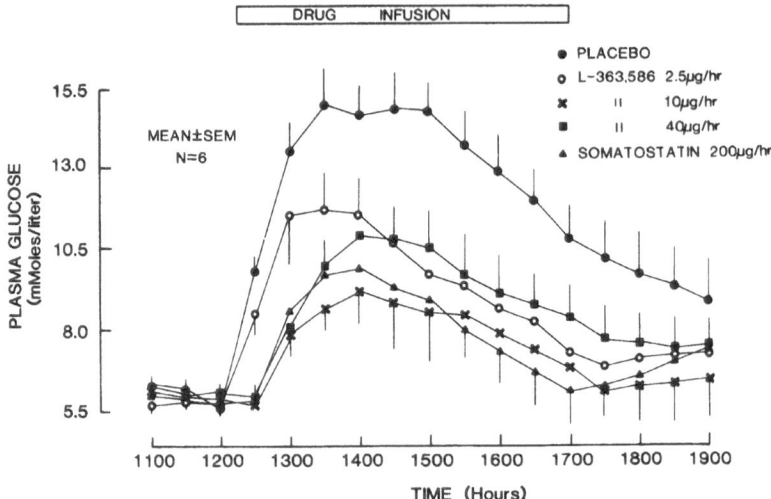

Fig. 5. Effects of L363,586 infusions at 3 concentrations and somatostatin (200 μg/hour) on postprandial plasma glucose levels in 6 IDDM patients compared to placebo.

A maximal reduction of only 35% was seen with the 40 μg/hour L363,586 and 200 μg/hour somatostatin infusions. Accordingly, these results provide indirect support of a role for excessive meal-stimulated glucagon secretion in the pathogenesis of postprandial hyperglycemia in IDDM patients (3).

All doses of L363,586 and somatostatin completely prevented any postprandial increase in plasma triglycerides (Fig. 7). The extent to which this suppression of postprandial increases in plasma triglycerides reflects the known effects of somatostatin on the small intestine, exocrine pancreas or gallbladder is not known at the present time.

All infusions were well tolerated without significant changes in heart rate, blood pressure, temperature, plasma electrolytes, SGOT, alkaline phosphatase, complete blood count or urinalysis. One subject developed mild indirect hyperbilirubinemia after the 10 μg/hour L363,586 and somatostatin infusions. One subject developed mild dyspepsia that resolved spontaneously during the 10 μg/hour L363,586 infusion, and one subject had a loose bowel movement the morning after both the 10 and 40 μg/hour L363,586 infusions.

Following these encouraging acute results, further experiments were undertaken examining the effect of a 3-day continuous infusion of L363,586 at a rate of 0.5 μg/hour in 8 volunteers with insulin-dependent diabetes mellitus. Twenty-four hour profiles of plasma glucose, glucagon, growth hormone and free insulin were determined on the third day of L363,586 and placebo infusions. In addition, stools were collected for determination of fat content. Without a change in insulin dose, there was a 32% decrease in mean 24-hour plasma glucose concentration (212 ± 21 vs. 145 ± 11

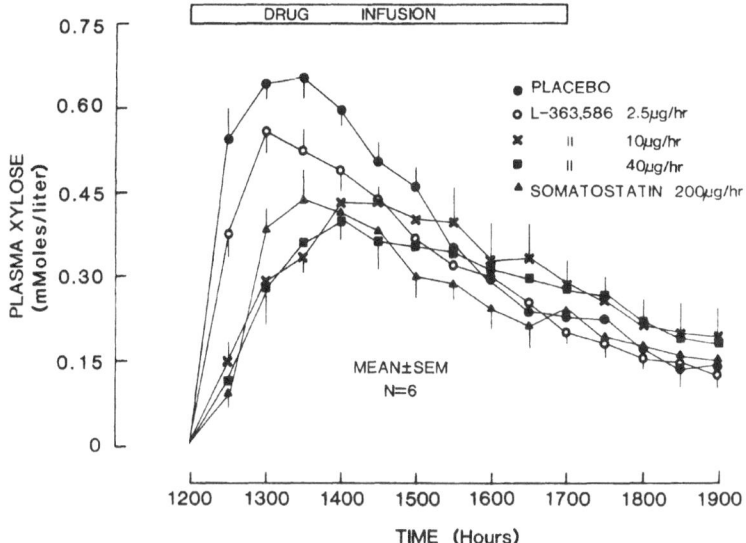

Fig. 6. Effects of L363,586 infusions at 3 concentrations and somatostatin (200 μg/hour) on postprandial plasma xylose levels in 6 IDDM patients compared to placebo.

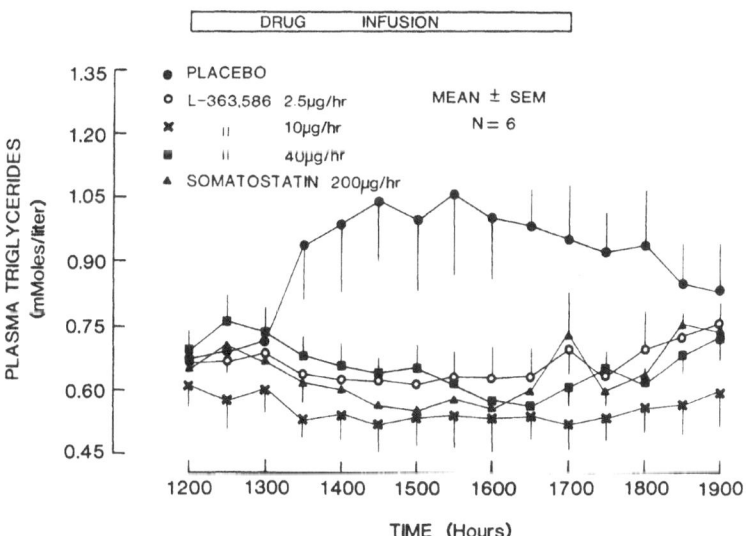

Fig. 7. Effects of L363,586 infusions at 3 concentrations and somatostatin (200 μg/hour) on postprandial plasma triglyceride levels in 6 IDDM patients compared to placebo.

mg/dl, P < 0.005). This occurred despite only modest reductions in 24-hour plasma glucagon and growth hormone levels (about 15 and 20%, respectively, both P < 0.05). Three-day stool fat increased in 6 of the 8 subjects from 5.3 ± 0.5 to 7.4 ± 1.9 gm per day but this was not statistically significant.

Again, the analog was well tolerated with no adverse signs or symptoms except transient mild dyspepsia and increased frequency of loose stools.

Since injections of L363,586 taken in addition to insulin might dissuade use of this analog, our next set of experiments was undertaken to determine whether the nasal route of administration was feasible, safe and effective.

Six subjects with IDDM were given 25, 100 and 400 μg of L363,586 by intranasal droplet one-half hour before a standard breakfast and supper with a standard lunch being taken in between. Subjects were admitted to the Clinical Study unit the night before experiments after having been withdrawn from their intermediate-acting insulin and treated with multiple subcutaneous injections of regular insulin for at least 24 hours. They were given a standard supper and connected to a closed-loop insulin infusion device (Biostator™ GCIIS, Life Science Instruments, Elkhart, Indiana), which maintained them euglycemic overnight. A mixture of regular and lente insulin was given one-half hour before breakfast.

The 25 μg dose produced no discernible effects on any of the parameters measured. With 100 and 400 μg doses, plasma glucose levels through the day were lower than those observed after placebo and the 25 μg dose. Both the 100 and 400 μg doses reduced postprandial plasma glucose concentrations 40-50% and completely prevented any increases in plasma triglycerides, glucagon and growth hormone. Plasma xylose concentrations were not affected by the 25 μg dose and were reduced comparably (~25%) with the 100 and 400 μg doses.

These studies thus showed that 100 μg L363,586 taken intranasally lasted at least 6 hours and therefore could be used on a twice daily basis to aid in the control of postprandial hyperglycemia in patients with IDDM. In general, the nasal route was well tolerated with only one subject complaining of transient nasal irritation, but this was also observed with placebo. Four subjects had a loose bowel movement after the 100 μg dose and 5 with the 400 μg dose. These episodes occurred between 8 and 18 hours after the second dose of the peptide.

Figure 8 shows the plasma levels of L363,586 after intranasal administration. Peak levels were reached within one hour, the first sampling time. The initial decrease in levels had a half-life of about 45 minutes, similar to that observed with intravenous infusion.

Since the intranasal administration appeared to be a feasible route of delivery for L363,586, we examined its effect on the dawn phenomenon when given by this route at bedtime (4). The dawn phenomenon is an early morning increase in insulin requirements occurring in patients with either IDDM or noninsulin-dependent diabetes mellitus (5) as well as in non-diabetic individuals (6).

Current evidence (7) indicates that nocturnal surges in growth hormone are the cause. In patients with diabetes mellitus and the inability to secrete additional insulin to compensate for the growth hormone-induced insulin resistance, marked hyperglycemia can develop in the early morning.

308

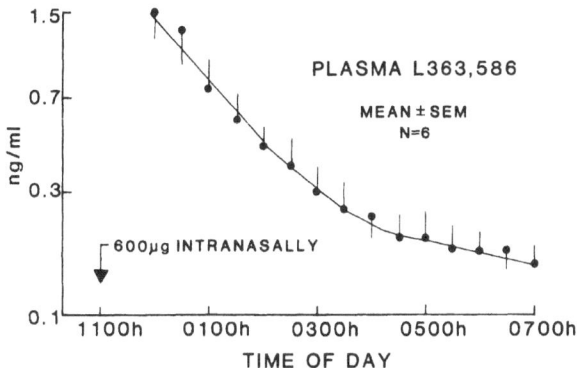

Fig. 8. Plasma L363,586 levels after intranasal administration of 600 μg of L363,586 in 6 IDDM patients.

One of the major problems in managing the dawn phenomenon is its variability which is presumably due to erratic growth hormone secretion. Production of consistent suppression of overnight growth hormone secretion should reduce this variability and make it easier to determine overnight insulin doses.

Therefore, to test the feasibility of treating the dawn phenomenon with a long-acting somatostatin analog like L363,586, 6 volunteers with IDDM, who had been withdrawn from their intermediate-acting insulin for 24 hours and managed solely by subcutaneous injections of regular insulin, were placed on a closed-loop insulin infusion device, rendered euglycemic after a standard supper and were infused with insulin at a constant rate from midnight to 7 a.m. on two occasions. On one occasion they received intranasal L363,586 (600 μg) and on the other, saline.

As shown in Figure 9, intranasal administration of L363,586 completely suppressed nocturnal surges in growth hormone secretion and reduced plasma glucagon levels throughout the night. Plasma cortisol and free insulin levels were not affected.

In control experiments, plasma glucose increased to over 250 mg/dl, whereas when L363,586 was administered plasma glucose did not increase until after 5 a.m. and then only to less than 150 gm/dl. These findings are illustrated in Figure 10. This increase presumably was due to the progressive decreases in plasma free insulin resulting from reduced delivery of insulin with the Biostator™ (8). None of the subjects experienced untoward effects from the intranasal L363,586. These studies, therefore, indicate that such administration of a long-acting analog might be feasible for managing the dawn phenomenon in patients in whom this cannot be done safely and effectively with mere adjustments in insulin doses.

In conclusion, in acute and relatively short-term studies, L363,586 was well tolerated when given by both intravenous and intranasal routes and was also effective in reducing both fasting and postprandial hyperglycemia in patients with insulin-dependent diabetes mellitus. Its main side effect was steatorrhea. Such an agent may be useful as an adjunct to

309

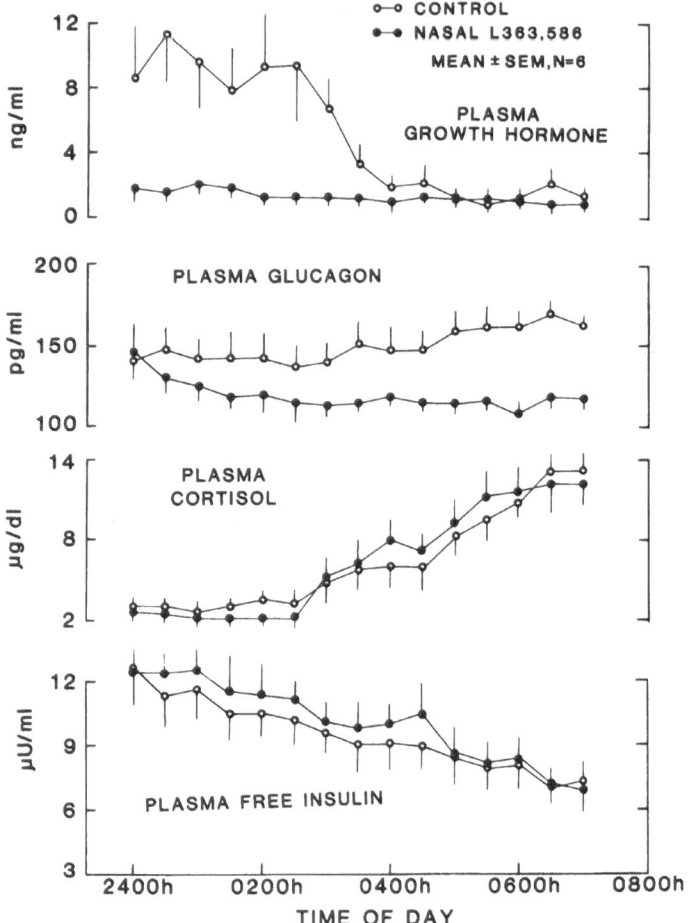

Fig. 9. Effects of intranasal L363,586 on overnight plasma growth hormone, glucagon, cortisol and free insulin levels in 6 IDDM patients receiving insulin infusions (0.15 mU/kg/min) compared to controls.

insulin in the treatment of diabetes mellitus, especially in patients unwilling or unable to take more than two daily injections of insulin in whom maintenance of near-normoglycemia is a therapeutic goal. Finally, because it appears to be safe, we wish to suggest that use of this agent in patients with rapidly progressive retinopathy that is unresponsive to laser treatment may deserve consideration as an alternative to hypophysectomy.

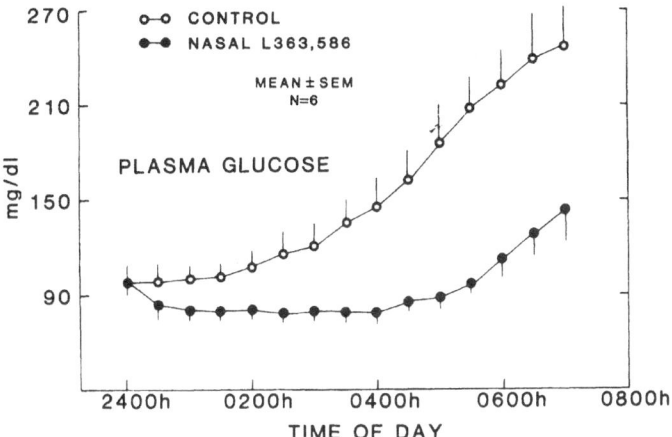

Fig. 10. Effects of intranasal L363,586 on development of early-morning hyperglycemia (dawn phenomenon) in 6 IDDM patients receiving insulin infusions (0.15 mU/kg/min) compared to controls.

ACKNOWLEDGMENTS

We are grateful to our colleagues at Merck, Sharp and Dohme Research Laboratories, our excellent laboratory personnel, and the staff of the Clinical Study Unit.

REFERENCES

1. Veber D, Saperstein R, Nutt T, et al. A superactive cyclic hexapeptide analog of somatostatin. Life Sci 1984; 35:1371.
2. Gottesman I, Tobert J, Vandlen R, Gerich J. Efficacy, pharmacokinetics and tolerability of a somatostatin analog (L363,586) in insulin-dependent diabetes mellitus. Life Sci (in press).
3. Gerich J, Lorenzi M, Karam J, Schneider V, Forsham P. Abnormal pancreatic glucagon secretion and postprandial hyperglycemia in diabetes mellitus. JAMA 1975; 234:159.
4. Campbell P, Bolli G, Gerich J. Prevention of the dawn phenomenon (early morning hyperglycemia) in insulin-dependent diabetes mellitus by a long-acting somatostatin analog. N Engl J Med (in press).
5. Bolli G, Gerich J. The dawn phenomenon—a common occurrence in both noninsulin-dependent and insulin-dependent diabetes mellitus. N Engl J Med 1984; 310:746.
6. Bolli G, De Feo P, De Cosmo S, et al. Demonstration of a dawn phenomenon in normal human volunteers. Diabetes 1984; 33:1150.
7. Campbell P, Bolli C, Cryer P, Gerich J. Pathogenesis of the dawn phenomenon in patients with insulin-dependent diabetes mellitus. N Engl J Med 1985; 312:1473.
8. Brennan J, Gebhart S, Blackard W. Pump-induced insulin aggregation: a problem with the Biostator™. Diabetes 1985; 34:353.

31

SOMATOSTATIN AND UPPER GASTROINTESTINAL HEMORRHAGE

Inger Magnusson

Department of Surgery
Karolinska Institutet at Sodersjukhuset
S-100 64 Stockholm, Sweden

INTRODUCTION

Somatostatin is a potent inhibitor of gastric secretion of acid, gastrin, pepsin and intrinsic factor (1,2). The peptide also increases gastric mucus production (3) and it decreases splanchnic blood flow (4). At an acid pH and in the presence of pepsin, platelet aggregation and plasma clotting are both abolished and previously formed platelet aggregates disaggregate (5). The inhibitory effect of somatostatin on gastric secretion might consequently be of benefit in the treatment of upper gastrointestinal bleeding.

About 75% of the patients with upper gastrointestinal hemorrhage will stop bleeding spontaneously. It is therefore important to identify the patients at risk for continuous bleeding or rebleeding. Stigmata of a bleeding lesion implies the occurrence of active bleeding, protruding vessel or clot. Foster et al. (6) found that 53% of the patients with peptic ulcers with stigmata needed emergency surgery whereas only one patient with a peptic ulcer without stigmata was operated upon. The other important factor in predicting the outcome for patients with massive upper gastrointestinal bleeding is the presence of hypovolemic shock or preshock on admission to the hospital (7).

METHODS

During a 28-month period a total of 95 patients were included in a double-blind randomized trial of somatostatin in the treatment of massive upper gastrointestinal bleeding (8). All patients included had had at least two of the following signs of shock or preshock: systolic blood pressure $\leq$ 100 mm Hg, pulse rate $\geq$ 100, a cold pale clammy skin, a history of fainting. Patients with diabetes mellitus or bleeding esophageal varices were not included in the study. Endoscopy was performed within eight hours of admission and the following day a control endoscopy was carried out.

After the initial endoscopy the patients were selected at random for treatment with either somatostatin or placebo. Forty-six patients were given an infusion of cyclic somatostatin-14 at a dosage of 250 μg/hour, after a bolus injection of 250 μg, and 49 patients were given placebo which was administered in the same manner as somatostatin. The infusions were given for 72 hours and no additional treatments except blood transfusions were given. Patients with rebleeding after the 72-hour infusion period were given an infusion of somatostatin for an additional 72-hour period.

The indications for surgical treatment were when the magnitude of bleeding necessitated more than 6 units of blood to keep stable circulation, or when cases of rebleeding necessitated transfusion of more than 4 units of blood.

RESULTS

The bleeding lesions found in the two groups are listed in Table 1. Peptic ulcer was the most common source of bleeding.

A total of 29 or 81% of the ulcer patients in the somatostatin group had lesions with stigmata. In the placebo group 36 or 86% of the ulcer patients had lesions with stigmata. On the day of admission, clinical or endoscopic signs of active bleeding were found in 36 patients in the somatostatin group and in 40 patients in the placebo group. On the following day, endoscopic examination revealed continuous bleeding in 8 patients in the somatostatin group and in 16 patients in the placebo group.

A total of 6 patients re-bled in the somatostatin group. One patient experienced a limited rebleeding during the somatostatin infusion which stopped spontaneously. Five patients re-bled after the somatostatin infusion. One of these patients stopped bleeding spontaneously. The remaining 4 patients were treated with somatostatin and one of them had to be operated upon.

In the placebo group 5 patients re-bled, 4 of them on the day following the admission. One of these patients had a continuous minor bleeding and was treated with somatostatin and he stopped bleeding. The other 4 patients with rebleeding in the placebo group were operated upon. In both groups all patients with rebleeding except one had lesions with stigmata.

In the somatostatin group a total of 5 patients were operated upon and 14 in the placebo group (Fisher's exact test, 2-tail, P = 0.04). All patients operated on except one in the placebo group had lesions with stigmata.

Table 1.

	Somatostatin group (no 46)	Placebo group (no 49)
Gastric ulcer	16	25
Duodenal ulcer	17	15
Stomal ulcer	3	2
Erosive bleeding	4	4
Miscellaneous	4	1
No diagnosis	2	2

314

In the placebo group as compared with the somatostatin group there was numerically but not statistically more patients with gastric ulcers. In this study the risk for operation was highest in patients with duodenal ulcer and the number of duodenal ulcers was equivalent in the two groups. The somewhat unequal distribution of patients with gastric ulcers has consequently not influenced the difference in number of emergency operations between the somatostatin and placebo groups (Table 2). One patient operated on in the somatostatin group had a stomal ulcer and one in the placebo group had multiple Mallory-Weiss tears.

The mean ± SD number of blood units given was 5.8 ± 5.3 units in the somatostatin group and 7.2 ± 6.5 units in the placebo group. The difference of 1.4 between the two groups was not significant because of the standard deviation.

The mortality rate in the study was 5.3% which included 4 patients in the somatostatin group and one in the placebo group. Two of the patients who died had been operated upon and their deaths were related to the upper gastrointestinal bleeding. Three of our patients died weeks after the bleeding had stopped from concomitant diseases but are included in the mortality rate.

No side effects of the somatostatin infusions were found regarding blood pressure and routine laboratory tests. One patient in the somatostatin group and two in the placebo group needed insulin administration.

DISCUSSION

The results in the present study are in conformity with those in the study by Kayasseh et al. (9) and Coraggio et al. (10) but differ from those presented by Somerville et al. (11).

In our trial (8) only patients with massive upper gastrointestinal bleeding have been included. In order to include all massive bleeders in a trial, it is necessary to perform endoscopy early as otherwise the risk will increase that some patients with severe bleeding will be excluded as their worsened condition might need immediate surgery. This statement is illustrated by the finding that in the present trial 3 patients were operated on within 8 hours after admission to the trial and 10 patients within 26 hours. All of these patients were on infusion with either placebo or somatostatin. Had the initial endoscopy been postponed, they would not have been included in our study.

In trials on upper gastrointestinal bleedings a control endoscopy should be performed. This second endoscopy implies more accurate diagno-

Table 2. Distribution of emergency operations
in both groups.

	Somatostatin group	Placebo group
Operation:		
Gastric ulcer, no (%)	2/16 (13%)	7/25 (28%)
Duodenal ulcer, no (%)	2/17 (12%)	6/15 (40%)

ses, verifies if the bleeding has stopped and should also be used to verify rebleedings. In trials, it is also important to have strict criteria for emergency operations as otherwise the number of emergency operations, which influences the mortality rate, cannot be properly estimated (12).

The importance of bleeding stigmata in predicting the outcome for patients with upper gastrointestinal bleeding was verified in the present study. Contrary to the finding by Griffiths et al. (13), in our study all patients with a protruding vessel at endoscopy were not operated upon because of recurrent or uncontrolled bleeding. In the present study, 17 patients had a protruding vessel at endoscopy and 4 of them were operated on. In our experience the presence of stigmata is the important finding and not the type of stigmata.

In conclusion, somatostatin significantly reduced the number of emergency operations. This reduction might be due to the inhibitory effect of somatostatin on gastric acid secretion and pepsin release which facilitate platelet aggregation and plasma clotting and prevent dis- aggregation of clots as the gastric pH is raised. This postulated mech- anism is supported by the finding that patients in the somatostatin group re-bled after termination of the somatostatin infusion whereas patients in the placebo group re-bled on the day following admission. The circulatory effects of somatostatin are probably of lesser importance as most ulcers bleed from large arteries.

REFERENCES

1. Schrumpf E, Vatn MH, Hanssen KF, Myren J. A small dose of somato- statin inhibits the pentagastrin stimulated gastric secretion of acid, pepsin and intrinsic factor in man. Clin Endocrinol (Oxf), 1978; 8:391.
2. Bloom SR, Mortimer CH, Thorner MO, et al. Inhibition of gastrin and gastric-acid secretion by growth-hormone release-inhibiting hormone. Lancet 1974; 2:1106.
3. Johansson C, Aly A. Stimulation of gastric mucus output by somato- statin in man. Eur J Clin Invest 1982; 12:37.
4. Bosch J, Kravetz D, Rodes J. Effects of somatostatin on hepatic and systemic hemadynamics in patients with cirrhosis of the liver: comparison with vasopressin. Gastroenterology 1981; 80:518.
5. Green FV, Kaplan MM, Curtis LE, Levine PH. Effect of acid and pepsin on blood coagulation and platelet aggregation. Gastroenterology 1978; 74:38.
6. Foster DN, Miloszewski KJA, Losowsky MS. Stigmata of recent haem- orrhage in diagnosis and prognosis of upper gastrointestinal bleed- ing. Br Med J 1978; 1:1173.
7. Bornman PC, Theodorou NA, Shuttleworth RD, Essel HP, Marks IN. Importance of hypovolaemic shock and endoscopic signs in predicting recurrent haemorrhage from peptic ulceration: a prospective evalua- tion. Br Med J 1985; 291:245.
8. Magnusson I, Ihre T, Johansson C, Seligson U, Torngren S, Uvnas- Moberg K. Randomised double blind trial of somatostatin in the treatment of massive upper gastrointestinal haemorrhage. Gut 1985; 25:221.
9. Kayasseh L, Keller U, Gyr K, Stalder GE, Wall M. Somatostatin and cimetidine in peptic-ulcer haemorrhage. Lancet 1980; 1:844.
10. Coraggio F, Scarpato P, Spina M, Lombardi S. Somatostatin and ranitidine in the control of iatrogenic haemorrhage of the upper gastrointestinal tract. Br Med J 1984; 289:224.

11. Somerville KW, Henry DA, Davies JG, Hine KR, Hawkey CJ, Langman MJS. Somatostatin in the treatment of haematemesis and melaena. Lancet 1985; 1:130.
12. Kim B, Wright HK, Bordan D, Fielding LP, Swaney R. Risk of surgery for upper gastrointestinal haemorrhage: 1972 versus 1982. Am J Surg 1985; 149:474.
13. Griffiths WJ, Neumann DA, Welsh JD. The visible vessel as an indicator of uncontrolled or recurrent gastrointestinal haemorrhage. N Engl J Med 1979; 300:1411.

32

SOMATOSTATIN AND ANALOGS IN THE MANAGEMENT

OF VARICEAL HEMORRHAGE

J. N. Baxter, S. A. Jenkins, and R. Shields

University Department of Surgery
University of Liverpool, U.K.

In most centers the emergency control of acute variceal hemorrhage is primarily nonsurgical using a combination of resuscitation, balloon tamponade and possibly vasoactive drugs. The main objective of these treatments is to arrest the variceal hemorrhage and improve the patient's condition until definitive treatment can be carried out, e.g., injection sclerotherapy, esophageal transsection or portal-systemic shunting.

However, conventional emergency procedures for the management of acute variceal hemorrhage are not always successful and are often associated with complications. Thus, balloon tamponade has a significant morbidity and mortality (1), especially in inexperienced hands. Similarly, although intravenous vasopressin has been used for many years for the emergency control of acute variceal hemorrhage, it is only successful in approximately 50% of patients presenting for treatment (2). Furthermore, vasopressin administration can be accompanied by serious side-effects such as coronary vasoconstriction, pulmonary edema and abdominal colic.

Therefore, there is a need to develop a treatment for acute variceal hemorrhage which is effective, simple and relatively free from side-effects, especially in the situation when inexperienced clinicians may be called upon to deal with the emergency. Following its isolation from the hypothalamus in 1972, somatostatin (SRIF), a 14 amino acid polypeptide, was shown to reduce wedged hepatic venous pressure in man (3,4). Indeed, in our own studies in cirrhotic rats we have found that an infusion of 4 μg/kg body weight/h SRIF preceded by a bolus of 4 μg/kg reduces portal pressure by approximately 30% (5). Furthermore, in patients with cirrhosis and portal hypertension we have consistently found that a bolus injection of 250 μg SRIF reduces wedged hepatic venous pressure by approximately 25%.

Initially we studied in a prospective randomized clinical trial, the relative efficacy of SRIF and vasopressin in the control of acute variceal hemorrhage (6). We studied patients with a significant endoscopically proven variceal hemorrhage. A significant variceal hemorrhage was defined as a systemic disturbance; heart rate >100, BP > 100 mm Hg for two consecutive hours requiring blood transfusion or the necessity to transfuse two or more units of blood in 24 hours to maintain vital signs. Patients who were excluded from the trial were those transferred from other centers with an esophageal balloon in situ or already receiving vasoactive drugs.

Patients were randomly allocated to receive either vasopressin (argipressin; Ferring Pharmaceutical Company) or SRIF (Serono Laboratories, U.K.). Patients randomized to receive vasopressin were infused at a rate of 0.4 U/min for 6 hours. If bleeding stopped the rate of vasopressin infusion was decreased to 0.2 U/min for the following 6 hours, then decreased to 0.1 U/min for a further 6 hours, and finally stopped if no further bleeding episodes occurred. Patients randomized to SRIF received. a bolus of 250 μg SRIF over 2 min and a constant infusion of 250 μg/h for 24 hours. Because of the very short half-life of SRIF (1.8 min), the bolus dose was always given after the infusion had been commenced in order to try and ensure that a "therapeutic" circulating level of the hormone was achieved and maintained during the treatment period. Furthermore, special precautions were taken to ensure that the SRIF infusion was continuous, e.g., overlapping of infusion bags. If there was any uncertainty regarding the continuity of the SRIF infusion, a further bolus dose of 250 μg was administered.

Success of the vasoactive therapy was defined as control of the variceal hemorrhage as evidenced by the absence of blood in the nasogastric aspirate, maintenance of the packed cell volume, and absence of other overt signs of continued bleeding while receiving the vasoactive drug.

Twenty-two patients were entered into the trial. Twelve patients received vasopressin and 10 SRIF. The reason for unequal numbers in the two arms of the trial was that randomization envelopes were initially prepared for the 30 patients. However, following an adverse editorial (7) on the efficacy of SRIF in the control of acute variceal hemorrhage, we performed an analysis of our results after 22 patients were entered into the trial. A highly significant result had been obtained and, therefore, we considered it unethical to continue with the trial.

The etiology of the portal hypertension, Child's grading, age, sex, and ratio of index to interval episodes of bleeding were similar in the two groups of patients (Table 1).

The overall success rate of SRIF and vasopressin in controlling acute variceal hemorrhage is shown in Table 2. Vasopressin was successful in controlling bleeding in only 4 of the 12 patients. In contrast, SRIF successfully controlled bleeding in all 10 patients. These differences were highly significant using Fisher's exact test (P = 0.003). Three of the patients in the SRIF group re-bled after the infusion was stopped and before definitive treatment could be instituted. In all these patients control of the variceal hemorrhage was regained by SRIF infusion. Therefore, when the total number of actual bleeding episodes controlled by SRIF is compared with those controlled by vasopressin, there is a very highly significant difference between treatments (P = 0.0002).

Considering the vasopressin group in more detail (Fig. 1), vasopressin was observed to be successful in controlling acute variceal hemorrhage in only 4 patients. These patients subsequently underwent injection sclerotherapy. In the remaining 8 patients initial control of the variceal hemorrhage was unsuccessful with vasopressin. In 2 of these patients, vasopressin infusion had to be stopped while they were actively bleeding because of undesirable side-effects: pulmonary edema in one patient and abdominal colic in the other. In both of these patients the variceal hemorrhage was controlled by balloon tamponade. In the remaining 6 patients, a combination of balloon tamponade and vasopressin was used in an attempt to control the hemorrhage. This was successful in 4 patients. However, 2 of these patients subsequently died as a result of complications of balloon tamponade: inhalation in one case and esophageal ulcera-

320

Table 1.   Clinical features of patients with acute
variceal hemorrhage entered into the trial.

	Vasopressin (n=12)	Somatostatin (n=10)
Cause of portal hypertension:		
Cirrhosis		
Alcohol related	6	5
Cryptogenic	3	3
Primary biliary cirrhosis	1	0
Sarcoidosis	1	0
Paroxysmal nocturnal hemo-globinuria	0	1
Extrahepatic block	1	1
Child's classification:		
A	2	2
B	4	2
C	6	6
Age (yrs)		
Mean (SEM)	51.5 (2.9)	55.8 (5.0)
Range	30-73	39-72
Number of men	6	6
Number of episodes of bleeding:		
Index	8	6
Interval	4	4

tion and perforation in the other.   In the remaining 2 patients the variceal hemorrhage was not controlled by balloon tamponade and vasopressin.   One of these patients underwent an emergency esophageal transsection but died one week later of liver failure.   The other patient died of a combination of hypovolemic shock and liver failure before any further treatment could be undertaken.

Looking at the SRIF group in more detail (Fig. 2), SRIF was successful in controlling the acute variceal hemorrhage in all 10 patients. Seven of these patients had no further bleeding episodes and went on to receive maintenance injection sclerotherapy.   However, 3 patients experienced further significant bleeding episodes before definitive treatment could be undertaken.   All these bleeding episodes, 7 in total, were again successfully controlled by further SRIF administration.

Table 2.   Results of vasopressin and somatostatin treatment
in controlling acute variceal hemorrhage.   Figures
indicate numbers of patients in whom treatment
was successful or unsuccessful with numbers
of episodes of bleeding in parentheses.

	Successful	Not successful
Vasopressin (n=12)	4	8
Somatostatin (n =10)	10 (17)	0

P = 0.003 (0.0002), Fisher's exact test.

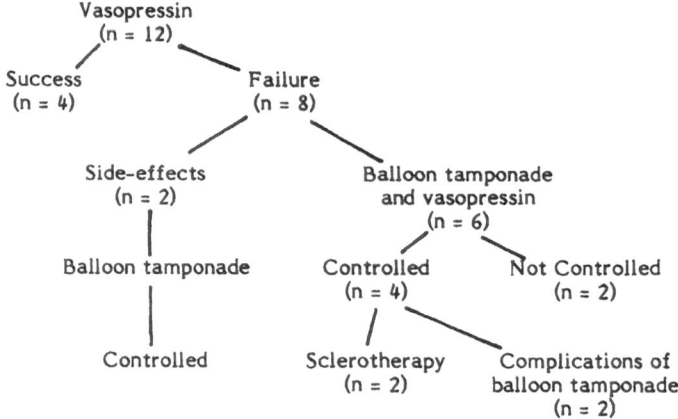

Fig. 1. Outcome of treatment with vasopressin in patients
with acute variceal hemorrhage.

To summarize, therefore, this randomized clinical trial clearly
indicates that: (i) SRIF is significantly more effective than vasopressin in controlling acute variceal hemorrhage, (ii) no complications could
be attributed to SRIF administration, and (iii) vasopressin administration
is relatively ineffective in controlling acute variceal hemorrhage and is
associated with complications. About the time we published our results of
this trial, Kravetz et al. (8) published their results of a similar study.
They found that there was no significant difference between SRIF and
vasopressin in the control of acute variceal hemorrhage and that administration of SRIF was associated with significantly fewer side-effects.
However, there were differences in the mode of administration of SRIF and
vasopressin which may explain the discrepancy between the two studies.
For example, their protocol allowed for an increase in the rate of administration of vasopressin, a choice which we did not have because we were
worried about side-effects from the vasopressin. Furthermore, a bolus of
only 50 μg SRIF was used and the precise details of when the bolus was
administered were not clear from their report. Our experimental work in a

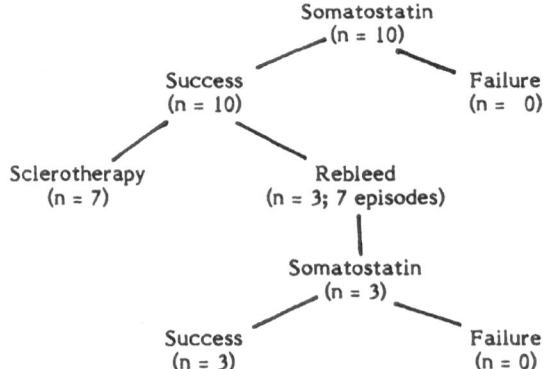

Fig. 2. Outcome of treatment with somatostatin in
patients with acute variceal hemorrhage.

322

cirrhotic rat model has suggested that a bolus dose of SRIF is necessary immediately before an infusion has been commenced in order to obtain a maximal drop in portal pressure (5). Thus, in our experience, we feel that bolus administration of SRIF is an important part of the regimen in order to obtain a therapeutic reduction in portal pressure. Therefore, if any doubt exists about the continuity of SRIF administration, a further bolus of 250 μg SRIF should be administered.

The efficacy of sclerotherapy in controlling acute variceal hemorrhage (85-95%) has led to the suggestion that this form of treatment should be the control against which newer forms of therapy should be judged (9). Therefore, in view of the promising results of our preliminary trial with SRIF, we have commenced a new randomized prospective controlled trial comparing SRIF with early injection sclerotherapy in the control of acute variceal hemorrhage. The hypothesis that this trial will test is whether SRIF is as good as or better than early injection sclerotherapy in controlling acute variceal hemorrhage.

Patients with a significant variceal hemorrhage (as defined previously) are randomized to receive SRIF or emergency injection sclerotherapy. Patients randomized to receive injection sclerotherapy are injected at the time of their initial endoscopy and again 5 days later. Those patients randomized to receive SRIF receive an IV infusion (250 μg/h) of the hormone for 5 days. A bolus dose of 250 μg SRIF is given as soon as the infusion is commenced and repeated at least every 12 hours.

Success of the treatment is defined using the criteria previously described for the control of hemorrhage in the preliminary trial. Rebleeding within the 5-day treatment period is regarded as a failure. In addition to comparing the efficacy of injection sclerotherapy and SRIF in controlling acute variceal hemorrhage, we are also comparing other possible beneficial effects of the treatment. For example, daily plasma amino acid profiles are performed on each patient during the 5-day study period together with assessment of the degree of encephalopathy. Further, daily blood samples are removed for endotoxin assay to assess the effects of the treatment on reticuloendothelial system activity. It is envisaged that these studies may indicate which treatment is more beneficial in terms of hepatic encephalopathy and reticuloendothelial system activity, two important considerations in the immediate post-bleed period.

To date 12 patients have been entered into the study, 6 of which have been randomized to receive SRIF and 6 injection sclerotherapy (Table 3). Injection sclerotherapy has been successful in all 6 patients while SRIF has been successful in 5 out of 6 patients. Interestingly, the one patient who was unsuccessful with SRIF had initial control of the hemorrhage with SRIF for 48 hours, then re-bled and thus is considered a failure.

Table 3. Outcome of patients with acute variceal hemorrhage receiving somatostatin or injection sclerotherapy.

	Injection sclerotherapy	Somatostatin
Number of patients	6	6
Initial control of hemorrhage	6	6
Rebleeding during trial period	0	1
Overall success	6	5

Since emergency endoscopic injection sclerotherapy is difficult and requires special expertise which is not always available, we consider that our trial will be of considerable interest to clinicians who do not have sclerotherapy facilities or the necessary skill to inject copiously bleeding varices. If SRIF is proved to be as effective as injection sclerotherapy in the control of acute variceal hemorrhage, the hormone may become an important therapeutic modality in hospitals which do not have the necessary facilities or expertise for injection sclerotherapy. In this situation variceal hemorrhage could be controlled by the administration of SRIF and the patient transferred to a specialized center under SRIF cover for definitive treatment.

With regard to the acute variceal bleed, SRIF has been found to be beneficial in three other clinical situations. Firstly, 5 days' SRIF treatment stopped bleeding in two patients who developed esophageal ulcers following injection sclerotherapy. Secondly, we have found SRIF to be useful in the management of 5 patients who re-bled 24-28 h following a course of injection sclerotherapy. Initially these patients were managed with 24 h of balloon tamponade but re-bled after compression was stopped. In all 5 patients the hemorrhage was successfully controlled with SRIF for 4-5 days when the patients underwent a further course of injection sclerotherapy. Finally, SRIF was successful in stopping recurrent hemorrhage in one patient who was bleeding from gastric varices.

In order to try and ascertain more precisely the mechanism of action of SRIF in lowering portal pressure, we have been studying the effects of bolus doses of 50 μg or 250 μg SRIF on wedged hepatic venous pressure and systemic cardiovascular hemodynamics in patients with cirrhosis and portal hypertension. In all patients so far studied, a bolus dose of 50 μg or 250 μg SRIF given over two minutes has reduced wedged hepatic venous pressure (corrected) approximately 25%. Furthermore, the reduction in wedged hepatic venous pressure is accompanied by an increase in arterial blood pressure and a bradycardia. These results, together with our studies in the cirrhotic rat (5) suggest that the systemic cardiovascular effects of SRIF, i.e., increase in arterial blood pressure and a reflex slowing of the heart are secondary to a marked splanchnic vasoconstriction. It is worthy of note that no patient so far studied has complained of any discomfort and no serious side-effects have been observed.

More recently we have been studying the effects of the long-acting analogue of SRIF, SMS 201-995 on hepatic hemodynamics in our cirrhotic rat model (10) and also in patients with cirrhosis and portal hypertension (11). The longer half-life and subcutaneous mode of administration of this drug may make it suitable for the long-term management of portal hypertension. In the cirrhotic rat, 2 μg/kg body weight SMS 201-995 produced a gradual and sustained decrease in portal pressure of approximately 28%. Moreover, in 9 patients with cirrhosis and portal hypertension a bolus dose of 50 μg SMS 201-995 IV reduced the intravariceal pressure approximately 38% (Fig. 3). Interestingly, in another 6 patients with cirrhosis and portal hypertension, 50 μg SMS 201-995 IV reduced wedged hepatic venous pressure only approximately 14%. Either wedged hepatic venous pressure is not a good measure of acute changes in hepatic hemodynamics (12) or the effect of SMS 201-995 is greater in the region of the gastroesophageal junction. In another patient who was undergoing an elective shunt procedure, a bolus injection of 50 μg SMS 201-995 IV reduced directly recorded portal pressure by 25%.

Encouraged by these results we have just commenced a randomized prospective controlled trial evaluating the efficacy of SMS 201-995 in preventing interval bleeding which occurs in 40% of patients undergoing maintenance sclerotherapy until the varices are obliterated. Immediately

324

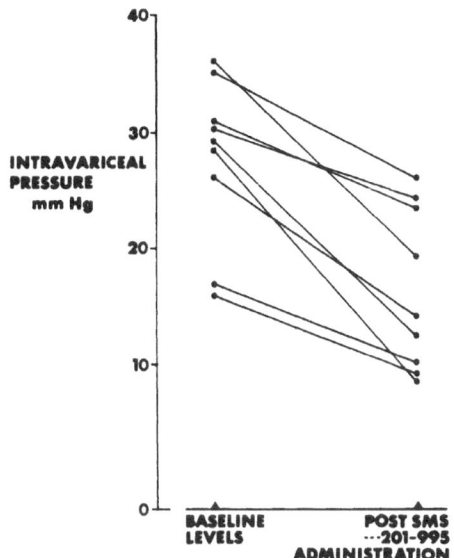

Fig. 3. Changes in intravariceal pressure
in 9 cirrhotic patients following a bolus
dose of 50 μg SMS 201-995

following control of the index bleed patients are randomized to receive
either 3 weekly injection sclerotherapy plus 50 μg SMS 201-995 sc b.i.d.
or 3 weekly injection sclerotherapy alone. Thus, we are testing the
hypothesis that SMS 201-995 administration will reduce the frequency of
interval bleeds during a program of sclerotherapy.

In conclusion, we believe that SRIF and possibly its analogue, SMS
201-995, have a role in the management of patients with portal hypertension who have bled from esophageal varices. Clearly, further studies
will determine whether these agents will have a central role in the
management of portal hypertension.

REFERENCES

1. Parbhoo S. The management of bleeding in liver disease. Br J Hosp
   Med 1975; 15:17-28.
2. Conn HO, Dalessio DJ. Multiple infusions of posterior pituitary
   extract in the treatment of bleeding oesophageal varices. Ann Intern
   Med 1962; 57:804-9.
3. Tyden G, Samnegard H, Thulin L, Friman L. Treatment of bleeding
   oesophageal varices with somatostatin (letter). N Engl J Med 1978;
   299:1466.
4. Bosch J, Kravetz D, Rodes J. Effects of somatostatin on hepatic and
   systemic haemodynamics in patients with cirrhosis of the liver and in
   normal subjects. Gastroenterology 1981; 80:526-32.
5. Jenkins SA, Devitt P, Day DW, Baxter JN, Shields R. Effects of
   somatostatin on hepatic haemodynamics in the cirrhotic rat. Digestion 1986; 33:126-34.
6. Jenkins SA, Baxter JN, Corbett WC, Devitt P, Ware J, Shields R. A
   prospective randomized controlled clinical trial comparing somato-

statin and vasopressin in controlling acute variceal haemorrhage.
Br Med J 1985; 290:275-8.

7. Editorial. Bleeding oesophageal varices. Lancet 1984; 1:139-41.

8. Kravetz D, Bosch J, Teres J, Bruix J, Rimola A, Rodes J. Comparison
   of intravenous somatostatin and vasopressin infusions in treatment of
   acute variceal haemorrhage. Hepatology 1984; 4:442-6.

9. Terblanche J, Kahn D, Campbell JH, et al. Failure of repeated
   injection sclerotherapy to improve long-term survival after oesophageal variceal bleeding. Lancet 1983; 2:1328-32.

10. Jenkins SA, Baxter JN, Corbett WA, Shields R. The effects of a
    somatostatin analogue SMS 201-995 on hepatic haemodynamics in the
    cirrhotic rat. Br J Surg 1985; 72:864-7.

11. Jenkins SA, Baxter JN, Corbett WA, Shields R. Effects of a somato-
    statin analogue SMS 201-995 on hepatic haemodynamics in the pig and
    on intravariceal pressure in man. Br J Surg 1985; 72:1009-12.

12. Valla D, Bercoff E, Menu Y, Bataille C, Lebrec D. Discrepancy
    between wedged hepatic venous pressure and portal venous pressure
    after acute propranolol administration in patients with alcoholic
    cirrhosis. Gastroenterology 1984; 86:1400-3.

33

SOMATOSTATIN IN THE TREATMENT OF HEMATEMESIS AND MELENA

Michael Langman

Department of Therapeutics
University Hospital
Nottingham NG7 2UH England

SUMMARY

Clinical trials generally show a trend towards reduced rebleeding rates in patients with hematemesis and melena due mainly to nonvariceal causes. Evidence of benefit to patients by reduced mortality is lacking. This may in part be due to the failure of investigators to accept that very large trials are needed if confident answers are to be obtained. Hardly any trials of any treatment are of adequate size.

In the United Kingdom about 1 in 2000 of the population is likely to suffer from upper gastrointestinal bleeding in an average year, or about 30,000 cases in all, and up to 10% will be likely to die. Improving treatment is therefore a worthwhile exercise. The possibilities include drug and electrophysical methods, but these are not mutually exclusive. Drug treatments also have the attraction that they are not dependent on clinical expertise for administration.

Available evidence suggests that useful improvements in outcome may be obtainable using histamine H_2 antagonists (1), and with tranexamic acid (2) although the evidence is not certain. As somatostatin has powerful actions in inhibiting gastric acid secretion and reducing blood flow, it has, logically, been examined as a treatment for upper gastrointestinal bleeding.

The Trials

To date results have been obtained in five groups of patients with primarily nonvariceal bleeding, and Table 1 compares the methods employed.

Size. Trials varied greatly, from the smallest which included 20 patients to the largest which included 630.

Methods. Studies were blinded but differed on inclusion criteria, the large including all comers, with randomization to test and control groups at the time of hospital admission while others only included patients once endoscopy had confirmed that there was active ulcer bleeding. One study was confined to patients with drug-induced bleeding. One study was also designed as a comparison in pairs of patients with equivalent clinical problems.

Table 1.

	Trial design	Total entered
Kayasseh et al. (4)	Paired sequential comparison in documented severe bleeding versus cimetidine	20
Magnusson et al. (5)	Randomized double-blind versus placebo severe bleeding (one hospital)	95
Somerville et al. (6)	Randomized double-blind two hospitals, all patients with diagnosed bleeding	630
Torres et al. (7)	Multicenter randomized	60
Coraggio et al. (3)	Triple comparison in drug-induced bleeding versus cimetidine and placebo	60

Outcome (Table 2)

Rebleeding. In all studies trends were seen towards reduced rebleeding rates, but the results diverged widely. Thus, in the analysis of outcome of drug-induced bleeding, results which were clear improvements on placebo treatment were observed in all the somatostatin recipients with no overlap whatsoever or unusual outcome. By contrast, in the largest study there was a 22% (but nonsignificant) decrease in overall rebleeding rates. These apparently conflicting results may be brought together by considering the 95% confidence limits round estimates, which, if they are plainly wide for the largest study, must be even wider for smaller studies. Taken overall the results are compatible with clinical effects of value though they may not be dramatic.

Operation. Data concerning operations have the disadvantage that they tend to reflect a combination of true need and physician prejudice. In two studies they suggest that there may be some clinical effect (although no trend at all was demonstrable in the largest study); confidence limits are very wide.

Death rates. The few deaths in the smaller series allow no sensible conclusions, and the trend against active treatment in the largest series argues that large treatment effects are unlikely although confidence limits are wide.

DISCUSSION

The varying results of somatostatin treatment may, at least in part, reflect the varying study methods adopted by investigators and the difficulty of defining suitable end points.

328

Table 2. Outcome of general trials of treatment with somatostatin for upper gastrointestinal bleeding.

	Bleeding			Somatostatin		
		95% confidence limits			95% confidence limits	
Kayasseh et al. (4)	Bleeding persistent	9/10	-	Bleeding persistent	2/10	-
	Operation	4/10	-		2/10	-
	Death	3/10	-		0/10	-
Magnusson et al. (5)	Total	49			46	
	Bleeding	%		Bleeding	%	
	persistent	32.6	(Not given)	persistent	17.4	(Not given)
	Operation	28.6	(Not given)		10.8	(Not given)
	Death	2.0	(Not given)		8.7	(Not given)
Somerville et al. (6)	Total	315			315	
	Bleeding			Bleeding		
	persistent	28.3	(23.4-33.6)	persistent	22.2	(17.8-27.3)
	Operation	10.8	(7.7-14.8)		11.1	(8.0-15.2)
	Death	7.9	(5.3-11.6)		9.8	(6.9-13.8)

NB—Results as published: In twelve cases the coding was misassigned but this did not alter the allocated number of operations or deaths but did mistransfer 2 cases of bleeding to placebo from somatostatin (i.e., true figure for placebo = 2 or less and true for somatostatin = 2 or more).

Torres et al. (7)	Total	30			30	
	Bleeding	%		Bleeding	%	
	persistent	33.3	(Not given)	persistent	10.0	(Not given)
	Operation	30.0	(Not given)		10.0	(Not given)
	Death	6.6	(Not given)		3.3	(Not given)
Coraggio et al. (3)	Rebleeding ceased earlier in all somatostatin-treated than in any of ranitidine or placebo recipients.					

Early entry trials, as conducted in Nottingham, have the virtue of including all comers and a trial conducted in this way is well-placed to answer the question: does treatment have any effect under the ordinary conditions of practice? On the other hand, treatment effects may be obscured because very severe bleeding not amenable to treatment is included as is trivial bleeding where the outcome will be uneventful. In addition an appreciable moiety of patients who ultimately prove not to have suffered from bleeding will be included.

Late entry (at endoscopy trials) have the advantage of removing patients ultimately considered not to have bled and can be used to select individuals with endoscopic stigmata suggesting a high risk of rebleeding. On the other hand the studies may fail to include patients with severe bleeding who do not come to endoscopy.

Table 3. Rebleeding episodes in patients receiving
at least two units of blood on day one.

Rebleeding	Yes	No	Total
Somatostatin	42	99	141
Placebo	57	75	132

$$x^2 = 4.73 \qquad P = 0.03$$

The definition of rebleeding is hindered because not all patients have visible hematemesis and melena and, even if they do occur, it is not easy to decide if they are substantial or are necessarily recent. Transfusion requirements appear more objective, but are affected by the severity of blood loss prior to the start of treatment and by physicians' beliefs about the size of transfusion ordinarily needed, which are likely to vary.

If rebleeding rates in the Nottingham trial are solely considered in those requiring at least two units of blood in the first 24 hours, then a "statistically significant" result emerges following this concentration upon cases where clinical evidence of hypovolemia was thought to be present (Table 3). However, this approach, which was made post hoc, must be weak in inferential terms.

Generally, high rebleeding rates should be associated with high operation rates, but clinically the decision to operate may in part be made on other considerations including patient age and previous history, which are plainly unrelated to the drug in use.

Death rates might then seem to be the logical arbiters, but few patients die, and those who do may do so because they suffer from complicating severe extra-gastrointestinal disease. As a consequence, it may be difficult to show any treatment effect.

To be sure of treatment effects it may therefore be sensible to show parallel improvements in rebleeding or transfusion rates, operation rates and mortality rates. That this search for parallel changes may be reasonable is suggested by considering the results of all 27 trials in 2760 patients who were randomly allocated treatment with histamine H_2 antagonists or placebo (1). The results suggested that rebleeding rates might be reduced by 11% with 95% confidence limits of minus 30% and plus 8%, operation rates by 21% with confidence limits of minus 39% and zero, and death rates by 30% with confidence limits of minus 50% and minus 41%.

The inability to come to a confident conclusion over the value of histamine H_2 antagonists emphasizes the very large numbers of patients required if firm conclusions are to be reached, and the position over somatostatin remains unsure.

REFERENCES

1. Collins R, Langman MJS. Treatment with histamine H_2 antagonists in acute upper gastrointestinal hemorrhage. Implications of randomized trials. N Engl J Med 1985; 313:660-6.

2. Barer D, Ogilvie A, Henry D, et al. Cimetidine and tranexamic acid in the treatment of acute upper gastrointestinal bleeding. N Engl J Med 1983; 308:1571-5.
3. Coraggio F, Scarpato P, Spina M, Lombardi S. Somatostatin and ranitidine in the control of iatrogenic haemorrhage of the upper gastrointestinal tract. Br Med J 1984; 288:244.
4. Kayasseh L, Gyr K, Keller U, Stalder GA, Wall M. Somatostatin and cimetidine in peptic ulcer haemorrhage. Lancet 1980; i:844-6.
5. Magnusson I, Ihre T, Johansson C, Seligson U, Torngren S, Uvnas-Moberg K. Randomized double-blind trial of somatostatin in the treatment of massive upper gastrointestinal haemorrhage. Gut 1985; 26:221-6.
6. Somerville KW, Henry DA, Davies JG, Hine KR, Hawkey CJ, Langman MJS. Somatostatin in treatment of haematemesis and melaena. Lancet 1985; 1:130-2.
7. Torres AJ, Landa I, Hernandes F, et al. Somatostatin (SS) in the treatment of upper gastrointestinal (GI) bleeding. A multicentre controlled trial [Abstract]. International Conference on Somatostatin, Washington, DC, May 6-8, 1986.

34

SOMATOSTATIN OCTAPEPTIDE IN THE MEDICAL TREATMENT

OF ACROMEGALY

G. M. Besser and J. A. H. Wass

Department of Endocrinology
St. Bartholomew's Hospital
London

SUMMARY

Somatostatin lowers growth hormone (GH) in patients with acromegaly but it has a short half life in the circulation and thus cannot be used for medical treatment. Recently an octapeptide analogue (SMS 201-995) of somatostatin has been developed with a much longer half-life and which has clear therapeutic potential in patients with growth hormone secreting tumors.

Somatostatin octapeptide causes the suppression of growth hormone for 3, 5 and 9 hours after 50, 100 and 200 µg respectively. 400 µg subcutaneously caused even longer growth hormone suppression but there were side-effects seen in some patients. Long-term treatment with 100 µg, subcutaneously, twice daily caused growth hormone suppression in all patients studied but some escape was seen at the end of the 12-hour study period. When bromocriptine responses were compared to those of somatostatin in the same patients, somatostatin caused better growth hormone suppression in 7 out of 8 patients studied; addition of bromocriptine to somatostatin did not cause better growth hormone suppression in 4 out of the 5 patients studied than somatostatin octapeptide alone.

We conclude that somatostatin octapeptide is a significant advance in the medical treatment of acromegaly.

INTRODUCTION

Somatostatin given parenterally suppresses growth hormone (GH) (1). Parenteral administration has been used in acromegalic patients (2), but long-term treatment is hampered by its short half-life of a few minutes in the circulation. A large number of longer acting somatostatin analogues have been produced since the first isolation of this tetradecapeptide. Some of these have a shorter peptide sequence which includes the main 4 amino-acids essential for its action in positions 7-10. Recently an octapeptide analogue (SMS 201-995, Sandoz Basel) has been developed and synthesized by conventional fragment condensation techniques and purified (3). Prolongation of activity is thought to result from D phenylamine substitution at the N terminus together with the C terminal alcohol sequence. Growth hormone inhibiting activity is greater than that of the native hormone and is associated with less prolonged inhibition of insulin and glucagon secretion (3). Furthermore, this analogue has a prolonged half-life in the circulation of 80-90 minutes and this has been confirmed in our specific radioimmunoassay for this compound. Thus, in vitro it is 3 times as potent at inhibiting growth hormone and in vivo, in rat and rhesus monkeys, is 20 times more active in suppressing growth hormone. Toxicity studies in 4 species of animals have shown no adverse effects.

Having confirmed that growth hormone levels were suppressed for a longer duration of time in acute intravenous studies, we set out to establish the optimum dose regime for use in long-term studies, to study patients on long-term treatment with somatostatin octapeptide, to see whether it was more effective than bromocriptine in suppressing growth hormone release, and, lastly, to establish whether simultaneous somatostatin and bromocriptine treatment were any more effective than somatostatin used alone.

PATIENTS AND METHODS

Eleven patients (aged 46-53 years) have taken part in 4 separate studies; 9 were male. All were documented to have acromegaly with a failure of growth hormone suppression during an oral glucose tolerance test. Five had had no previous treatment and 5 had had external pituitary irradiation (10-12 years prior to the study). One had had both external pituitary irradiation and a transsphenoidal hypophysectomy in the year prior to the study. Despite these treatments acromegaly persisted. All patients had been off dopamine agonist therapy for at least a month prior to the study. Serum GH was sampled hourly for 12 hours between 09:00 and 21:00 hours during treatment. Long-term treatment was continued between 2 weeks and 9 months.

RESULTS

Dose Response Study

In contrast to administration of saline, single subcutaneous doses of 50, 100 and 200 μg somatostatin octapeptide caused a suppression of growth hormone, and levels began to rise after 3, 5 and 9 hours respectively.

When 200 and 400 μg sc were compared with control injections in the same patients, growth hormone levels remained suppressed throughout the 12-hour study period. Two of these patients, however, complained of abdominal pain on the higher dose.

Long-term Administration

When compared to the pretreatment 12-hour profile of serum GH levels, GH was suppressed in all patients. Individual minimum growth hormone ranged from less than 1 to 6.5 mU/l. Before treatment, mean growth hormone levels (mean of 12) ranged from 19.5-135 (mean ± 1 SEM, 70 ± 13). On treatment with somatostatin octapeptide mean growth hormone levels ranged from 4.5-36 mU/l (mean ± 1 SEM 14 ± 3). Only one patient had a mean growth hormone level on treatment of greater than 20 mU/l. The minimum levels were reached between 3 and 5 hours after the administration.

Glucose tolerance was assessed by monitoring glucose levels through the 12-hour study periods on normal food intake. These did not deteriorate and were not significantly altered.

Five patients noted side-effects. Four of these noted diarrhea (bowels open up to 4 times a day) and one, abdominal pain for 10 minutes after the injection when the injection was given on an empty stomach.

Comparison of the Effects of Somatostatin Octapeptide and Bromocriptine

In the 8 patients studied off treatment, mean growth hormone levels through the 12-hour period ranged from 30-135 (mean 75 ± 13). On bromocriptine (20-40 mg daily) in these patients growth hormone values ranged from 13-22 (mean 32 ± 6). On somatostatin octapeptide, 100 µg every 12 hours, growth hormone values ranged from 4-36 (14 ± 3 mU/1). In 7 of the 8 patients somatostatin produced better growth hormone control than bromocriptine, given in doses known to maximally suppress growth hormone secretion. Addition of bromocriptine to the established somatostatin regimes did not further suppress GH levels in these patients.

DISCUSSION

Somatostatin octapeptide clearly causes prolonged growth hormone suppression in patients with acromegaly. As such it is a useful advance in the medical treatment of this condition (4). It is clear from these studies that 50 µg administered subcutaneously causes growth hormone suppression that is too short in duration. We chose for the long-term studies to use 100 µg twice daily, because even this dose caused mild side-effects of diarrhea and abdominal pain and we reasoned that using a higher dose would increase the incidence of side-effects further as indeed was the case when single doses of 400 µg were studied. Nevertheless, escape of growth hormone levels was seen using this dose for periods of 2 weeks and we now recommend that patients on long-term treatment administer their injections every 8 hours. Despite the theoretical problems of carbohydrate intolerance due to suppression of insulin secretion, long-term treatment was not associated with worsening of carbohydrate tolerance. Indeed, mean blood glucose levels improved in 3 patients. Presumably, this was associated with suppression of growth hormone levels, although when taken overall, the changes in glucose levels did not reach statistical significance. Three patients on somatostatin octapeptide treatment for 9 months have shown no escape of growth hormone suppression and there have been no side-effects. It is already clear that acromegaly is better controlled in most patients with twice daily somatostatin octapeptide injections than on maximally suppressive doses of bromocriptine taken orally.

Somatostatin suppresses exocrine function of the pancreas and 4 patients have developed diarrhea on treatment. This did not lead to cessation of treatment in any case. Fecal fat excretion was raised above normal in 2 patients. It is clear that in long-term treatment, malabsorption might be troublesome.

The prolonged action of somatostatin octapeptide in suppressing growth hormone values in part relates to its prolonged half-life in the circulation. It is possible also that it has a prolonged action at receptor sites on the anterior pituitary and this may account for the lack of rebound. Rises in growth hormone are seen after native somatostatin injections.

We consider that long-term studies of this compound in the treatment of acromegaly are merited as no serious side-effects have been seen.

REFERENCES

1. Brazeau P, Vale W, Burgus R, et al. Hypothalamic polypeptide that inhibits the secretion of immunoreactive pituitary growth hormone. Science 1973; 178:77-9.
2. Besser GM, Mortimer CH, McNeilly AS, et al. Longterm infusion of growth hormone release inhibiting hormone in acromegaly: effects on pituitary and pancreatic hormones. Br Med J 1974; 4:620-7.
3. Bauer W, Briner U, Doepfner W, et al. Somatostatin 201-995: a very potent and selective octapeptide analogue of somatostatin with prolonged action. Life Sci 1982; 31:1133-40.
4. Ch'ng LJ, Sandler LM, Karenzlin ME, Burrin JM, Joplin GF, Blood SR. Longterm treatment of acromegaly with a long acting analogue of somatostatin. Br Med J 1985; 1:284-5.

35

EFFICACY AND SAFETY OF A SOMATOSTATIN ANALOGUE IN

ACTIVE ACROMEGALY

George Tolis, Angelos Yotis, Emilio del Pozo,
and Alan Harris

Hippokrateion Hospital, Athens, GR 11527 and
Sandoz Ltd., Clinical Research, Basle, CH 4002

INTRODUCTION

Acromegaly has been associated, in the past, with chronic discomfort leading from invalidism to death. Partial or complete removal of the pituitary gland has been the preferred mode of therapy but if the growth hormone (GH) secreting tumor cannot be totally removed GH oversecretion will persist. Radiotherapy may be needed to further suppress GH serum levels, but even this may prove to be ineffective. Efforts to develop medications that suppress the secretory capacity of the pituitary tumor cells have succeeded in providing drugs mimicking neurotransmitter-dependent secretory processes.

L-dopa, bromocriptine, lisuride and pergolide have been used both as the initial step of therapy as well as after other modes of treatment have failed. Unfortunately the results that have been obtained were less satisfactory than expected. It is possible that this relates either to the dependence of drug efficacy upon suprahypophysical intact mechanisms—which may not be the case in acromegaly—or to lack of high affinity receptors on tumor surface for the various dopaminomimetic agents. The knowledge that somatostatin receptors are present in GH secreting human pituitary tumors (1-3) has led to the idea of synthesizing various somatostatin analogues with a longer half-life than the natively occurring tetradecapeptide (4).

The recent development of an 8-aminoacid somatostatin analogue, octeotride, which could effectively suppress GH secretion both in animals and man prompted us to evaluate its efficacy in active acromegaly.

METHODS—PATIENTS

Octeotride or H-(D)Phe-Cys-Phe-(D)Trp-Lys-Thr-Cys-Thr(ol) code-named SMS 201-995 was synthesized by use of conventional fragment condensation technique. Vials with various concentrations were stored at 4°C prior to injection. The patients were taught to inject themselves subcutaneously (sc) once to three times daily. The initial dose was 25 μg twice daily.

Prior to the onset of therapy all patients had computerized axial tomography and the following dynamic testing:

(a) Oral glucose tolerance test: 100 gm intake with sampling for blood sugar (BS) insulin (IRI) and GH at 0', 30', 60', 90', 120'.

(b) GRF testing: 1 μg/kg body weight IV injection and sampling for GH at 0', 30', 60'.

(c) TRH testing: 200 μg IV bolus and sampling for TSH, PRL and GH at 0', 30', 60'.

(d) SMS 201-995 testing: 25 or 50 μg sc and sampling for GH, BS, IRI at 0', 30', 60', 120', 180', 240'.

(e) Combined SMS 201-995 and GRF or TRH testing: SMS 201-995 was injected at 0' whereas GRF or TRH were given at 2 hours after SMS 201-995.

Fourteen patients (8 male, 6 female, age range 20-57 years), half of whom had been treated previously with surgery and/or radiotherapy with no success and in whom GH levels were elevated while on bromocriptine (exceeding 5 ng/ml after an oral glucose load), participated in the study. All signed an informed consent form provided by the Greek FDA (EOF).

Prior to the onset of therapy, a list of subjective and objective signs was prepared and the various findings were tabulated and rated with an arbitrary scale of 0-4; this rating was subsequently followed at weekly visits for 6 weeks and at monthly periods thereafter. Repeat GH testing and CAT scanning were done after the initial 6-week therapy.

RESULTS

Hormonal

Basal serum GH levels ranged from 7-320 ng/ml; two patients had 7 and 10 ng/ml fasting values whereas the mean of the rest was 83 ng/ml (range 16-320 ng/ml). None of the above patients suppressed serum GH to normal (<5 ng/ml) after a glucose load. A rise of serum GH to more than 50% of random fluctuation occurred in 3 out of 8 tested. All four patients who were on bromocriptine 7.5-35 mg/daily had fasting and 3-hour GH values in excess of 10 ng/ml. The acute SMS 201-995 administration resulted in an acute decline of serum GH which reached normal values in 11 out of 14 patients; in the rest three GH values suppressed as follows: 210 → 155, 320 → 200 and 110 → 16 ng/ml respectively. GRF and TRF induced GH rise was in part inhibited after preceding SMS 201-995 injection by a net of 40-110 ng/ml, after GRF and 5-15 ng/ml after TRF; these figures represent a mean of 79.6% for GRF and 56% for TRF.

Following the acute SMS 201-995 injection nadir GH values were reached within 60-140 minutes and the return to pre-injection blood levels required 4-10 hours. A repeated injection of SMS 201-995 reproduced the same response pattern; this phenomenon was seen at 1 week, 1 month and 1 year during chronic therapy. Although a significant drop in serum GH followed each injection, the 24-hour GH profile was still abnormal unless SMS 201-995 was injected in a total not less than 100 μg and at 3 divided doses. Patients with the highest basal values required larger SMS 201-995 doses (150-300 μg); even then a complete suppression of serum GH could not be obtained.

Basal serum T4, T3, PRL, sex steroids and plasma cortisol did not change with chronic SMS 201-995 therapy. A mild elevation of blood sugar and a drop in circulating insulin levels was seen with the initial acute SMS 201-995 injection.

338

Clinical

Significant improvement in soft tissue swelling, reduction in ring size, disappearance of carpal tunnel syndrome, impressive relief from headaches and perspiration were cardinal features of benefit during SMS 201-995 therapy. Some of the symptoms, i.e., headache, were influenced within the first 4 days of therapy while other symptoms and signs required 2-4 weeks. An improvement, but of lesser degree, was seen even in those patients in whom serum GH decreased but did not normalize. In addition to these specific GH related complaints, patients noticed an improvement in their performance status and a decrease in their somnolence and depression; sexual function was improved in those with normal pituitary LH reserve and no evidence of diabetic neuropathy. Menstruation was unaffected. Galactorrhea decreased in one and disappeared in another.

Radiological

A shrinkage of the pituitary tumor was evidenced in two out of 8 evaluable patients whereas in the rest pituitary tumor size was unchanged.

Side Effects

Three of the patients developed abdominal cramps at different times of therapy; one of 3 who was known to have a gallbladder lithiasis, experienced a colic attack during therapy. None of the patients developed diarrhea, allergic reactions or glycosuria.

Effects of Therapy Discontinuation

Following discontinuation of therapy there was a gradual return of practically all symptoms and signs which again improved upon re-initiation of treatment. Serum GH levels did not show any rebound phenomenon after therapy was discontinued; the decline of its levels after re-initiation of treatment with SMS 201-995 was easy to establish.

DISCUSSION

The administration of the long-acting stable somatostatin analogue octeotride or SMS 201-995 in our patients, resulted in an impressive and rapid clinical improvement. These data are consistent with earlier work of ours and other investigators who treated patients from a minimum of 3 days to 6 months (5-13).

The amelioration of symptoms even in patients who had been failures to both invasive and medical forms of therapy is of particular interest since such a population of patients exists in not small numbers. The ability of SMS 201-995 to bind to pituitary tumor receptors with high affinity may predict that this analogue could have an effect on GH secreting cells. Certainly, in vitro studies comparing dopamine agonist drugs and SMS 201-995 would be of interest, if they were to show a correlation between in vivo and in vitro concordance of modulation of GH secretion by these agents. The ability of SMS 201-995 to suppress effectively GH secretion even in those patients who did not benefit from bromocriptine indicates that somatostatin-analogues may be a very promising tool for treatment of acromegaly. Our finding of tumor-shrinkage in some patients is in accordance with experience by others. It should be mentioned, however, that the decrease in tumor size is far less impressive than that obtained with bromocriptine in prolactinoma patients. The inability of SMS 201-995 to suppress GH completely in all patients studied is of some concern. It is possible that higher doses could do that but we avoided it because of possible side effects on other hormonal parameters, intestinal motility and fat absorption (14). In such patients it has been proposed to combine SMS 201-995 with bromocriptine but long-term efficacy studies have not been reported as yet. Of interest to us was also the effects of SMS 201-995 on nonspecific associated features such as headache, decreased libido or vitality, somnolence and depression. Although one could theorize that with the return of function of daily activities (thanks to the relief of specific complaints, i.e., resumption of tennis playing in a patient with carpal tunnel syndrome), there is a nonspecific benefit to the patient, the fact that the improvement in the above symptoms occurred rapidly may suggest other mechanisms. Indeed, sites that bind to radiolabeled SMS 201-995 are widely distributed in the brain and SMS 201-995 can influence catecholamine turnover and opiate dependent central and peripheral processes (15-18). The interaction of decreased GH and SMS 201-995 with central neuroactive substances should be explored in the future.

In conclusion, it appears that long-term therapy of patients with active acromegaly is feasible with the use of this long-acting analogue of somatostatin. Although failures of conventional therapeutic maneuvers represent the first choice for such a therapy, the possibility remains for patients that have never been treated to benefit from this new mode of therapy.

REFERENCES

1. Reubi JC, Landolt AM. High density of somatostatin receptors in pituitary tumors from acromegalic patients. J Clin Endocrinol Metab 1984; 59:1148-51.
2. Lamberts SWJ, Verleun T, Oosterom R. The interrelationship between the effects of somatostatin and human pancreatic growth hormone-releasing factor on growth hormone release by cultured pituitary tumor cells from patients with acromegaly. J Clin Endocrinol Metab 1984; 58:250-4.
3. Reubi JC, Perrin M, Rivier J, Vale W. Pituitary somatostatin receptors: dissociation at the pituitary level of receptor affinity and biological activity for selective somatostatin analogs. Regul Pept 1982; 4:141-6.
4. Bauer W, Briner U, Doepfner W, et al. SMS 201-995: a very potent and selective octapeptide analogue of somatostatin with prolonged action. Life Sci 1982; 31:1133-40.
5. Plewe G, Beyer J, Krause W, Neufeld M, del Pozo E. Long-acting and selective suppression of GH secretion by SMS 201-995 in acromegaly. Lancet 1984; 2:782-4.
6. Tolis G, Pitoulis C, Yotis A, et al. Therapy of acromegaly with a mini somatostatin. Program, Endocrine Society, 1984:488.
7. Tolis G. SMS 201-995: long term use in active acromegaly. Neuroendocrinology Letters 1985; 7:119.
8. CH'NG, LJC, Sandler LM, Kraenzlin ME, Burrin JM, Joplin GF, Bloom SR. Long term treatment of acromegaly with a long acting analogue of somatostatin. Br Med J 1985; 290:284-5.
9. Lamberts SWJ, Oosterom R, Neufeld M, del Pozo E. The somatostatin analogue SMS 201-995 induces long-acting inhibition of GH secretion without rebound hypersecretion in acromegalic patients. J Clin Endocrinol Metab 1985; 60:1161-5.
10. Lamberts SWJ, Vitterlinden P, Verschoorm L, Van Dongen KT, del Pozo E. Long-term treatment of acromegaly with the somatostatin analogue SMS 201-995. N Engl J Med 1985; 313:1576-80.
11. Tolis G, Malachtari S, Mortoglou A, et al. Therapy of acromegaly with SMS 201-995: long-term studies. Scand J Gastroenterol 1986

(in press).

12. Tolis G, Yotis A, del Pozo E, Pitoulis S. Long-term therapeutic efficacy of a somatostatin analogue (SMS 201-995) in active acromegaly. J Neurosurg 1986 (in press).
13. Tolis G, Yotis A, Malachtari S, et al. Follow-up of acromegalic patients treated with an octapeptide somatostatin analogue for over a year. Program, Endocrine Society Annual Meeting, 1986.
14. del Pozo E, Kutz K. Pharmacological properties and effects on glucose homeostasis of a somatostatin derivative (SMS 201-995): studies in human. In: Ludecke D, Tolis G, eds. Growth hormone and acromegaly. New York: Raven Press, 1986 (in press).
15. Reubi JC. Evidence for two somatostatin-14-receptor types in rat brain cortex. Neurosci Lett 1984; 49:259-63.
16. Maurer R, Gaehwiler BH, Buescher HH, Hill RC, Roemer D. Opiate antagonistic properties of an octapeptide somatostatin analog. Proc Natl Acad Sci USA 1982; 79:4815-7.
17. Kiang JG, Wei ET. Inhibition of an opioid-evoked vagal reflex in rats by naloxone, SMS 201-995 and ICI 154, 129. Regul Pept 1983; 6:255-62.
18. Beal MF, Martin JB. The effect of somatostatin on striatal catecholamines. Neurosci Lett 1984; 44:271-6.

36

TREATMENT OF GUT-ASSOCIATED NEUROENDOCRINE TUMORS WITH THE LONG-ACTING SOMATOSTATIN ANALOG, SMS 201-995

Gareth Williams, John V. Anderson, and Stephen R. Bloom

Department of Medicine, Royal Postgraduate Medical School

Hammersmith Hospital, Du Cane Road, London W12 OHS, U.K.

INTRODUCTION

Neuroendocrine tumors associated with the gut are very rare (affecting only about 1/100,000 of the population), but are of exceptional interest from two major points of view. The first is that they infringe many of the classical rules of "malignancy," in that patients may remain in relatively good health and survive for several years even in the presence of multiple metastases. This raises questions about the nature of malignancy itself and the mechanisms through which tumors damage and ultimately kill the host; differences in the secretion of tumor products analogous to the recently-described tumor necrosis factor may be responsible.

The second point of interest is the pathophysiological and endocrine effects which these tumors may produce. Neuroendocrine tumors have proved to be a cornucopia of biologically-active regulatory products, whose exaggerated effects lead to characteristic clinical syndromes and so provide clues as to their more subtle physiological actions in health. In recent years, greater understanding of the factors regulating the secretion of these peptides and of their actions has allowed us to begin to manipulate these same regulatory mechanisms to the advantage of patients with neuroendocrine tumors.

Despite their relatively "benign" course, these tumors are often difficult to treat (1,2). Palliative attempts to reduce the tumor mass —whether by surgical debulking, arterial embolization (which causes devascularization and necrosis) or cytotoxic drugs—may initially alleviate symptoms, but in general have a poor long-term record of success (1-4). On the other hand, the slow growth of these tumors means that survival for many years with relatively high quality of life is possible, if tumoral hormone secretion can be switched off or if the biological effects of the hormones can be countered.

The discovery of somatostatin and the appreciation of its wide range of actions have had immense therapeutic potential in the management of secreting neuroendocrine tumors. The actions of somatostatin have already been described in detail (Section II). In addition to its well-known inhibition of growth hormone release, somatostatin suppresses the secretion of insulin, glucagon and a battery of gut peptide hormones, notably vasoactive intestinal polypeptide (VIP), gastrin, gastric inhibitory peptide (GIP), pancreatic polypeptide and motilin (5). Somatostatin may also antagonize the biological actions of certain gut hormones: for example, it directly suppresses gastric acid secretion in addition to inhibition of gastrin release. A third way in which somatostatin and its analogs may be therapeutically useful in the neuroendocrine syndromes is by interfering with the growth of the tumor itself. Certain experimental animal tumors, such as hamster insulinomas, carry receptors to somatostatin which can inhibit and retard tumor growth (6). However, it must be pointed out that as yet there is no firm evidence for such an action in man.

Many different somatostatin analogs have now been synthesized, exploiting structural changes to confer various pharmacological advantages over native somatostatin-14, whose destruction in the circulation is so rapid that it is only therapeutically effective when infused intravenously. One such analog, SMS 201-995 (Sandoz), is outstandingly resistant to enzymatic degradation, resulting in a long circulating half-life (70-100 minutes) and the ability to suppress peptide hormone secretion for some hours after a single subcutaneous injection (7,8).

During the last three years, we have used this analog to treat several patients with various neuroendocrine tumors including VIPomas, gastrinomas, glucagonomas and a pancreatic tumor secreting growth-hormone releasing factor (GRF). The results of SMS 201-995 treatment were particularly encouraging in VIPomas, where symptomatic remission of up to 18 months was achieved after the failure of other, more invasive forms of treatment.

TREATMENT OF VIPOMAS WITH SMS 201-995

VIP and VIPomas

Vasoactive intestinal polypeptide (VIP) is found in neurons widely distributed throughout the gastrointestinal tract and the central and peripheral nervous systems (9). Its main physiological action may be as a neurotransmitter and perhaps as a "paracrine" regulator, affecting cells adjacent to its point of release. Its important biological actions, and those which give rise to the clinical "VIPoma" syndrome, are summarized in its name. It is a powerful vasodilator, with a prolonged action in both peripheral and splanchnic vasculature. Its main intestinal action is to stimulate watery secretion from the small and large bowel, rich in bicarbonate and potassium. VIP also directly inhibits gastric acid secretion, and may cause hypercalcemia and carbohydrate intolerance (9). Functioning neuroendocrine tumors producing VIP are mostly derived from pancreatic islet cells but may also arise in the gut wall, and in children are mostly ganglioneuroblastomas.

The clinical syndrome caused by excessive VIP secretion is known descriptively as "pancreatic cholera," or less dramatically as the "Watery Diarrhea Hypokalemia Achlorhydria" (WDHA) syndrome (10). The clinical features are explicable by its known actions and indeed have been reproduced in normal volunteers by intravenous infusion of VIP (11). The copious intestinal secretion depletes the body of water, potassium and bicarbonate, causing hypovolemia, hypokalemia and metabolic acidosis. The tumors are generally malignant, and metastases are present in most cases at the time of diagnosis.

Patients often report two to three years of intermittent symptoms with occasional acute exacerbations before the diagnosis is established.

344

If successfully resuscitated from dehydration and electrolyte disturbance, survival for some years is the rule.

A number of methods of treatment has been employed. Streptozotocin, especially in combination with 5-fluorouracil, can produce useful symptomatic improvement in 40-70% of cases, although clinical relapse usually follows in 1-2 years (3). Embolization of the arterial supply of the tumor with a suspension of dura mater fragments or microspheres can also induce remission for several months, but its success is crucially dependent on the vascular anatomy of the tumor (4). Simply reducing the tumor mass by surgical debulking may also be helpful (1). High-dose steroids may temporarily reduce diarrhea in about half of the patients (1). A new pharmacological approach was prompted by the observation that native somatostatin and a somatostatin analog were found to inhibit secretion of VIP from pancreatic tumors (12,13). Since 1983, we have treated four VIPoma patients with SMS 201-995.

VIPoma Patients and Responses to SMS 201-995

The clinical features of the patients are shown in Table 1. Three were male and one was female, and they were in their mid-30s to 50s at the onset of symptoms. The relatively indolent course of the disease is underlined by the long duration of symptoms, present for six years in one case at presentation to the Hammersmith Hospital. The primary tumor was pancreatic in three cases and in the wall of jejunum in the female patient. The diagnosis was established by high plasma VIP concentrations, by the CT demonstration of hepatic metastases in every case (see Fig. 1), and by histological examination with immunocytochemistry in two cases. All the patients had previously received prolonged courses of streptozotocin, combined in two cases with 5-fluorouracil; in one case, the drugs had been infused directly into the hepatic artery as well as systemically. Three patients had undergone arterial embolization of hepatic metastases, and attempts to remove the primary tumor surgically had been made in two cases. Generally, these treatments had temporarily reduced VIP and produced symptomatic relief, although relapse had followed some weeks or months later; both the transient nature of these remissions and the general tendency for VIP levels to rise are illustrated by patient no. 4 (Fig. 2). When referred to the Hammersmith Hospital, all were disabled by severe diarrhea with up to eight watery stools totalling 2-8 1/day, and by

Table 1. Clinical features of VIPoma patients
before treatment with SMS 201-995.

Pt. no.	Sex, age	Duration of symptoms	Tumor anatomy		Previous treatments
			Primary	Metastases	
1	M,40	6 years	pancreas	liver +++	ptl. pancrx STZ, embol.
2	M,55	6 months	pancreas	liver +++	STZ + 5-FU embol.
3	M,47	1 year	pancreas	liver +++	STZ
4	F,47	3.5 years	jejunum	liver +++	1° resected STZ + 5-FU embol.

ptl. pancrx. = partial pancreatectomy; STZ = streptozotocin; 5-FU = 5-fluorouracil; emb = arterial embolization.

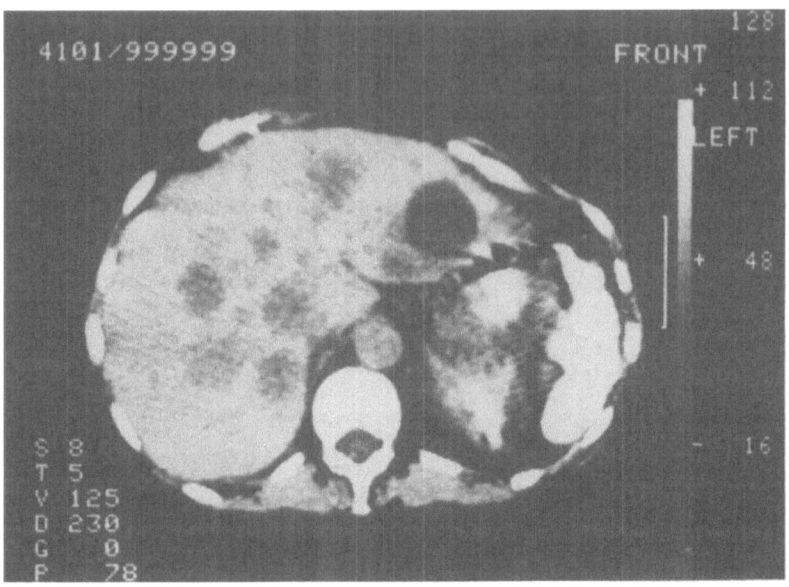

Fig. 1.   Unenhanced abdominal CT scan in patient no. 4, showing
multiple, polymorphic hepatic metastases.   The primary tumor, in
the wall of the jejunum, had been excised three years previously.

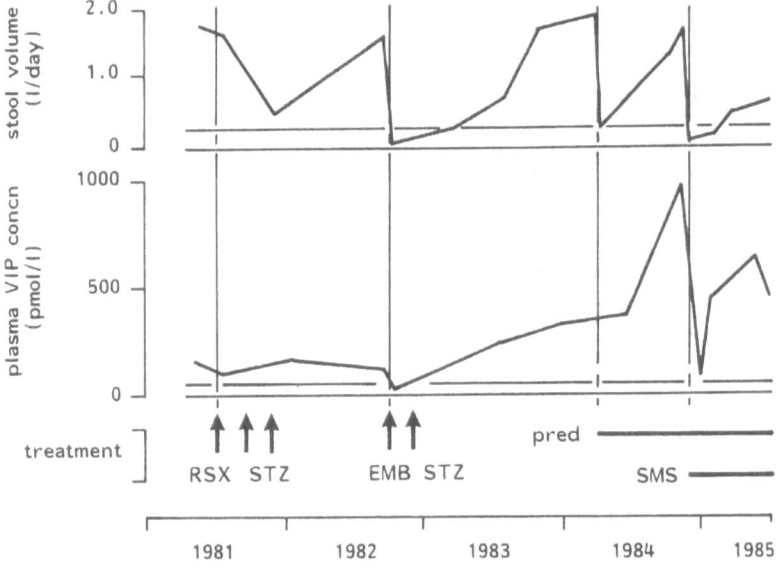

Fig. 2.   Clinical course and responses to treatment of patient no. 4,
1981-1985.   Top panel: stool volumes (normal range, < 300 ml/day).
Middle panel: plasma VIP concentrations (normal range, < 30 pmol/l).
Lower panel: treatment used.   RSX = resection of primary tumor; STZ =
streptozotocin; EMB = arterial embolization of hepatic metastases;
pred = prednisolone (20-40 mg/day); SMS = SMS 201-995 (100-300 µg/day).

nocturnal incontinence in patient no. 3. All were receiving high doses of antidiarrheal agents (codeine, loperamide) and patient no. 2 was taking methysergide. High-dose prednisolone (up to 40 mg/day) had achieved a temporary remission in patient no. 4, but attempts to reduce the dosage to below 20 mg/day had provoked severe diarrhea and she had developed the clinical complications of steroid excess. All the patients had recently suffered serious exacerbations of diarrhea with profound dehydration and hypokalemia (plasma potassium concentration, 1.0-2.5 mol/l), requiring intensive intravenous fluid repletion (up to 10 l/day).

SMS 201-995 produced immediate biochemical and clinical improvement in all cases, with particularly dramatic responses in patients no. 1 and 2. The acute suppression of plasma VIP concentrations to a single test dose of SMS 201-995 (50 μg) injected subcutaneously 30 minutes before a standardized test breakfast (530 cal), is illustrated by patient no. 3 in Figure 3 (upper panel). Plasma VIP concentrations fluctuated widely, but all values in the preceding days were considerably greater than the normal range of 30 pmol/l. After SMS injection, VIP levels fell rapidly to within or close to the normal range. The other three patients also showed significant suppression of VIP concentrations, into the normal range in one other case (Fig. 3, lower panel).

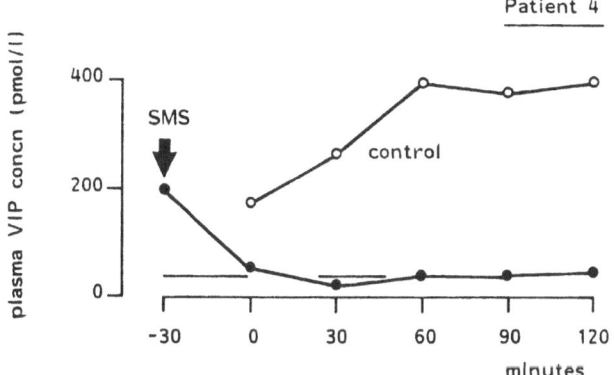

Acute fall in plasma VIP levels after SMS 201-995 (50 μg).

Pt. no.	Plasma VIP level before SMS (pmol/l)	Plasma VIP level during SMS (pmol/l)
1	361 ± 19	207 ± 25 *
2	120 ± 2	60 ± 2 *
3	68 ± 2	13 ± 2 **
4	332 ± 45	38 ± 4 **

Fig. 3. Initial plasma VIP responses to SMS 201-995. Upper panel: plasma VIP concentrations in patient no. 4, on a control day (hollow symbols) and showing prompt suppression after 50 μg SMS (solid symbols). A standardized test breakfast was eaten at time 0 on each day. Lower panel: mean (+ SEM) plasma VIP levels in the VIPoma patients, during the 3 days before and 3 days after starting SMS treatment. *:P < 0.05; **:P < 0.01.

347

Figure 4 shows the effects on stool volume and frequency of three days of SMS treatment (100-300 µg/day, given as 8- or 12-hourly subcutaneous injections; individual doses are indicated in Fig. 8). Stool volumes could not be accurately documented in patients no. 1 and 2 due to incontinence. Stool frequency and volumes fell markedly and stool texture changed from watery to well-formed. Nocturnal incontinence was alleviated in patient no. 4, whose prednisolone dosage was gradually reduced over the next few weeks to a maintenance level dose of 2-5 mg/day, allowing considerable resolution of her iatrogenic Cushing's syndrome. Experimental withdrawal of SMS in patient no. 1 was followed immediately by the return of torrential watery diarrhea. What is not apparent from these figures, and is indeed impossible to quantitate, is the huge impact which SMS treatment initially had on quality of life in every case, by stopping the diarrhea which had threatened both their dignity and their lives.

For 6-12 weeks, SMS effectively suppressed the VIP levels throughout the day, an effect which was still discernible before the morning dose of SMS (Fig. 5). Thereafter, however, VIP levels tended to rise in patients no. 1, 2 and 4, and had exceeded 200 pmol/l by 3 months after starting treatment. In contrast, VIP levels in patient no. 3 remained just above normal. Despite the rising VIP levels, diarrhea did not recur for some time, perhaps suggesting a direct, inhibitory effect of SMS on gut secre-

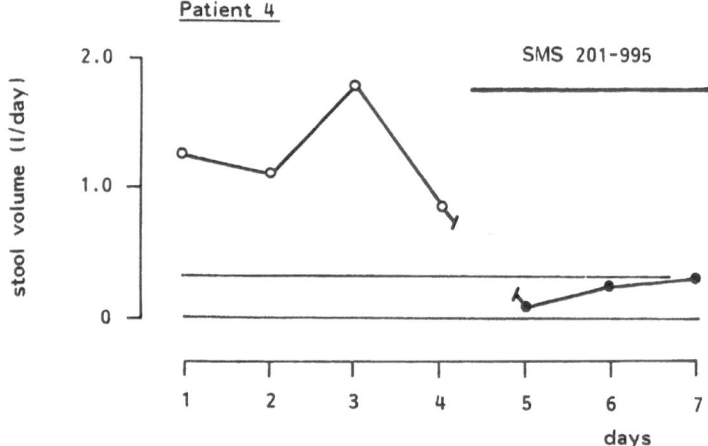

Reduced stool frequency and volumes during initial SMS treatment.

Pt. no.	Stool frequency/day		Stool volumes (ml)	
	pre-SMS	with SMS	pre-SMS	with SMS
1	5-6	1	~8000	500
2	5-6	1-2	~4000	500
3	4-6	1-2	1200	280
4	7-8	1-2	1160	220

Fig. 4. Changes in stool volume and frequency during initial SMS treatment. Upper panel: stool volumes in patient no. 4 on successive days before and after starting SMS (100 µg/day). Lower panel: ranges of stool frequency/day and mean stool volumes in the VIPoma patients during 3 days before and 3 days after starting treatment.

tion. After 6 months, intermittent diarrhea returned in patient no. 4, despite increasing the SMS dosage to 1000 μg/day and the prednisolone to 15 mg/day. Patient no. 2 relapsed symptomatically after 15 months, and patient no. 1 after 18 months; increased SMS dosages (up to 1500 μg/day) failed to suppress either the rising VIP concentrations or diarrhea (Fig. 6), and both have subsequently undergone further treatment (embolization of the primary pancreatic tumor and further streptozotocin in patient no. 1; streptozotocin in patient no. 2). Figure 7 shows that the ability of SMS (even at increased dosage) to suppress VIP levels in patients no. 1, 2 and 4 apparently declined after several months of treatment. Patient no. 3 remains SMS-responsive, with suppressed VIP levels and no diarrhea after 15 months of treatment.

The side-effects of SMS treatment were few. The injections are uncomfortable (probably because of the low pH of the injection vehicle), but in view of the impressive symptomatic relief, all the patients were more than willing to inject themselves 2 or 3 times per day at home. Effective insulin suppression resulted in slight deterioration of carbohydrate tolerance: fasting blood glucose concentration remained normal, but the 2-hour postprandial value was elevated (9.0-14.0 mmol/l). No specific antidiabetic treatment was required. There was no biochemical or clinical evidence of anterior pituitary dysfunction.

Any effect of SMS on tumor bulk was difficult to assess, due to the technical problems of volume measurement even on thin-slice CT scanning, the possible effects of other treatment such as embolization and chemotherapy, and the fact that the natural growth rate of these tumors is not known. However, careful measurement suggests that the hepatic metastases have expanded slightly in patients no. 1, 2 and 4 during the period of follow-up. In patient no. 3, there has been obvious growth of hepatic metastases (Fig. 8), which is at variance with his continued biochemical and clinical remission during SMS treatment.

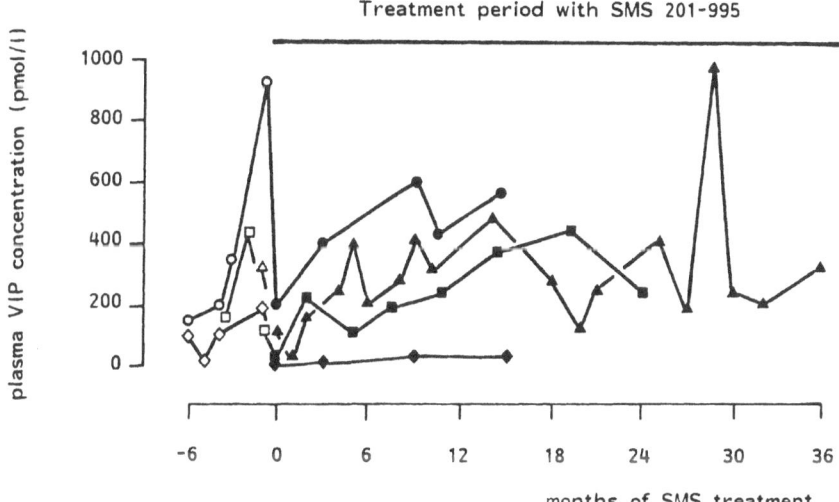

Fig. 5. Fasting plasma VIP levels in the VIPoma patients, before (hollow symbols) and after (solid symbols) starting SMS, demonstrating "escape" of VIP levels in 3 cases but persisting VIP suppression in patient no. 3 (♦).

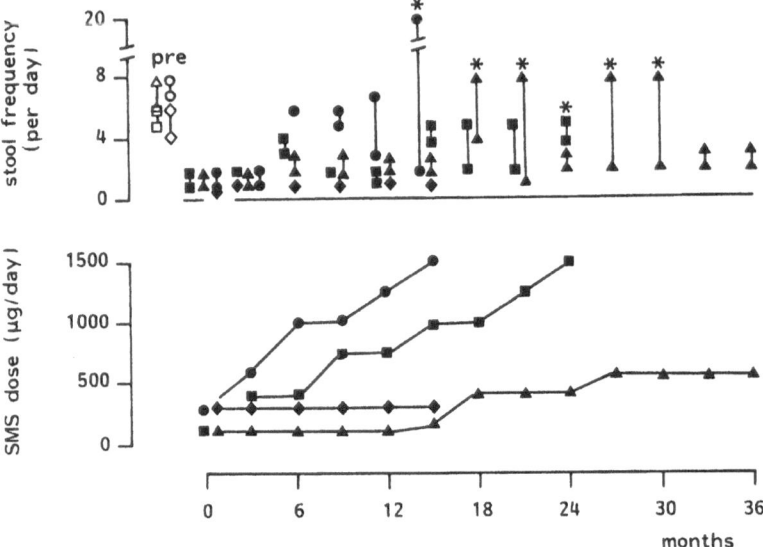

Fig. 6. Upper panel: range of daily stool frequencies in
the VIPoma patients, before ("pre") and at 3-month intervals during SMS treatment. * = acute diarrheal exacerbations requiring hospitalization. Lower panel: daily SMS
dosages (µg) in the VIPoma patients. Only patient no. 3
(♦) remains in clinical remission with low SMS dosages
(see Fig. 5).

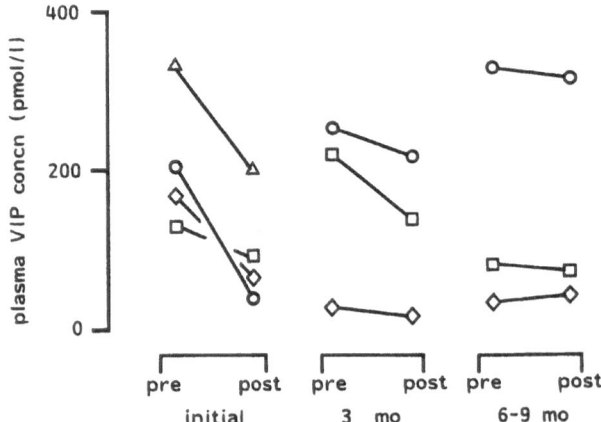

Fig. 7. Plasma VIP concentrations before and 2
hours after SMS injection, initially and after 3
and 6-9 months of continuous SMS treatment,
demonstrating reduced suppression of VIP.

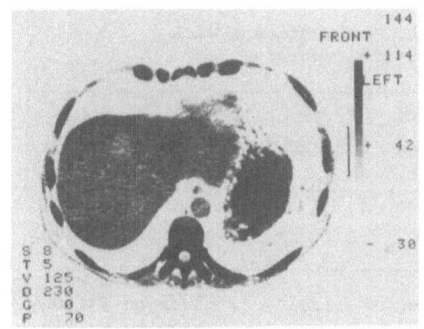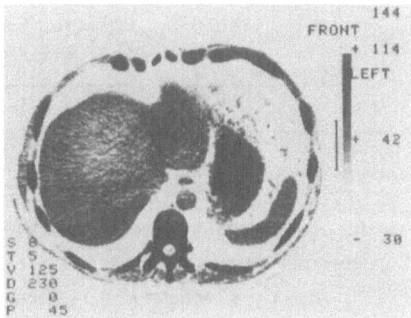

Fig. 8. Unenhanced abdominal CT scan in patient no. 3, showing gross expansion of a metastasis in the left lobe of the liver after 15 months of SMS treatment. The contrast-filled stomach is seen on the right of each photograph.

Discussion

In these 4 patients, SMS 201-995 effectively suppressed VIP levels, relieved incapacitating diarrhea, and allowed a return to a normal life for 6-18 months. Three of the patients had previously undergone many attempts at treatment and were considered clinically "end-stage." After 3 months, however, VIP levels tended to rise again in these three patients, although useful clinic remission extended for many weeks or months beyond this. Possible mechanisms of "escape" of VIP levels could include down-regulation of the somatostatin receptor or perhaps simply tumor expansion, of which there was evidence in each case; paradoxically, the patient with the most obvious tumor expansion remains in biochemical and clinical remission. We previously reported that the hepatic metastases in patient no. 1 apparently shrank during initial treatment with SMS 201-995 (17). However, as described above, recent CT scans performed after a longer period of follow-up suggest that the metastases have subsequently expanded. The cause for the persisting suppression of diarrhea despite rising VIP levels is not clear. A direct antisecretory effect of SMS on the gut is possible, as is the selective suppression by the SMS of "small," biologically-active VIP with persistence of immunoreactive precursor molecules of higher molecular weight but lower biological activity (14).

SMS 201-995, therefore, has induced useful clinical remission of several months, which is at least as long as other interventions. The drug was well tolerated and had few side-effects. Somatostatin analogs may be useful in the treatment of VIPomas where other forms of treatment are refused, have failed, or are contraindicated; arterial embolization is contraindicated by portal vein thrombosis, and may technically be impossible or ineffective if the tumor vascular anatomy is unfavorable (4).

OTHER NEUROENDOCRINE TUMORS AND SMS TREATMENT

SMS 201-995 has also been evaluated in a number of other patients with a variety of gut-associated endocrine tumors (Table 2). Two had gastrinomas, with multiple hepatic metastases in patient no. 5, and had a history of epigastric pain and diarrhea lasting some years. Both were receiving high-dose cimetidine (3-4 g/day) and patient no. 1 had previously undergone hepatic artery embolization. Both were currently symptomatic with grossly elevated plasma gastrin concentrations.

Table 2. Clinical features of patients with
other gut endocrine tumors.

Pt. no.	Sex, age	Diagnosis	Duration of symptoms	Previous treatments	Plasma peptide levels (pmol/l)	
5	M,73	gastrinoma	5 years	embol.	gastrin =	130
6	M,50	gastrinoma	4 years	-	gastrin =	200
7	M,73	glucagonoma /gastrinoma	5 years	embol.	glucagon = gastrin =	1200 110
8	M,66	glucagonoma /gastrinoma	5 years	embol., STZ	glucagon = gastrin =	800 70
9	M,70	glucagonoma	3 years	-	glucagon =	450
10	F,60	GRF-oma	4 years	embol.	GRF >	3000

Treatment key as for Table 1. Normal ranges of gut peptides:
gastrin < 40 pmol/l; glucagon < 50 pmol/l; GRF < 250 pmol/l.

Two patients, both elderly males, had mixed pancreatic tumors with
multiple metastases secreting both glucagon and gastrin. One had insulin-
treated diabetes and both had the migratory necrolytic rash characteristic
of the glucagonoma syndrome (15) shown in Figure 9, which had been present
intermittently for over 5 years in each case. Oral zinc sulphate treatment had partially improved the rash. Another elderly male had a "pure"
glucagonoma with severe generalized rash; he had declined invasive methods
of treatment and was only taking oral zinc sulphate.

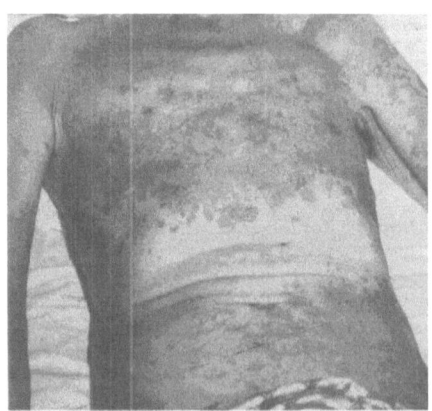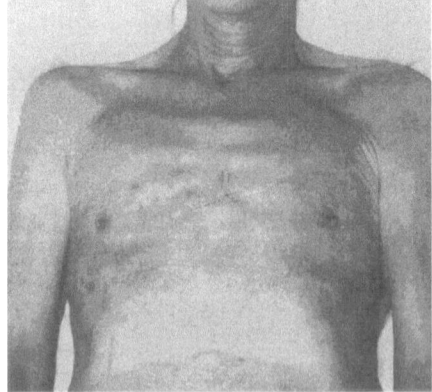

Fig. 9. Extensive migratory necrolytic erythematous rash characteristic of glucagonoma in patient no. 8 (mixed gastrinoma-
glucagonoma), before SMS treatment (a). After 3 weeks of SMS
treatment (b), the rash has largely cleared.

The sixth patient was a 60-year-old female with acromegaly of some years' standing, who was subsequently found to have multiple hepatic deposits from a pancreatic tumor which was secreting growth hormone releasing factor (GRF). Her main complaints were of the facial changes of acromegaly and excessive sweating; her fasting growth hormone concentrations were over 20 mIu/1 (normal range, < 4 mIu/1).

In each case, SMS 201-995 was found to suppress excessive secretion of peptide hormones (Fig. 10) for several hours after subcutaneous injection. In the case of the mixed glucagonoma-gastrinoma patients, both hormones fell substantially to just above the normal range.

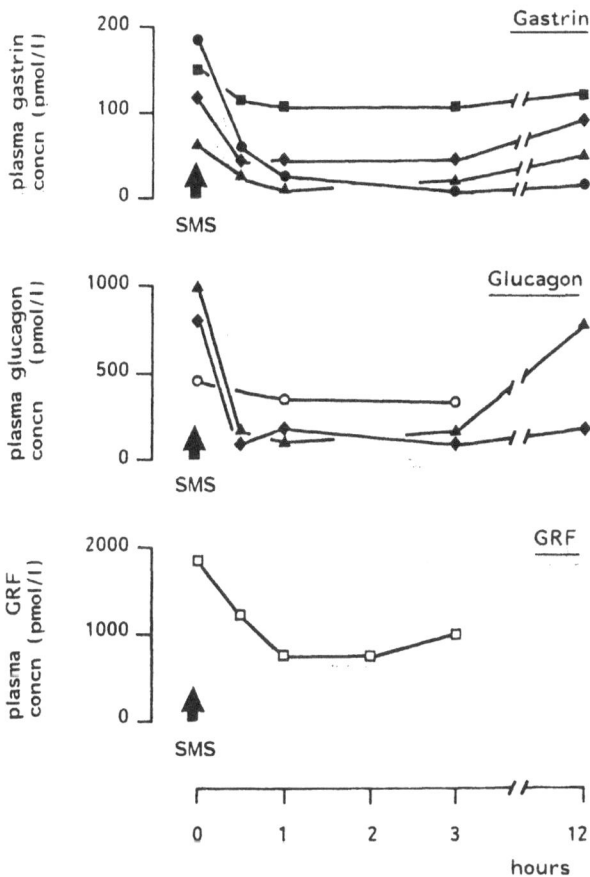

Fig. 10. Acute responses of gut peptides (upper panel, gastrin; middle panel, glucagon; lower panel, growth hormone releasing factor) to SMS 201-995 (50 μg) in 2 cases of gastrinoma (■ ●), 2 cases of gastrinoma-glucagonoma (♦ ▲), one pure glucagonoma (○, middle panel), and a GRFoma (□, lower panel).

Long-term SMS treatment was undertaken in one glucagonoma-gastrinoma patient (no. 4, treated for nearly 2 years), the "pure" glucagonoma patient (no. 5, 3 months of treatment), and the woman with the GRFoma (no. 6, 6 months of treatment). In the glucagonoma-gastrinoma patient, mean plasma glucagon levels fell slightly after starting SMS treatment (from 340 to 332 pmol/l), but tended to rise in the following few weeks (Fig. 11). The necrolytic rash improved considerably during this period (Fig. 11), although it is not clear whether this was spontaneous, as is characteristic of the syndrome, or due to SMS treatment. Similarly, apparent improvement of the rash in the autumn of 1984 after increasing the dose of SMS may or may not have been related to treatment. Diabetic control and subcutaneous insulin requirements improved during SMS treatment. In the glucagonoma patient, mean plasma glucagon levels fell significantly from 458 to 364 pmol/l and there was a sustained improvement in the rash and also in the hypoproteinemia and the anemia which this patient suffered. The woman with the GRFoma showed a fall in the fasting growth hormone levels to 10 mIu/l and her excessive sweating improved.

Discussion

The effect of SMS 201-995 in this second, heterogeneous group of patients is harder to gauge. Although effective acute suppression of abnormal peptide hormone secretion was demonstrated, long-term trials yielded less impressive results than in VIPomas. The fluctuating course of glucagonomas makes objective assessment difficult, although intravenous infusions of native somatostatin have caused extremely rapid resolution of

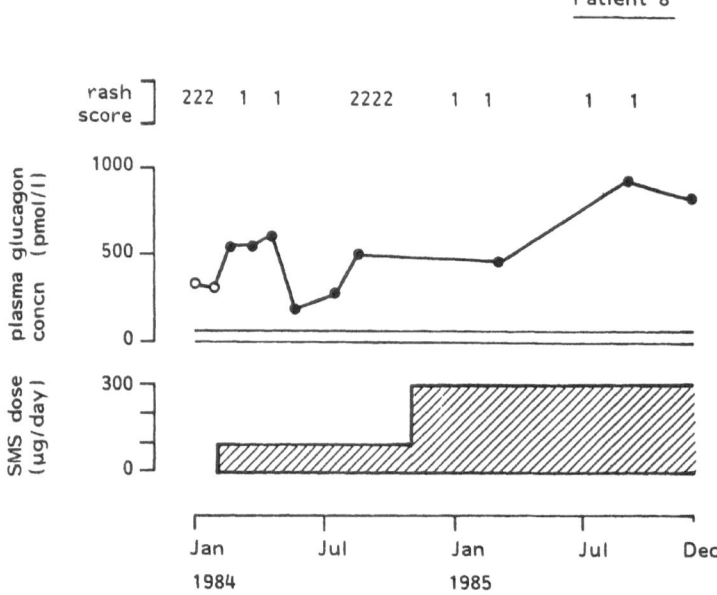

Fig. 11. Clinical course of patient no. 8 (mixed gastrinoma-glucagonoma), 1984-1985. Upper panel: rash, scored as 1— limited to perineum; 2—extensive on trunk and elsewhere; no score—quiescent. Middle panel: plasma glucagon levels before (hollow symbols) and during (solid symbols) SMS treatment. Lower panel: daily SMS dosage (μg).

the necrolytic rash (16). The GRFoma patient showed significant and sustained drops in both GRF and growth hormone levels and concomitant symptomatic clinical improvement.

CONCLUSIONS

These tumors disrupt and threaten life through their excessive production of regulatory gut hormones. In somatostatin and its analogs, we have the means to turn off excessive hormone secretion. Using a long-acting, subcutaneously injectable somatostatin analog, useful symptomatic remissions lasting many months were achieved in VIPoma patients. These trials have raised their own questions, particularly relating to the mechanism underlying the escape of VIP levels, and have added to the continuing controversy as to whether somatostatin has any direct effect on tumor bulk (17). These question will no doubt be answered by further trials of somatostatin analogs, which may also find a place in the treatment of other neuroendocrine tumors including insulinoma (18) and carcinoid (19).

ACKNOWLEDGMENTS

We are very grateful to the Sister- and staff nurses of the Metabolic Unit for their help, to Miss Susan Williams, BSc, for performing the peptide assays, and to Mrs. Jacqui Chatterton for her customary secretarial skill in the preparation of this manuscript.

REFERENCES

1. Friesen SR. Tumors of the endocrine pancreas. N Engl J Med 1982; 306:580-90.
2. Sabate MI, Carlei F, Bloom SR, Polak JM. Endocrine tumours of the gut and pancreas. In: Polak JM, Bloom SR, eds. Endocrine tumours. The pathobiology of regulatory peptide-producing tumours. Edinburgh: Churchill-Livingstone, 1985.
3. Moertel CG, Hanley JA, Johnson LA. Streptozotocin alone compared with streptozotocin plus fluorouracil in the treatment of advanced islet-cell carcinoma. N Engl J Med 1980; 303:1189-94.
4. Allison DJ. Therapeutic embolization. Br J Hosp Med 1978; 20:707-15.
5. Adrian TE, Barnes AJ, Long RG, et al. The effect of somatostatin analogues on secretion of growth, pancreatic and gastrointestinal hormones in man. J Clin Endocrinol Metab 1981; 53:675-81.
6. Reubi JC. A somatostatin analogue inhibits chondrosarcoma and insulinoma tumour growth. Acta Endocrinol 1985; 109:108-14.
7. Bauer W, Briner U, Doepfner W, et al. A very potent and selective octapeptide analogue of somatostatin with prolonged action. Life Sci 1982; 31:1133-40.
8. Kraenzlin ME, Wood SM, Neufeld M, Adrian TE, Bloom SR. Effect of long acting somatostatin-analogue SMS 201-995 on gut hormone secretion in normal subjects. Experientia 1985; 41:738-40.
9. Said SI, ed. Vasoactive intestinal peptide (Advances in peptide hormone research series). New York: Raven Press, 1982.
10. Verner JV, Morrison AB. Islet cell tumour and a syndrome of refractory watery diarrhoea and hypokalemia. Am J Med 1958; 25:374-80.
11. Kane MG, O'Dorisio TM, Krejs GJ. Production of secretory diarrhoea by intravenous infusion of vasoactive intestinal polypeptide. N Engl J Med 1983; 309:1482-5.
12. Ruskone A, Rene E, Chayvialle JA, et al. Effect of somatostatin on

diarrhoea and on small intestinal water and electrolyte transport in a patient with pancreatic cholera. Dig Dis Sci 1982; 27:459-65.

13. Long RG, Barnes AJ, Adrian TE, et al. Suppression of pancreatic endocrine tumour secretion by long acting somatostatin analogue. Lancet 1979; 2:764-7.

14. Wood SM, Kraenzlin ME, Adrian TE, Bloom SR. Treatment of patients with pancreatic endocrine tumours using a new long-acting somatostatin analogue: symptomatic and peptide responses. Gut 1985; 26:438-44.

15. Mallinson CN, Bloom SR, Warin AP, Salmon PR, Cox B. A glucagonoma syndrome. Lancet 1974; 2:1-5.

16. Sohier J, Jeanmougin M, Lombrail P, Passa P. Rapid improvement of skin lesions in glucagonomas with intravenous somatostatin infusions. Lancet 1980; 1:40.

17. Kraenzlin ME, Ch'ng JLC, Wood SM, Carr DH, Bloom SR. Long-term treatment of a VIPoma with somatostatin analogue resulting in remission of symptoms and possible shrinkage of metastases. Gastroenterology 1985; 88:185-7.

18. Osei K, O'Dorisio TM. Malignant insulinoma: effects of somatostatin analog (compound 201-995) on serum glucose, growth, and gastroenteropancreatic hormones. Ann Intern Med 1985; 103:223-5.

19. Dharmsathaphorn K, Sherwin RS, Cataland S, Jaffe B, Dobbins J. Somatostatin inhibits diarrhoea in the carcinoid syndrome. Ann Intern Med 1980; 92:68-9.

37

SOMATOSTATIN IN THE TREATMENT OF ACUTE PANCREATITIS

Ulrich Leuschner, Karl Uberla, Klaus-Henning Usadel

University Hospital
Medical School of Frankfurt/M
Munchen, Heidelberg/Mannheim, FRG

INTRODUCTION

The treatment of acute pancreatitis has markedly improved within the last 80 years. The lethality rate receded from 60% to a mean of 15-20%. However, this improvement was not due to any specific pancreatitis therapy but to intensive care measures alone.

Therapeutic Mode of Action

To date the rationale of a specific therapy of acute pancreatitis was based on the principle to inhibit secretion of proteolytic enzymes and kinines. Activated pancreatic enzymes induce tissue necrosis, vasoactive substances cause circulatory shock syndromes, respiratory and renal failure (1,2). The administration of secretion inhibitors, however, or measures to neutralize the effect of substances secreted, represents no causative but symptomatic treatment only.

Measures to calm the process are fasting, aspiration of duodenal pancreatic juice (3), administration of carboanhydrase inhibitors, of the callikrein antagonist aprotinine (4,5), of hormones such as glucagon (6), salmon-calcitonin (7) and recently somatostatin (8). The use of protease inhibitors, of inhibitors of phospholipase A and elastase (EACA, AMCA, PAMBA) (9) is an attempt at enzyme inhibition. The effect of the low molecular proteinase inhibitor gabexate-mesilate (FOY) is under investigation at present. Investigations of pancreatic polypeptide, TRH, ACTH, vasopressin and prostaglandins have not been completed to date.

Hormone Therapy

When infused intravenously calcitonin will inhibit basal and stimulated gastric secretion and stimulated pancreatic secretion (10). Two double-blind trials with synthetic salmon-calcitonin (7,11) comprising 101 patients (plus 96 patients on placebo) showed a positive effect concerning pain and normalization of amylase values. However, there was no difference of lethality rate. It amounted to 8.9 (verum) and 9.4% (placebo). Nevertheless, salmon-calcitonin was recommended as admixture to infusion solutions in a dosage of 60 μg=300 MRC (Medical Research Council) units/24 hours for 6 days.

Glucagon too inhibits the basal and stimulated gastric secretion and the stimulated pancreatic secretion. After preliminary uncontrolled studies had suggested a positive effect on the course of the disease, these results could not be confirmed by three further double-blind trials with a total of 165 patients (6,12,13). The question whether or not at least individual parameters of the disease could be improved by glucagon, as by salmon-calcitonin, has not been elucidated.

SOMATOSTATIN IN ACUTE PANCREATITIS

Hypothetical Mode of Action

The tetradecapeptide somatostatin could be demonstrated in the central nervous system, gastric mucosa cells, in pancreatic tissue, in the urinary bladder, in the retina and even in the thyroid gland (14,15). However, only the cyclic 14 amino acid-containing somatostatin, but not the linear form of the peptide, is effective. Somatostatin-28 is efficient as well; possibly it is a prohormone. When somatostatin-14 is administered in a dosage of 125-600 µg/hour, it shows an inhibitory effect in man and animal on insulin, glucagon, growth hormone and the gastrointestinal hormones gastrin, secretin and CCK (16,17).

The inhibition of pancreozymin and secretin which results in inhibition of exocrine pancreatic secretion as a sequel, represents the first hypothetical therapeutic principle of somatostatin in the treatment of pancreatitis.

Besides inhibition of secretion, somatostatin is believed to have cytoprotective properties, same as prostaglandin PGE_2. A positive effect, for example, could be demonstrated in ethanol-induced erosive gastritis, cysteamin-induced duodenal and stress-induced gastric ulcers in rats (18, 19), in phalloidin injury of rat liver (20), isolated rat liver cells and in galactoseamin hepatitis. In 1977 and 1978 our own team could show that feeding of cysteamin to rats will induce severe perforating duodenal ulcers afflicted with a dose-dependent mortality. Somatostatin could statistically significantly reduce symptoms and lethality rate. Hereby we found that the positive effect was neither due to acid-output nor to inhibition of gastrointestinal hormones, since these parameters were found changed only to a minor degree (18).

Therefore, cytoprotection represents the second hypothetical therapeutic principle in the treatment of acute pancreatitis.

Somatostatin in Pancreatitis of Animal Experiments

In 1977 Lankisch et al. (21) reported that somatostatin obviously exerted no beneficial effect on acute, experimental pancreatitis in rats when injected subcutaneously, which contradicted preliminary investigations of our unit with dogs, where we had administered somatostatin intravenously. As we could further show in 21 female beagle dogs with a body weight of 11-12 kg in 1979 (22) administration of 62.5 µg somatostatin/hour not only exerted a therapeutic but obviously even a prophylactic effect on bile-induced pancreatitis (6 ml auto-bile). We administered a bolus of 250 µg 15 minutes before and 2 hours after induction of pancreatitis; a constant infusion of 62 µg/hour followed. The control animals developed all signs of acute hemorrhagic pancreatitis, whereas the somatostatin-treated dogs were in a significantly better state of health. Lipase and amylase elevations were noted in all groups after bile injection. Within the next 42 hours there was no reduction of values either in the group with prophylactic or in the group with therapeutic administration of somatostatin. The somewhat milder elevation in the somatostatin dogs compared to controls was statistically not significant. Serum gastrin and secretin levels remained unchanged after induction of pancreatitis; CCK rose mildly. There was no change under treatment. In the controls autopsy revealed massive morphologic alterations. In the somatostatin group edema, severe hemorrhage and abscess formation were rare. Thus even in bile-induced pancreatitis of the dog the behavior of biochemical parameters on one hand and morphologic findings on the other hand point to the fact that somatostatin, besides its influence on hormone secretion, has direct organ protective properties.

In 1985 Baxter and co-workers (23) reported in 18 rats a beneficial effect of not only somatostatin, but of its long-acting analogue SMS 201-995 as well in acute pancreatitis due to prepapillary bile duct ligation. Somatostatin was given in a dosage of 4 µg/kg body weight in form of bolus prophylactically and after ligation in a constant infusion for 12 hours, SMS 201-995 in one dose of 2 µg/kg sc and in another dose 12 hours later. This regimen produced a significantly higher survival rate, the amount of ascites was reduced, serum levels of amylase and lipase were lower than in controls. According to this result, not only somatostatin but SMS 201-995 as well is said to be beneficial in the treatment of acute pancreatitis in man.

Somatostatin in Pancreatitis of Man

In man the therapeutic effect of somatostatin was investigated in three groups: (1) in patients with acute pancreatitis; (2) in operated patients, to prevent postoperative pancreatitis; (3) in patients past endoscopic retrograde cholangio-pancreaticography (ERCP).

Schlegel and co-workers showed in 1977 (24) in 3 patients regression of hyperamylasemia due to somatostatin. In 1978 Raptis and co-workers (25) reported a positive influence in 9 of 12 patients, and in 1979 our own group observed a beneficial therapeutic effect in a total of 30 patients with acute pancreatitis. In 1980 Limberg and Kommerell (8) treated 14 patients with a bolus injection of 250 µg somatostatin/hour and a subsequent constant infusion of the same dosage. Besides fasting and addition of fluid they refrained from any other therapy. Pains receded, analgetics consumption was unnecessary, muscular defense in the abdomen vanished. Under therapy serum lipase and amylase levels returned to normal rapidly. After termination of therapy some patients showed anewed mild elevation of values.

In 1979 (26) Klempa and co-workers found that prophylactic and postoperative administration of somatostatin in the aforementioned dosage maintained serum amylase levels of 10 patients with pancreas surgery within normal range, whereas there was elevation of values of 500-1000 U/ml in two untreated patients. Treatment duration was 5 days in each case. Here, too, additional fasting, fluid substitution and antibiotics were the only regimen.

In all studies quoted classification of acute pancreatitis in serousinterstitial, hemorrhagic-necrotizing and apoplectic pancreatitis had not been performed. Since control collectives subjected to conventional treatment were lacking too, a definitive assessment on actual somatostatin effect is impossible.

After 1978 Tamas and co-workers (27) rendered probable that somatostatin could prevent even the ERCP-induced pancreatitis, or at least that it was capable of preventing elevation of serum transaminase levels, in 1980 we initiated a multicenter double-blind trial of two years' duration wherein 18 centers from the Federal Republic of Germany, Switzerland and Greece participated (Table 1). The aim of the study was to elucidate which effect a standardized 7-day treatment with somatostatin would have with regard to mortality, survival rate, clinical course and biochemical data.

All patients with acute pancreatitis were registered in a logbook. Only those patients entered the study whose pancreatitis was not of longer duration than 48 hours. The following criteria had to be met: serum amylase or lipase levels had to exceed the threefold of the normal range, spontaneous abdominal pain was required. In order to exclude mild cases, at least three of the following parameters had to be present: muscular defense of the right upper abdomen, ileus or subileus shock syndrome (systolic blood pressure below 100 mgHg, pulse rate above 100/min), leukocytosis above 12,000/mm^3, and blood glucose level above 150 mg/dl. In case of detection of acute pancreatitis at laparotomy, none of the three criteria had to be fulfilled.

Exclusion criteria included complaints for longer than 48 hours, prior therapy with aprotinine, calcitonin, glucagon, atropine, carboanhydrase inhibitors, insulin-dependent diabetes, renal failure, relapsing pancreatitis, age below 18 years, pregnancy, mental disorders. Randomization of placebo and verum groups was done according to the method of Billewitz and Deeley.

Therapy consisted of a bolus injection of 250 µg somatostatin and a constant infusion of the same dosage/hour. Additional regimen included only fasting, substitution of fluids and a gastric tube in case of ileus. Analgetics were permitted in form of pentazozine (Fortral®) or pethidine (Dolantin®).

The beneficial effect of somatostatin was assessed by the lethality rate 3 weeks after admission to the study, by the behavior of laboratory data, consumption of fluids and analgetics and by the ultrasonographic findings during the 7 treatment days.

Table 1. APTS study: 77 complete protocols (11 out of 18 centers).

Hospital	Somato-statin	Placebo	Total
1 Frankfurt	3	4	7
Frankfurt NW	2	2	4
3 Marburg	1	1	2
5 Gottingen	5	5	10
6 Freiburg	7	7	14
9 Basel	2	3	5
10 Heidelberg	3	4	7
11 Berlin	4	5	9
12 Bremen	1	3	4
13 Furth	2	1	3
15 Mainz	2	2	4
18 Athen	4	4	8
Total	36	41	77

Out of 77 patients who had entered the study, 22 men and 14 women (n=38) were allocated to the verum group (Group A) and 27 men and 14 women (n=41) to the placebo-group (Group B). Fifteen of the 77 patients had gallstone disease either in their case history or at the time of the study. Data on alcohol consumption are indistinct. Treatment with somatostatin revealed in none of the numerous parameters monitored any statistically significant difference compared to the placebo group. Figure 1 shows the course of analgetics consumption, Figure 2 of calcium and Figure 3 of lipase concentration in the serum.

Summary

In this multicenter prospective double-blind study out of 77 patients with partially necrotizing pancreatitis 63.6% were men and 46.3% were women. 9.5% of them had gallstones, 3.9% had already undergone cholecystectomy; that means 13.4% had history of gallstone disease. Sixteen percent of the patients reported gastric or duodenal ulcer in their history. Lethality rate of partially necrotizing pancreatitis amounted to 14.3%; there was no difference between placebo and verum group (group A, 4 patients; group B, 7 patients). The therapeutic measures were identical in both groups with respect to quality and quantity.

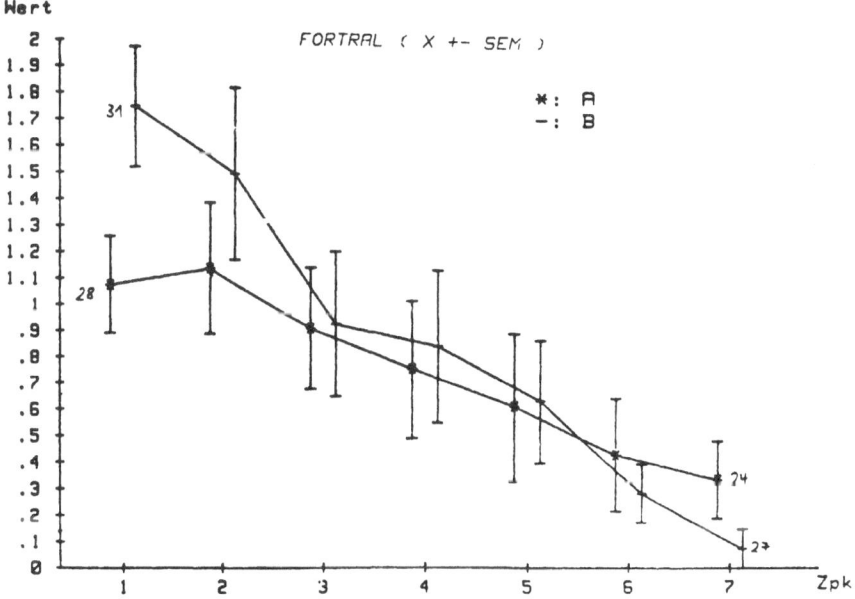

Fig. 1. APTS-Study: Consumption of analgetics (Pentazozin = Fortral®) in the verum (A) and placebo (B) group during 7 days of treatment with somatostatin.

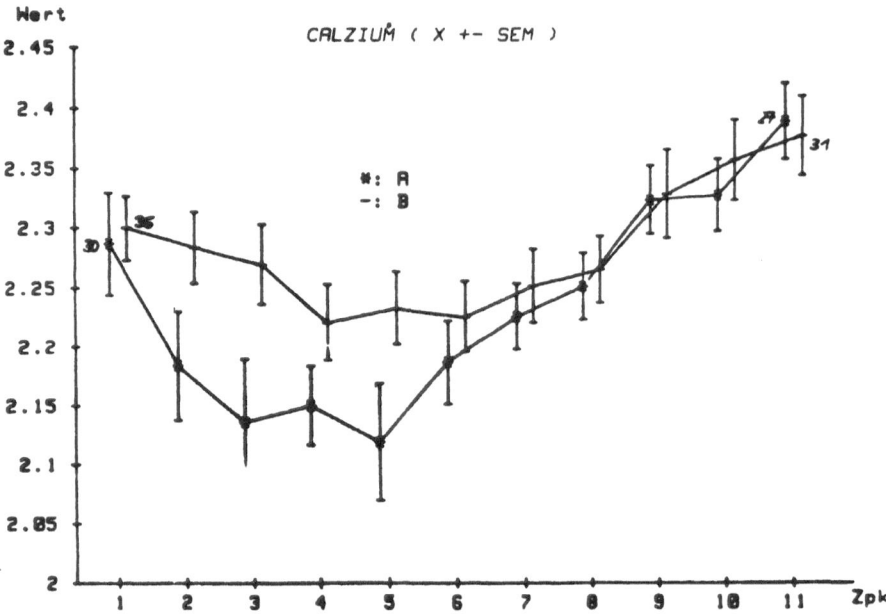

Fig. 2. APTS-Study: Serum Ca^{++}-levels of group A (somato-statin) and B (placebo) during 11 days of treatment with somato-statin.

CONCLUDING REMARKS

This study leaves us with the following questions to answer:

(1) Why did somatostatin in animal experiments show a beneficial effect on bile-induced pancreatitis not only when administered prophylactically but therapeutically as well?

(2) Why did pilot studies reveal positive results in approximately 70 patients with acute pancreatitis?

3) Does inhibition of secretion represent a therapeutic principle in the treatment of acute pancreatitis at all?

(4) If not, why did cytoprotection, believed to be one of somatostatin's properties, prove to be without effect?

(5) Was somatostatin administered at the right time and in the right dosage in our double-blind study in 77 patients?

These questions still wait to be answered. Based on the results obtained from our study we have to admit at present that somatostatin, same as glucagon and salmon-calcitonin, is unsuitable for the treatment of hemorrhagic-necrotizing pancreatitis. Since serous pancreatitis does not call for any treatment at all, we have to confess that we still do not have any specific pancreatitis medication.

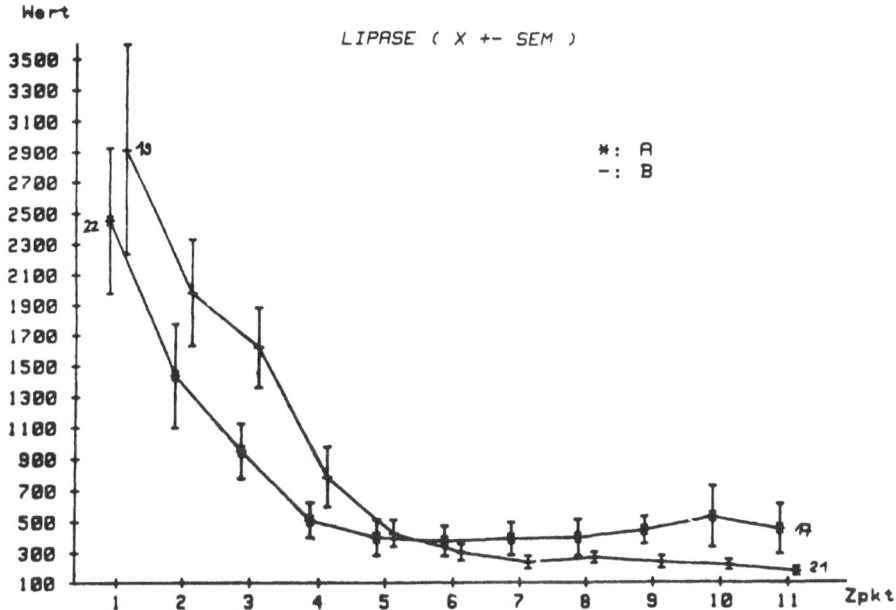

Fig. 3. APTS-Study: Lipase concentration in the serum of group A (somatostatin) and B (placebo) during 11 days of treatment with somatostatin.

REFERENCES

1. Papp MD, Nemeth EP, Horvath EJ. Pancreaticoduodenal lymph flow and lipase activity in acute experimental pancreatitis. Lymphology 1971; 4:48.
2. Werner MH, Hayes DF, Lucas CE, Rosenberg IK. Renal vasoconstriction in association with acute pancreatitis. Am J Surg 1974; 127:185.
3. Levanth JA, Secrist DM, Resin H, Sturdevant RAL, Guth PM. Naso-gastric suction in the treatment of alcoholic pancreatitis. JAMA 1974; 229:51.
4. Anderson MC. Review of pancreatic disease. Surgery 1969; 66:434.
5. Trapnell JE, Rigby CC, Talbot CH, Duncan EHL. A controlled trial of trasylol in the treatment of acute pancreatitis. Br J Surg 1974; 61:177.
6. Medical Research Council. Multicenter trial glucagon and aprotinin. Death from acute pancreatitis. Lancet 1977; II:632.
7. Goebell H, Ammann R, Akovbiantz A, et al. Calcitonin in der Behand-lung der akuten pankreatitis [Abstract 86]. Eine doppelblindstudie. Z Gastroenterol 1977 (suppl).
8. Limberg B, Kommerell B. Treatment of acute pancreatitis with somato-statin. N Engl J Med 1980; 303:284.
9. Konttinen YP. Epsilon-aminocaproic acid in treatment of acute pancreatitis. Scand J Gastroenterol 1971; 6:715.
10. Goebell H, Hotz J. Effects of calcitonin and somatostatin on the gastrointestinal tract and pancreas. Sympos Wien 1975, Verhbd 10, K. Demeter, Grafelfing 1976.

11. Paul F, Ohnhaus EE, Hesch RD, et al. Behandlung der akuten Pankreatitis mit Salm-Calcitonin. Ergebnisse einer multicenter-doppelblind-studie [Abstract 87]. Z Gastroenterol 1977 (suppl).
12. Durr HK, Maroske D, Zelder O, Bode JC. Glucagon therapy in acute pancreatitis. Gut 1978; 19:175.
13. Olazabal A, Fuller R. Failure of glucagon in the treatment of alcoholic pancreatitis. Gastroenterology 1978; 74:489.
14. Falkmer S, Elde RP, Hellerstrom C, Peterson B. Phylogenetic aspects of somatostatin in the gastroenteropancreatic (GEP)-endocrine system. Metabolism 1978; 27:(Suppl 1)1193.
15. Polak IM, Pearse AGE, Grimelius L. Growth hormone release-inhibiting hormone in gastrointestinal and pancreatic D cells. Lancet 1975; I:1220.
16. Boden G, Sivitz MC, Owen OE. Somatostatin suppresses secretin and pancreatic exocrine secretion. Science 1975; 190:163.
17. Konturek SJ, Tasler J, Obtulowicz W, Coy DH, Schally AV. Effect of growth hormone-release inhibition hormone on hormones stimulating exocrine pancreatic secretion. J Clin Invest 1976; 58:1.
18. Schwedes U, Usadel KH, Szabo S. Cysteamine induced duodenal ulcer: prevention by somatostatin (SRIEF). Eur J Pharmacol 1977; 44:195.
19. Schwille PO, Putz F, Thun R, Schellerer W, Draxler G, Lang G. Anti-stress ulcer and anti-secretory effect of somatostatin in rats failure to suppress serum gastrin. Acta Hepatogastroenterol 1977; 24:259.
20. Wdowinski JM, Schwedes U, Faulstich H, et al. Beneficial effect of somatostatin in phalloidin intoxicated rats. Influence on survival rate, biochemical and morphological data, and H-Demethylphalloidin absorption rate by the liver. Res Exp Med 1981; 178:155.
21. Lanksich PG, Koop H, Winkler K, Folsch UR, Creutzfeldt W. Somatostatin therapy of acute experimental pancreatitis. Gut 1977; 18:713.
22. Schwedes U, Althoff U, Klempa I, et al. Effect of somatostatin on bile-induced acute hemorrhagic pancreatitis in the dog. Horm Metab Res 1979; 11:655.
23. Baxter JN, Jenkins SA, Day DW, et al. Effects of somatostatin and a longacting somatostatin analogue on the prevention and treatment of experimentally induced acute pancreatitis in the rat. Br J Surg 1985; 72:382.
24. Schlegel W, Raptis S, Harvey RF, Oliver JM, Pfeiffer EF. Inhibition of cholecystokinin-pancreozymin release by somatostatin. Lancet 1977; II:166.
25. Raptis S, Schlegel W, Lehmann E, Dollinger HC, Zoupas CH. Effects of somatostatin on the exocrine pancreas and the release of duodenal hormones. Metabolism 1978; 27:1321.
26. Klempa I, Schwedes U, Usadel KH. Verhutung von postoperativen pankreatischen Komplikationen nach Duodeno-pankreatektomie durch Somatostatin. Chirurg 1978; 50:427.
27. Tamas GY, Tulassay ZS, Papp J, et al. Effect of somatostatin on the pancreatitis-like biochemical changes due to endoscopic pancreaticography: preliminary report. Metabolism 1978; 27:1333.

AUTHOR INDEX

Peptide
  hormone, 3-12
    gene expression, 3-13 <u>see</u>
      Gene
    intestinal,vasoactive(VIP),
        122,137,153,186,231,280,
        344
      inhibition by SMS <u>201-995</u>
        see SMS <u>201-995</u>
    listed, 225
    prosomatostatin-derived, 40-47
    release and radioimmunoassay,
        149
    somatostatin-derived, 33-50
Peptone, 249,285-289
Pergolide, 337
Pertussis toxin, 125-129,131,
        138,139,143,255-257,261
Phage lambda, 15
Phallotoxin, 194
Phentolamine, 230,231
Phenylalanine ring,aromatic, 84,
        86
Phaeochromocytoma of rat, 25,26
Phorbol ester, 137,141,232,255
Phosphatidyl inositol, 232
Phosphoenolphruvate carbox-
        ykinase, 29,31
Phospholipase C, 122,233
Phospholipid, 152
Pineal gland in medium, 74-77
Piribedil, 188
Pituitary gland
  in acromegaly, 337
    treatment, 337-341
  tumor, 256
Pituitary hormone, 151-152
  release inhibited by somato-
        statin, 121-135
  see Growth hormone
P/K substance, 6
Plasma membrane, 73,105-107
  depolarization, 74-75
  preparation, 103
Plasmids, 17,18,22,24,25
Plexus
  myenteric, 253,254,256,267
  submucosal, 267
PMSF, 37
Polypeptide,intestinal,vaso-
        active, 21,29
  pancreatic, 202,213
Potassium, 151,152,254
  ion gradient across membrane,
        130,137
Potassium chloride, 22,23
Preprosomatostatin, 7,33,34,40,
        41,45-47,51-70
  I, 59-70
  II, 59-70
Proenkephalin, 29,31

Proglucagon, 6
Proglumide, 240,260
Prohormone, 5
Prolactin, 5,121,127
Proliferin,placental, 5
Proline, 84-86
Promoter of response, 9
Pro-opiomelanocortin, 6
Propranolol, 230,231,262
Prosomatostatin, 7-8,33-50,
        59-67
Prostaglandin, 242,261,288,358
Protein,trophic, 73
Protein kinase
  C, 137,138,140,141,231-233,
        255
  type <u>2</u>, 29
Pseudoobstruction,colonic, 269

Quinine, 112

Rabbit, 269,362
Radioimmunoassay, 26,53,54,157,
        209,221
Radioligand, 90
Rat, 22,39-47,158,174,177,
        210-213,239-241,245,246,
        268,269,319,358
Receptor of somatostatin, 83-102
Regulation of gene expression,
        3-12
Relaxin, 5
Reporter gene, 17
Repressor, 8,9
Reserpine, 76
Response
  element, 8,10
  promoter, 9
RNA, 3,22,23
Rous sarcoma virus, 17,28
  promoter, 17,28
Rubidium flux, 113-114

Saccharomyces cerevisiae
  alpha factor, 52
  somatostatin secretion by,
        51-58
Salivary gland, 74
Schizophrenia, 163,184-188
Sclerosis,multiple, 183
Sclerotherapy by injection,
        323-325
Secretion, 5,111,231,275,276,
        280,358
Seizure, 188
Serotonin, 151,159
Short bowel syndrome, 269
Signal
  peptide cleavage, 60-61
  transduction cascade, 3,4
    mechanism, 131